Quick Reference to

Adult Nursing Procedures

J. B. Lippincott Company Philadelphia/Toronto

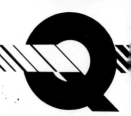

Quick Reference to

Adult Nursing Procedures

Eunice M. King R.N., M.Ed., F.A.A.N.
Administrator, Division of Special Patient Services and
Education, Amarillo Hospital District, Amarillo, Texas
Assistant Clinical Professor of Nursing, University of
Texas at Arlington School of Nursing, Arlington, Texas

Lynn Wieck R.N., B.S.N.
Assistant Director, Clinical Nursing, Special Projects
Assistant, Northwest Texas Hospital, Amarillo, Texas

Marilyn Dyer R.N., M.S.N.
Director and Instructor, Northwest Texas Hospital
School of Nursing, Amarillo, Texas

Illustrated by Janice F. Wojcik

Sponsoring Editor: Paul R. Hill
Manuscript Editor: Megan E. Thomas
Indexer: Donna Dickert
Art Director: Tracy Baldwin
Production Supervisor: N. Carol Kerr
Production Assistant: Susan A. Caldwell
Compositor: TriStar Graphics
Printer/Binder: R.R. Donnelley & Sons Company

Library of Congress Cataloging in Publication Data

King, Eunice M.
  Quick reference to adult nursing procedures.

  (Lippincott's quick references)
  Reprint. Originally published: Illustrated manual of nursing techniques.
Philadelphia : Lippincott, 1977.
  Bibliography
  Includes index.
  1. Nursing—Handbooks, manuals, etc.
I. Wieck, Lynn. II. Dyer, Marilyn. III. Illustrated manual of nursing tech-
niques. IV. Title. [DNLM: 1. Nursing care—In adulthood—Outlines. WY 18
K5li]
RT51.K54 1982   610.73   81–20945
ISBN 0–397–54409–X   AACR2

The authors and publisher have exerted every effort to ensure that drug selection and
dosage set forth in this text are in accord with current recommendations and practice at the
time of publication. However, in view of ongoing research, changes in government
regulations, and the constant flow of information relating to drug therapy and drug reactions,
the reader is urged to check the package insert for each drug for any change in indications
and dosage and for added warnings and precautions. This is particularly important when the
recommended agent is a new or infrequently employed drug.

To my daughters, Janet and Kathy, who
have encouraged and inspired me in
my professional endeavors.

E.M.K.

To my wonderful parents,
Mr. and Mrs. J. B. Fish,
whose love and confidence
I treasure.

L.W.

To Mindi, Cheri, Mark, Keith,
Trent, and Brooke, who enjoy
having a nurse for a mother,
and to my dear pediatrician
husband who is genuinely
interested in nursing and
nursing education.

M.D.

Contents

Unit 2
Techniques for Adult Patients

Unit 3
Techniques for Critically Ill Patients

Unit 4
Techniques for Obstetric Patients

Preface

Adult Nursing Procedures was created in response to the requests of nurses and nursing students for an accessible pocket-sized reference that could be carried to the bedside. This manual was compiled from the chapters on adult nursing care in the first two editions of *Illustrated Manual of Nursing Techniques*. The original edition has been translated into four languages and is now being used as a textbook supplement, reference manual, procedure manual, and review text.

Great care has gone into strengthening the concepts related to the nursing process and to effective nursing intervention. The manual focuses on the unique needs of the adult patient in implementing total patient care, including the technical aspects. We believe that the "skills" component of care is a very important element in the nursing process.

This manual has been developed as a basic guide and ready reference, and is designed to complement and supplement the basic texts in each clinical area. The carefully outlined presentation of each technique provides essential content for safe and therapeutic care. Four major headings, corresponding to the steps of the nursing process, have been utilized.

I. ASSESSMENT OF SITUATION

A. Definition

B. Terminology

C. Rationale for Actions

II. NURSING PLAN

A. Objectives

B. Patient Preparation

C. Equipment

III. IMPLEMENTING NURSING INTERVENTION

A. Therapeutic Aspects

B. Communicative Aspects
1. Observations
2. Charting
3. Referrals

C. Teaching Aspects

IV. EVALUATION PROCESS

The use in this book of the feminine pronouns to describe the nurse is not intended to imply that all nurses are women. For convenience, the pronoun "she" is used to differentiate the nurse from the patient, who is referred to as "he."

We believe that *Adult Nursing Procedures* adds a major dimension to the technical skills area of nursing practice. Feedback and comments from those who use it will provide valuable assistance in future editions.

We wish to thank our colleagues in nursing education and nursing service who have collaborated with us and shared their expertise in the various clinical areas. We also wish to express our appreciation to David T. Miller and Paul Hill and the staff of the J. B. Lippincott Company for their continued support.

Eunice M. King, R.N., M.Ed., F.A.A.N.
Lynn Wieck, R.N., B.S.N.
Marilyn Dyer, R.N., M.S.N.

Illustration Credits

Unless credited otherwise, the illustrations in this manual are selected from units of the Lippincott Learning System, a self-instructional audiovisual program. The following units are represented:

**Anatomical Terminology,
  Joint Classification,
  and Range of Motion
  Asepsis
*Body Mechanics
**Bowel Elimination
*Care of the Mouth

*Care of the Skin
*Making a Bed
*Oral Medication
*Parenteral Medication
*Vital Signs
  Wound Care
**Urine Elimination

A single asterisk indicates units for which the copyright is held by the Regents of the University of Wisconsin/Milwaukee, whose permission to reproduce them here is gratefully acknowledged. A double asterisk indicates that copyrights are held by both the Regents of the University of Wisconsin/Milwaukee and the J. B. Lippincott Co. The absence of an asterisk indicates that the J. B. Lippincott Co. is the sole copyright holder.

The figures listed below were selected from the motion picture series, *Procedures in Patient Care* © J. B. Lippincott Co.:

Figures 44-1, 44-2, 49-1, 49-2, 49-3, 49-4, 49-5, 58-1, 58-2, 58-3, 58-4, 58-5, 58-6, 58-7, 58-8, 58-9, 58-10, 58-15, 58-16, and 98-2.

The figures listed below were selected from the film series, *Experiences in Clinical Nursing* © J. B. Lippincott Co.:

Figures 8-1 and 49-6.

Quick Reference to
Adult Nursing Procedures

The Nursing Process in the Presentation of the Nursing Techniques

Nursing is currently undergoing dynamic changes. These changes are the result of many educational, socioeconomic, psychological, and health care factors that have exerted pressure in varying degrees on all of the health professions. One of the important new approaches in nursing today is the provision of nursing care that is geared to meet the needs of the individual patient. This approach is embodied in the nursing process, which ensures that care given to patients will be systematic, scientific, deliberate, and individualized.

In order to correlate this manual with the nursing process concept, the authors have reviewed a variety of nursing processes with different types and numbers of steps. The nursing process most appropriate for the purposes of this book is that developed by Yura and Walsh, which is composed of four major steps: assessment, planning, implementation, and evaluation. The categories used in presenting the various nursing techniques in this manual are organized according to the four steps of the nursing process and reflect its principles.

ASSESSMENT PHASE

The assessment phase involves a process that requires the ability to make decisions and judgments. These judgments are based on data collected by the nurse about the state of the patient's health. The collection of data is accomplished by such methods as observation, physical examination, and the interviewing process (or history-taking). This information is then organized and analyzed so that the nurse is able to identify the patient's problem or problems.

The nurse must bring to the assessment phase a basic understanding of the situation, the terminology associated with it, and the nursing actions demanded by it. Hence, in this book, the assessment phase includes a definition of the specific nursing technique, a glossary of terms, and a specific rationale for each nursing action. A basic example is this list of the eight identifiable rationales for an enema:

A. To cleanse or remove accumulated solids or gases from lower bowel
B. To stimulate peristalsis in bowel
C. To soothe and treat irritated mucosa
D. To supply fluids and nourishment to the patient

E. To decrease body temperature through coolant contact with the proximal vascular system

F. To stop local hemorrhage

G. To decrease cerebral edema

H. To introduce medication into the system

PLANNING PHASE

The planning phase is a guide for the nursing care actions of the nurse. Based upon the assessment, the nurse can set priorities, identify objectives, outline specific nursing actions for the achievement of the objectives, state expected outcomes, and formulate a written plan.

In this manual, the nursing objectives specific to each nursing technique are clearly stated. Since carefully written objectives are important in establishing goal direction and clarity for the nurse, the following guidelines are observed: each objective describes the specific behavior of the nurse, is written with action verbs, and is clear, concise, and measurable. Short-term, intermediate, and long-term goals are identified.

These characteristics are illustrated in the nursing objectives written for the prevention and treatment of pressure sores (decubitus ulcers), which follow:

1. To maintain clean, dry skin
2. To examine bone prominences and skin folds regularly
3. To observe and note factors that may interfere with the healing process
4. To prevent or reduce infection and promote healing

Another aspect to be considered in formulating a plan for administering nursing techniques is the need to identify all of the equipment that will be required. Hence, as part of the planning phase, a detailed equipment list is provided for each nursing technique.

Patient preparation, both physical and psychological, is included as an integral part of the nursing plan stage. The therapeutic nurse–patient relationship should be established prior to the implementation of any nursing technique. The nurse should identify the physical and psychological needs of the patient as a part of the preparation for the nursing technique.

IMPLEMENTATION PHASE

The implementation phase is the action phase of the nursing process. During this phase the nurse also identifies the responses of the patient to nursing care. To be successful, implementation or intervention should involve the patient in his own care as much as possible; this emphasis contributes both to the patient's sense of satisfaction and to the quality of nursing care. If the patient is enabled to become more independent in meeting his own needs, the entire nursing process will have been highly effective in every aspect of the nursing care. This manual identifies the following categories under nursing intervention:

1. Therapeutic aspects
2. Communicative aspects
   a. Observation
   b. Charting
   c. Referrals
3. Teaching aspects

The therapeutic aspects identify the scientific principles that underlie the specific nursing technique. The emphasis of the technique becomes "why" rather than just "how-to." The nurse then has a valid basis for the nursing care she intends to perform. Principles from chemistry, anatomy, physiology, physics, and microbiology are applied in this section. An example of a physics principle that applies to the administration of enemas is the following: "*Gravity course*—the solution to flow from the reservoir into the rectum; the higher the elevation of fluid, the faster the rate of flow and the greater the pressure in the rectum." Such information helps to eliminate the problems of memorizing techniques and of half-learned information.

The communicative aspects include observations and charting. Observation as an element of nursing intervention can help the nurse to identify patient responses to nursing care. When the nurse reviews the nursing objective for the specific nursing technique, she can more effectively identify responses that indicate change has occurred. Charting is an essential component of communication. The book gives standardized examples of charting for the specific nursing techniques. Although charting is done in many ways, in all types of hospitals, the emphasis in this manual is on the charting of observations made during the implementation of the nursing technique. Information regarding referrals as a part of the implementation of nursing techniques is of value to all practicing nurses; it also serves to emphasize continuity of care for the patient.

Teaching aspects complete the nursing intervention category. In each nursing technique, emphasis is placed on instruction given to the patient and his family. Such information can be given only after the nurse has established the therapeutic nurse–patient relationship previously discussed. It is hoped that the nurses using this book will employ various teaching methods and aids as they care for the patient.

EVALUATION PHASE

The fourth and final step of the nursing process is evaluation, although it is taking place throughout the process. Through evaluation the nurse can determine the effectiveness of the care given, how well the nursing objectives were met, and the changes brought about in the condition of the patient.

Nursing the Older Person

In the United States there are some 26 million people over the age of 65, and 10 million over 75 years of age; this is the fastest growing segment of the population. The elderly population is increasing in the United States, and by the year 2020, elderly persons may constitute one-fifth of the total population. It is evident that the scope of the field of geriatrics is expanding rapidly, and this phenomenon has many implications for the health professions. Adequate health care for the elderly, the senescent, and the senile will require special knowledge and skills on the part of the medical profession and other health professions. What is the role of nursing? Like any other highly specialized area of nursing, the care of the older person requires a unique body of knowledge.

The approach that has been prevalent in the past, that is, medical care primarily directed toward maintenance and the status quo, will no longer suffice because of the body of knowledge and the scientific developments that have evolved in the last several decades. Degeneration in many elderly persons can be reversible, and the links between the social, psychological, and physical disorders that are usually found have not been fully explored or understood. The relationships and interaction of these systems should receive special consideration by nursing personnel.

The dynamics of aging have been the focus of considerable study and research in recent years. What is normal aging? What are some of the common problems associated with the aging process, and how can these problems be effectively dealt with in administering nursing care? This brief chapter is written with the intent of placing special emphasis on the care that is provided the elderly, keeping in mind their special needs.

THE AGING POPULATION

Many hypotheses about the aging process and the psychosocial dynamics associated with it have been presented by both psychologists and sociologists. Nurses will find results from these studies meaningful and useful in caring for the elderly. The causes of aging are multidimensional, encompassing physiological, psychological, social, and cultural factors. Literature available in the area identifies some general characteristics of aging, as follows:

1. Susceptibility to stress increases. This is a critical area; authors generally agree that stress can cause illness, and that vulnerability to stress-induced disease increases in old age.
2. Loss is more prevalent among the elderly, who often, and inevitably,

experience drastic life changes, such as loss of spouse, lifelong friends, job, and home.
3. Many suffer from low self-esteem because of cultural neglect.
4. Loneliness has been identified as the most common mental health problem.
5. Chronological age is not a valid indicator of aging. Individual differences are great, and a total assessment of each individual is needed to determine the degree of aging and the physiological, sociological, and psychological changes that have occurred.
6. The elderly are not a homogeneous group. Each person is unique in background and current health status.
7. Change is gradual; persons age at vastly different rates.
8. Elderly people have generally been characterized as hostile, inflexible, senile, prejudiced, and set in their ways.
9. A small percentage of the elderly are in institutions (5%); for many, old age is a satisfying time of life with minor physical or mental impairment.
10. Old age is not synonymous with disease, yet age increases susceptibility to disease, and disease usually intensifies the aging process.
11. A major need of the elderly is the desire to be involved and not isolated or neglected. Noninvolvement usually leads to rapid mental and physical deterioration.
12. Personality is a key factor in the person's response and adjustment to the aging process.
13. Activity is important, and new avenues should be developed; when lifelong activities must be given up, substitutes should be found.
14. A major cause of emotional disorders in the elderly is the loss of self-esteem and lowered social status.

COMMON PHYSICAL CHANGES

The physical changes that occur with aging vary markedly among different persons, and they may appear at varying points along the life span continuum. Some of the commonly found changes are: weight loss, progressive structural decline of the body, graying of the hair, loss of teeth, loss of hearing, loss of eyesight, and wrinkling and discoloration of the skin.

Diseases commonly found in the elderly are osteoporosis, atherosclerosis, cardiovascular diseases, stroke, cancer, severe or mild organic brain disease, arthritis, arteriosclerosis, rheumatoid arthritis, and diabetes mellitus.

A major problem in physical illnesses is that elderly patients do not report physical symptoms and frequently resort to self-treatment. Many physical diseases impair mental ability. Drug tolerance is lower in older persons and must be monitored closely. Antihypertensive drugs can decrease the cerebral blood flow, diuretics may change the electrolyte balance, and digitalis may cause adverse reactions in the central nervous system.

COMMON EMOTIONAL CHANGES

Functional mental disorders in the elderly affect at least 15% of the older age group. An in-depth diagnostic study should be undertaken to distinguish emotional changes or problems due to stress and loss from the more severe functional disorders. Organic disorders result from physical causes. Organic brain syndrome is often found in the elderly. The first sign of mental impairment is usually the loss of memory or a state of confusion. However, elderly persons commonly show signs of slow thinking, irritability, and hostility, and experience grief, loneliness, and anxiety.

Our attitudes in caring for the elderly are most important. We need to remember that aging is not necessarily accompanied by a decline in mental abilities; in fact, much can be done to prevent this, and studies have demonstrated that this decline can be reversible in many cases. When an elderly person feels that he is losing his memory, he may become very anxious, and the severe distress that results predisposes to physical and psychological problems. Multiple losses, such as those of status, income, home, spouse, friends, and self-image, in addition to the fear of death, often intensify mental stress.

The most prevalent functional disorders found in elderly persons are depression, paranoid states, and late-life schizophrenia. Depression, which is widespread, is characterized by feelings of helplessness and sadness, poor self-image, lack of interest, and emotional withdrawal. Physical symptoms are fatigue, constipation, sleeplessness, and loss of appetite.

NURSING IMPLICATIONS

A very important part of the nurse's task is to help the elderly person maintain his independence. The older patient should be encouraged to take part or assist as much as possible in his own care. The need to conserve his physical strength must not be overlooked.

A basic need of the elderly person is the need to talk to someone. The nurse should allot time to spend with the patient, encouraging him to verbalize and express his feelings. All nursing measures and treatment should be thoroughly explored, and time should be provided for the person to ask questions.

Isolation and loneliness can result in depression, loss of purpose, loss of willpower, and, finally, both physical and mental deterioration. Therefore, the older person should be encouraged to visit with other patients, participate in recreational and social activities, read, watch TV, and participate in arts, crafts, or other activities that appear to interest him.

The needs of the elderly are much more than mere day-to-day physical needs; aging persons have deep-seated needs for security, dignity, self-esteem, independence, and respect. The whole person must be understood; the nurse's awareness of the special needs of the elderly is as important as it is for any other age group.

DEVELOPMENTAL TASKS OF THE AGING

1. To clarify, explore, and find depth in what has already been attained in a lifetime of learning and adapting

2. To conserve one's inner strength for the enjoyment of the finished product

3. To accept and adjust to the losses that occur along the life cycle, which are usually inevitable during later years: loss of health, loved ones, financial security, independence, and social activity

4. To maintain the lifelong processes of inner growth and development

5. To sustain one's self-image or self-view and the sense of ongoing usefulness

6. To reassess one's priorities, setting new goals to maximize the use of time and resources

7. To adjust to retirement with a new and positive focus on life

8. To adjust to reorganized family patterns

9. To accept new limitations affecting physical ability, energy, intellectual resources, and health

10. To accept the aging process and the inevitability of death with serenity

Psychosocial Aspects of Nursing Care

Psychosocial aspects in the care of patients include all of the intrapersonal and interpersonal processes that stimulate and modify behavior. Illness very often alters a person's usual behavior pattern, as well as his ability to cope with the new and sometimes unpleasant situations that face him. It is the nurse's responsibility to assist the patient in adjusting to his new situation and, at the same time, retaining his self-image and sense of worth as an individual.

The format of this book is focused on patients, not on procedures or diseases. The core of the nursing process is the nurse–patient relationship. Florence Nightingale in her *Notes on Nursing* (1859) referred to the behavioral aspects of illness and the effect of the body on the mind. Thus, the inclusion of the behavioral sciences in nursing care is not a new concept.

CONCERN FOR INDIVIDUAL NEEDS

Procedures should never be viewed as "routine"; rather, nursing intervention should be viewed as an individual process concerned with the total needs of the patient. Within this framework, therapeutic procedures become an integral part of total patient care. It is the responsibility of the nurse to continuously strive to increase her knowledge and understanding of human needs and their relationship to the preservation of the individual's psychosocial and physiological equilibrium, or state of balance. A broad view of the psychosocial aspects of human behavior is presented in this introduction; content specific to nursing technique is included in each chapter.

The Need for Security

One basic human need is to feel safe, comfortable, and accepted in any situation that may occur. Confrontation with an illness at home or admission to a hospital can cause a certain amount of fear and anxiety. As humans, we fear the unknown and the idea that our role in the family may change or that we may lose our identity and become a case or a number instead of a person. The ways in which the health care provider responds to these fears and worries will greatly influence the individual's experience during illness.

The Need for Knowledge and Reassurance

The best method of allaying fear of the unknown is adequate explanation. This builds trust and security, promotes comfort and safety, and greatly enhances interpersonal relationships. Explanation of physical care procedures also helps in advancing the nurse–patient relationship by establishing trust and two-way communication. Allowing the patient to ask questions and express his feelings gives him security and comfort in a strange or frightening situation.

A person who is fearful will react with increased anxiety if those caring for him show doubt or lack of concern. The nurse must maintain a calm attitude and convey competence through her actions. Because of her close association with her patient, the nurse can do more to enhance his security and well-being than any other member of the health care team.

Self-esteem and Self-image

In addition to being a fear-provoking experience, illness represents a threat to a person's self-esteem and self-image. He suddenly finds himself in a state of utter dependency, even for his most basic needs, such as food and elimination. The nurse should dwell on the positive aspects of treatment and expected therapeutic results in order to combat negative feelings on the part of the patient. She should perform tasks carefully and confidently and maintain an attitude of acceptance. Of extreme importance in enhancing self-image is attention to the patient's privacy and modesty. The need for adequate use of screening and draping techniques cannot be overemphasized.

Encouraging Independence

If the patient is allowed to participate in his own care as much as he is able, he feels less helpless and dependent. He is also likely to be more cooperative if he is allowed to follow his established behavior patterns as closely as is feasible in the hospital setting. For example, if he is accustomed to retiring at a late hour, he will feel less threatened and more secure if he is allowed to follow this practice in the hospital, provided there are no medical contraindications.

The nurse must be aware of any physical restrictions and ensure that the patient remains within the set limits. If he understands the reasons for the restrictions, he will be more cooperative. Maintaining limits not only gives the patient a feeling of security but bolsters his self-esteem, since he sees that others care about him.

Relieving Anxiety

Tension and anxiety increase one's perception of pain. Measures which can be taken to relieve the anxiety level, and thus reduce the need for pain medication, include two-way communication, backrubs, explanations, and reassurance. Hospitalized patients may have untoward emotional reactions to their conditions. Emotions may be controlled or manipulated by such diversionary techniques as reading, television, etc. Inclusion of the patient's family in therapy and teaching will enrich the therapeutic atmosphere and aid in the patient's acceptance of what is happening to him.

Fear of Disfigurement or Bodily Injury

Patients should be prepared in advance if there is a possibility of alteration in body image due to treatment, surgery, or medications. A person's perception of his body image has developed from childhood and is usually firmly established. If his body image is changed as a result of illness or treatment, the patient's adjustment to the alteration will come about slowly. The nurse must avoid unnecessary or premature demands for adjustment, since the patient needs time to get used to his altered body image.

Fear of Illness and Death

Every society holds attitudes and beliefs about illness and death that guide the behavior of its members. The nurse must allow the patient to verbalize these feelings. She should answer questions truthfully and reinforce explanations given by the physician. This will help show the patient that he is accepted as a valued member of society without regard to his physical condition. The way in which a person perceives his current situation is directly related to his past experiences in the same or similar situations. If he has had a previous unpleasant experience when ill, he may need extra prompting, explanation, and encouragement from the nurse.

Aesthetic Needs

The American people place high values on beauty and cleanliness. Each patient should be clean and comfortable, with particular attention paid to personal hygiene. If the patient feels clean and fresh, his entire outlook is better. Each person is an individual, and one of the most personal and valued possessions is the image of self. Nurses owe it to their patients to help them leave the hospital with their self-images intact.

Environmental Needs

People tend to constantly evaluate and modify their environments to protect themselves against potential danger. The nurse can aid in this process by removing unpleasant stimuli, such as bright lights, sudden noises, and temperature extremes, and by showing concern for the patient's safety in such ways as raising side rails and giving adequate instructions.

The Need to be Valued as a Person

A hospitalized patient is sensitive to verbal and nonverbal communication; difficulties arise when inconsistencies are noted. If the nurse says she cares for the patient, she must also communicate this attitude nonverbally, by a gentle touch or attentive listening. Before a patient can accept himself and his altered physiological condition, he must feel that he is accepted by others.

Health Teaching

The nurse has many opportunities for health teaching in the hospital setting. Motivation is a prerequisite to learning; hence, the patient must be able to see some correlation between what the nurse is saying and how it affects him. The patient learns when he understands what the health problem is and what he can do about it. The person's educational and intellectual levels also influence his ability to understand. The nurse should be cognizant of her patient's level of knowledge and gear her explanations to it.

Psychosocial Resources

If a person is to receive optimal medical and nursing care, the area of psychosocial functioning must receive as much attention as the patient's physiological needs. Nurses will need to draw on knowledge and skills from the social science disciplines, sociology, psychology and anthropology, in treating the "whole" person. It is the hope of the authors that nurses will utilize the unlimited reference materials available in this area, and that the application of principles from the social sciences will be a major objective in planning patient care.

1

Techniques for Diagnostic Studies

1

Barium Enema

I. ASSESSMENT OF SITUATION

A. Definition

X-ray visualization of the large intestine after rectal instillation of contrast medium

B. Terminology

1. *Fluoroscopy:* use of a fluorescent screen to visualize shadows in body cavities

2. *Polyp:* a tumor with a pedicle commonly found in vascular areas such as the nose, uterus, and rectum

3. *Hemorrhoid:* a dilated blood vessel in the anal region

C. Rationale for Actions

1. To reveal the presence of polyps, tumors, or other lesions of the large intestine

2. To demonstrate any malfunction or abnormal anatomy of the bowel

II. NURSING PLAN

A. Objectives

1. To prepare the patient thoroughly and ease his anxiety

2. To prepare the bowel adequately to assure maximum radiologic results

B. Patient Preparation

1. A thorough explanation is essential to gaining patient cooperation. Knowledge of the bowel preparation as well as what will occur during the x-ray procedure is important. The patient should be assured that the barium is insoluble and will not be absorbed by his system.

2. Bowel preparation must be thorough and complete if adequate visualization is to be accomplished. Usually on the evening before the x-ray examination, the patient receives a liquid supper and a strong laxative, such as castor oil. The patient may also receive an enema the night before the examination x-ray (see Technique 45, Enema [lower bowel irrigation] and Rectal Tube). On the morning of the x-ray examination, the patient may receive enemas until the return is clear, signifying that no fecal matter remains in the bowel to interfere with the x-ray. To reduce the possibility of nausea or of fecal material accumulating, the patient is usually NPO after midnight.

C. Equipment

Enema setup

III. IMPLEMENTING NURSING INTERVENTION

A. Therapeutic Aspects

1. X-rays are a form of radiant energy that penetrate according to the density of the tissue. In order for soft tissues to be visualized, a substance that appears opaque on an x-ray film is used to fill the organs and cause them to cast an outline shadow on the film. Barium sulfate, a fine, white, odorless, tasteless bulky powder, insoluble in water and impermeable to the x-ray beam, is used to outline the GI tract. In the x-ray department the patient is placed on his side on the x-ray table. A tube is inserted into the rectum, and, with the aid of a fluoroscope, the barium is run into the large intestine. If the patient has been adequately prepared, the contour of the colon (including cecum and appendix) is clearly visible. The motility of each portion can also be observed. Films are made with the barium in place and after it has been evacuated. Occasionally, air may be inserted to inflate the bowel. In this way, the outline is better illuminated to show polyps. The procedure usually takes 1 to 2 hours.

2. Upon returning to the nursing unit, the patient will probably be very tired. Barium enema is an exhausting procedure. Fluids should be encouraged until all of the barium is evacuated; this may take 2 to 3 days. A cleansing enema may be administered to facilitate barium evacuation.

B. Communicative Aspects

1. *Observations*

   a. The patient should be carefully observed during the bowel cleansing procedure in order to avoid overfatigue.

   b. Laxatives and enemas can irritate hemorrhoids and cause a small amount of rectal bleeding. Any rectal bleeding should be checked carefully and reported to the physician.

   c. After the x-ray examination, the patient should report when he has a bowel movement so that the nurse can verify that the barium is passing satisfactorily and further evacuation assistance is unnecessary.

2. *Charting*

DATE	TREATMENT	TIME	OBSERVATION	SIGNATURE
4/7	Enemas until clear in prep. for BE	0600	Cleansing enemas X 4 given. Last enema returned clear. Pt. encouraged to rest until time for x-ray. No rectal bleeding.	C. Allen, R.N.

3. *Referrals*

Not applicable

C. Teaching Aspects

1. The patient must be cautioned about expelling all of the barium after the x-ray examination. He should understand that failure to evacuate the barium could lead to impaction. The importance of fluids and high-fiber foods to elimination should be discussed.

2. The period before and after the barium enema may provide the nurse with an excellent opportunity to give the patient sound nutritional guidance, practical information about exercise and activity, and guidelines for judicious use of over-the-counter medications for relief of minor gastrointestinal disturbances. The nurse can also help the patient to develop a positive, flexible attitude about elimination patterns.

IV. EVALUATION PROCESS

A. Did the patient understand the need for the bowel preparation?

B. Did the patient accept the need for the x-ray examination?

C. Did the patient understand how to ensure that all barium is evacuated?

D. Were abnormalities or pathology visualized on the colon film?

E. Was the patient able to retain the barium? ·

F. Was the bowel adequately cleansed?

G. Did the patient pass all of the barium and begin having normal stools?

2

Blood Samples, Arterial and Venous

I. ASSESSMENT OF SITUATION

A. Definition

Removal of a small amount of blood from an artery or vein for laboratory analysis

B. Terminology

1. *Radial artery*: the artery located in the forearm at the wrist
2. *Brachial artery*: the artery located at the bend of the arm
3. *Femoral artery*: the artery located in the groin area
4. *Antecubital area*: the area around the elbow on the forearm

C. Rationale for Actions

1. To analyze blood gases in determining the effectiveness of ventilation
2. To obtain a blood specimen for laboratory analysis of normal constituents
3. To assess the blood to detect the presence of foreign substances in making a diagnosis

II. NURSING PLAN

A. Objectives

1. To minimize the trauma at the puncture site
2. To allay the nervousness of the patient
3. To preserve the specimen appropriately

B. Patient Preparation

1. A careful explanation should precede arterial puncture or venipuncture. The reason for the procedure, as well as an explanation of what will happen, is necessary. It is also important to mention that although the amount of blood removed may seem excessive, in reality it is a very small amount. Explaining that the body is continually manufacturing new blood even when none is lost may also allay the patient's apprehension about the amount of blood taken.
2. Usually no physical preparation is necessary, other than availability of the puncture site. Some blood tests require abstinence from food or ingestion of certain substances.

C. Equipment

1. Venipuncture
   a. Tourniquet
   b. Alcohol sponge
   c. Needle (usually 20-, 21-, or 23-gauge)
   d. Cotton ball and tape
   e. Syringe or vacuum container
2. Arterial puncture
   a. Five- or 10-ml syringe (preferably glass)
   b. Heparin (1,000 U/ml)
   c. 20-gauge needle

    d. Blood gas syringe cap (metal or cork)

    e. Alcohol sponge

    f. Cup of ice

III. IMPLEMENTING NURSING INTERVENTION

A. Therapeutic Aspects

1. *Venipuncture*

    a. Withdrawal of blood by venipuncture depends on differences of pressure. Blood in the vein is put under greater than normal pressures by the damming action of the tourniquet, which is placed several inches above the desired site of venipuncture. Microorganisms normally found on the skin may be pathogenic if allowed to enter the bloodstream. The site of venipuncture should be cleaned with an alcohol sponge.

    b. The vein can be located by site (bluish appearance) or by feel (a firm, rubbery rebound sensation). Usually the vein of choice is located in the antecubital area. Pumping of the fist may help to distend the vein.

    c. The skin should be held taut. The pressure needed to pierce the skin is sufficient to force the needle into the vein. The needle with syringe attached should be held at a 45° angle with the bevel up. When the needle enters the vein, venous return is visible immediately in the syringe because of the negative pressure. The blood specimen may be obtained by gently drawing back on the plunger of the syringe. If a vacuum container is used, the external needle on the adapter is inserted into the vein. Once venous return is visible, the vacuum container is pushed down onto the needle and the tube fills with blood. If more than one tube is needed, the first tube can be replaced with a second tube without removing the needle.

    d. After venipuncture is accomplished, the tourniquet should be released and the needle should be withdrawn. A dry cotton ball should be held firmly on the venipuncture site for several minutes. An adhesive strip is then placed on the site to prevent oozing.

2. *Arterial Puncture*

    a. Direct puncture of the artery may be accomplished for a variety of reasons, but the most common is to ascertain the effectiveness of ventilation. This is evidenced by study of the blood gases. A glass syringe is preferable because gases can permeate the plastic syringe, causing inaccurate readings.

    b. The site of the puncture is any artery in which the pulse is easily palpable—usually the radial, brachial, or femoral artery. Before the radial artery is punctured, an ulnar pulse must be palpable.

c. Since an unclotted specimen is needed, the syringe is lubricated with 0.5 ml of heparin. After the barrel has been coated, the remaining heparin is ejected.

d. After the area is cleaned with an alcohol sponge, the artery is palpated with the middle and index finger of the free hand. When the pulsation is felt, the needle is inserted at a 90° angle between these two fingers into the artery. The wrist may be anchored on the surface near the puncture site for finer needle control. Once the artery is pierced, pressure will force the blood into the syringe, displacing the plunger. Usually, 2 to 4 ml of blood are needed.

e. After the desired amount is obtained, the needle is withdrawn and pressure is applied to the site for at least 5 minutes. The specimen should be cleared of any air bubbles, capped, and placed on ice at once. An iced specimen is good for several hours, whereas an uniced specimen is good only for 10 minutes.

B. Communicative Aspects

1. *Observations*

   a. The site of arterial puncture or venipuncture must be observed for signs of oozing or leaking into the tissue, resulting in hematoma. Small hematomas are common, but excessive bleeding may indicate a clotting deficit.

   b. Ulnar circulation must be present before radial venipuncture is attempted. To check for this, the radial artery is compressed tightly while the patient makes a tight fist. Maintaining compression of the radial artery, the nurse instructs the patient to relax his fist. It should return to normal color.

   c. The patient should not be receiving oxygen, positive pressure breathing treatments, or other ventilatory assistance when blood gases are drawn unless the purpose is to measure the effectiveness of the assistive apparatus.

2. *Charting*

DATE	TREATMENT	TIME	OBSERVATION	SIGNATURE
1/5	Arterial puncture of radial artery for blood gases	0600	Adequate ulnar collateral circulation present. Iced specimen to lab for stat blood gases. Pressure to radial artery for 7 min.	F. White, R.N.

3. *Referrals*

Not applicable

C. Teaching Aspects

1. Inform the patient that the blood specimens may be done very early in the morning. Blood drawn before a patient has eaten breakfast is usually more chemically uniform.
2. There may be a momentary, deep throbbing pain when arterial puncture is accomplished.

IV. EVALUATION PROCESS

A. Did the patient comply during the procedure?

B. Did the patient understand what was happening?

C. Did hematoma develop?

D. Was adequate arterial pressure applied?

E. Did the specimen get to the laboratory in proper condition?

F. Were the results of blood tests within normal range?

3

Bone Marrow Aspiration

I. ASSESSMENT OF SITUATION

A. Definition

Puncture and withdrawal of marrow from thin flat bones; *e.g.*, sternum, spinous process of vertebra, iliac crest; also called sternal puncture, bone tap

B. Terminology

1. *Dyscrasia:* abnormality
2. *Periosteum:* the outer layer of the bone

C. Rationale for Actions

1. To determine the presence of blood dyscrasias
2. To assess the progression of serious blood diseases such as leukemia
3. To determine the level of immunity

II. NURSING PLAN

A. Objectives

1. To allay the fear and nervousness of the patient regarding the procedure

2. To prevent complications after the puncture

3. To expedite the procedure by being thoroughly prepared

4. To transfer properly labeled specimen to the laboratory promptly

5. To maintain the mental and physical comfort of the patient

B. Patient Preparation

1. The patient will need a great deal of reassurance and explanation because the procedure itself is uncomfortable, and the fear of the results may be overwhelming to the patient. A complete explanation should be offered before the puncture is done. A surgical consent form should be signed by the patient or his legal guardian.

2. Withholding food and fluids is unnecessary. However, the patient may be given a sedative, tranquilizer, or pain medication before bone-marrow aspiration is begun.

C. Equipment

1. Cotton balls or gauze swabs

2. Antiseptic cleaning solution

3. Bone-marrow puncture tray containing syringe, bone-marrow needles with stylets, additional sterile swabs, and drapes

4. Glass slides with covers, test tubes, and labels

5. Syringe, needle, and local anesthetic

6. Band-Aid or tape for pressure dressing

III. IMPLEMENTING NURSING INTERVENTION

A. Therapeutic Aspects

1. In addition to a complete explanation before the test is begun, an ongoing explanation during the procedure should be offered. Constant reassurance is also necessary.

2. Specimens may be obtained from the sternum, ilium, or vertebrae. The site will determine the patient's position; if the sternum is used, he will be flat on his back. If the ilium is used, he may sit on the side of the bed and lean forward (Fig. 3-1). For vertebral puncture, the patient should be on his side with his knees drawn up to his chest.

3. The unbroken skin offers a natural barrier to pathogenic organisms. The normal microorganisms present on the skin may be pathogenic when introduced into the bloodstream or tissues. The puncture site is cleaned with an antiseptic solution. A local anesthetic is administered through all skin layers to the periosteum.

4. The area is draped to provide a sterile field. The bone-marrow needle with stylet in place is inserted by the physician through the cortex of the bone into the marrow. The stylet is then removed, the syringe is attached, and aspiration is accomplished. The actual aspiration may cause a brief moment of pain which the patient should expect.

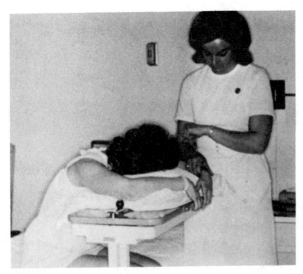

FIGURE 3.1

5. The bone marrow should be placed on sterile slides, covered by a cover slip, and sent directly to the lab. Proper labeling is essential.
6. Pressure should be applied to the puncture site for 5 to 10 minutes after aspiration. If there is any indication of bleeding, a pressure dressing should be applied and watched carefully. If no oozing is apparent after pressure has been applied, a Band-Aid may be used but must be checked frequently. The patient may be asked to remain in bed for a while after the procedure.

B. Communicative Aspects

1. *Observations*
   a. The puncture site must be carefully observed for oozing.
   b. There is a slight chance of hemorrhage after marrow aspiration. Vital signs should be checked every 15 minutes for 2 hours; significant changes warrant immediate attention.

2. *Charting*

DATE	TREATMENT	TIME	OBSERVATIONS	SIGNATURE
6/21	Bone marrow puncture of sternum done.	1115	Pt. seemed relaxed throughout procedure. Some discomfort during aspiration. Pressure applied for 7 min. No indication of tendency to bleed. Specimen to lab.	F. White, R.N.

3. *Referrals*

Not applicable

C. Teaching Aspects

1. The patient and family should understand the need for this diagnostic test.

2. An interpretation of the physician's explanation of the test results may allay the patient's anxiety.

IV. EVALUATION PROCESS

A. Did the patient understand and cooperate during the procedure?

B. Did the patient understand the test results?

C. Were the test results positive?

D. Did the puncture site seal readily with no oozing?

4

Bronchoscopy, Assisting With

I. ASSESSMENT OF SITUATION

A. Definition

Direct visualization of the trachea and bronchial tree by means of a rigid or flexible tube called a bronchoscope for the purpose of diagnosis, removal of a foreign body, or specimen collection.

B. Terminology

1. *Bronchoscope:* a rigid, hollow metal instrument that is passed into the upper portions of the bronchi to visualize the respiratory tract

2. *Tracheobronchial tree:* the trachea, bronchi, and bronchial tubes

3. *Bronchi:* the major branches of the respiratory tract leading from the trachea to the lungs

4. *Bronchioles:* the smaller subdivision of the bronchi

5. *Fiberoptic bronchoscope:* a flexible instrument of smaller diameter than the metal bronchoscope used for visualization of the respiratory tract

C. Rationale for Actions

1. To visualize the tracheobronchial tree for diagnostic purposes

2. To obtain a tissue specimen

3. To remove a foreign body
4. To assist the physician by promoting maximum efficiency and minimal time expenditure

II. NURSING PLAN

A. Objectives

1. To prepare the patient adequately to ensure maximum compliance during the procedure
2. To be aware of and continually observe for adverse reactions or complications

B. Patient Preparation

1. Thorough preparation is essential because patient compliance will aid greatly in the success of the procedure. Many patients fear that they will be unable to breathe with the bronchoscope in place. The patient should be instructed about and should practice breathing through his nose with his mouth open. Assurance that breathing will not be inhibited during the examination may help the patient relax his neck muscles and breathe regularly.
2. The patient should not eat or drink for several hours prior to bronchoscopic examination. The respiratory tract is lined with mucous membranes, and fluid is essential to the production of the watery mucus that is normally present. Insertion of a foreign body such as the bronchoscope stimulates mucus secretion which is undesirable during this procedure. Limiting fluids and administering a mucus-inhibiting agent may decrease the amount of mucus secretion and the danger of vomiting.
3. Either local or general anesthesia may be used. If local anesthesia is chosen, the patient should understand that this will be uncomfortable, since it will stimulate the gag reflex when administered by spray, swab, or drip through cannula.
4. Dentures and partial plates should be removed and mouth care given prior to the examination.

C. Equipment

1. Bronchoscope setup from surgery
2. Anesthetic agent
3. Syringe and cannula or swabs (local anesthestic)
4. Suction pump and tubing
5. Suction catheters or aspirating tubes
6. Specimen container, biopsy forceps
7. Tissues
8. Emesis basin

9. Lubricating jelly
10. Basin with sterile saline solution
11. Sterile slides with cover (for smear)

III. IMPLEMENTING NURSING INTERVENTION

A. Therapeutic Aspects

1. Endoscopic examination of the respiratory tract is usually done with the lights dimmed to provide maximum visualization. A towel is placed over the patient's eyes.

2. The local anesthetic inhibits the gag and swallow reflex. For this reason, the patient should not receive anything by mouth for several hours after the procedure until the gag reflex returns. A feeling of swelling of the tongue and throat may follow application of the anesthetic. This is a false sensation, as is the feeling of the inability to swallow. The patient should be reassured that these sensations are normal and that actually there is little or no swelling present. Suctioning will eliminate the drooling that results from the patient not swallowing.

3. The nurse should remain with the patient to offer him continual reassurance and reminders to relax and breathe normally. The more the patient relaxes, the less pressure he will feel.

4. Severe complications may follow bronchoscopy. For this reason the patient must be carefully observed for respiratory distress (which may indicate laryngeal edema) and for frank bleeding (indicating hemorrhage).

B. Communicative Aspects

1. *Observations*

   a. Observe for the patient's ability to relax and comply with directions.

   b. Signs of laryngeal edema include dyspnea, cyanosis, and restlessness.

2. *Charting*

DATE	TREATMENT	TIME	OBSERVATIONS	SIGNATURE
9/1	Returned to room following bronchoscopy	1000	Swallow reflex still diminished. Placed on right side to facilitate drainage of saliva. Slight blood-tinged mucus from coughing. B/P 110/88 P 90 R 20. Daughter states she understands complications to watch for and will call if help is needed.	F. White, R.N.

3. *Referrals*

If an abnormality or disease of the respiratory tract is discovered, referral to the American Lung Association may be appropriate.

C. Teaching Aspects

1. The patient should be taught to utilize tissues to catch expectoration so that the presence of blood can be noted, as well as for cleanliness. Tissues should be disposed of in a receptacle or paper bag near the bedside.

2. The patient should report any blood in the mucus. A small amount is expected, but frank bleeding indicates a serious complication.

3. The patient may have a sore throat for several days and should avoid further irritation (caused by smoking, talking, or coughing) as much as possible.

IV. EVALUATION PROCESS

A. Did the patient cooperate during the procedure?

B. Does the patient understand the importance of reporting complications and the need to refrain from smoking, coughing, and talking until the irritation subsides?

C. Did the bronchoscope pass easily?

D. Is there any evidence of laryngeal edema or hemorrhage?

E. Are the pulse and respiration rates within acceptable ranges?

5

Cholangiogram, Oral and IV

I. ASSESSMENT OF THE SITUATION

A. Definition

X-ray visualization of the bile ducts and gallbladder

B. Terminology

1. *T-tube:* a T-shaped tube that is sutured into the wound after cholecystectomy to allow the drainage of bile

2. *Cholecystectomy:* surgical removal of the gallbladder

C. Rationale for Actions

1. To determine the presence of stones or other pathology blocking the bile duct

2. To rule out the gallbladder as a possible cause of gastric upset and abdominal pain

II. NURSING PLAN

A. Objectives

1. To provide an adequate x-ray film upon which sound diagnostic judgment may rely

2. To allay the patient's anxiety

3. To prevent allergic complications

B. Patient Preparation

1. The patient should understand that there is no pain involved in radiological examinations and that the exposure to radiation is so minimal as to warrant no concern.

2. The patient may receive fatty meals for a few days prior to the test; bile emulsifies fat. Therefore, the increased intake in fat will cause the gallbladder to empty prior to the test. The meal on the evening before the cholangiogram is usually low in fat to avoid contracture of the gallbladder.

3. An x-ray is a form of radiant energy that penetrates according to the density of tissue. The stomach and bowel should be empty so that they will not interfere with the gallbladder x-ray. Food may be withheld for 12 hours prior to the test, and a laxative or enema or both may be ordered to precede the x-ray study.

4. A complete history of the patient's allergies is essential prior to cholangiography. The oral dye contains iodine. After the initial films are taken, the patient is fed a fatty meal containing eggs to test the gallbladder's contractibility and ability to empty completely. Therefore, patients who may be allergic to eggs or dairy products must be carefully screened.

5. If the gallbladder is not visualized the first time, the test is often repeated. If it is not visualized the second time, pathology is considered and surgical intervention is usually required. The patient should understand that the examination may have to be repeated.

C. Equipment

1. Oral dye tablets

2. Wheelchair or stretcher for transport

III. IMPLEMENTING NURSING INTERVENTION

A. Therapeutic Aspects

1. After the oral tablets are ingested, the dye takes about 13 hours to reach the liver where it is excreted in the bile and passes through the gallbladder. This makes the duct and gallbladder radiopaque. If, after two examinations, there is no visualization, the duct is assumed to be blocked and surgery is usually necessary.

2. In IV cholangiogram, the dye is injected directly into a vein. Usually a small amount is injected first to check for allergic reaction; the rest of the dye is then injected slowly.

3. The initial x-ray film and subsequent films may take several hours to complete. Nurses should be certain that no more follow-up films are necessary before feeding the patient.

4. Reactions to the contrast medium range from no reaction to nausea, vomiting, and hives, or anaphylactic shock. The nurse should observe the patient carefully for any signs of a reaction.

5. After cholecystectomy, a T-tube may be left in place for a short time to allow for the drainage of bile. Dye may be inserted through the T-tube to ascertain whether more stones are present.

B. Communicative Aspects

1. *Observations*

   a. The patient must be observed for any reaction to the contrast medium, such as nausea, vomiting, hives, shortness of breath, or cyanosis. A reaction calls for immediate attention.

   b. The patient's compliance with the x-ray procedure should be noted.

2. *Charting*

DATE	TREATMENT	TIME	OBSERVATIONS	SIGNATURE
1/5	IV Cholangiogram completed	1145	No itching, nausea, vomiting, or respiratory distress. Alert and requesting food.	G. Ivers, R.N.

3. *Referrals*

   Not applicable

C. Teaching Aspects

1. The patient should be assured that x-ray studies are safe and of significant diagnostic value.

2. The signs and symptoms of an allergic reaction should be described to the patient so that he can assist in early detection of problems.

IV. EVALUATION PROCESS

A. Did the patient cooperate during preparation and x-ray?

B. Did the patient exhibit anxiety concerning the procedure?

C. Was the gallbladder visualized?

D. Did the patient suffer an allergic reaction?

Electrocardiogram (ECG, EKG)

I. ASSESSMENT OF SITUATION

A. Definition

A graphic record of the normal heart beat

B. Terminology

1. *P wave:* the first graphic wave of the electrocardiograph (ECG) caused by contraction of the atria

2. *Q, R, S, and T waves:* the second series of waves of an ECG related to contraction of the ventricles

3. *Atrium (pl. atria):* the upper chamber of each half of the heart

4. *Ventricle:* the lower chamber of each half of the heart which propels blood into the arteries

5. *SA node (sinoatrial node; normal pacemaker):* the area where the electrical impulse stimulating a heartbeat begins; located in the superior aspect of the right atrium

6. *AV node (atrioventricular node):* the area of the heart through which the electrical impulse travels prior to initiating ventricular contraction; located between the atria and the ventricles

C. Rationale for Actions

1. To provide grounds for the diagnosis of cardiac arrhythmias, arteriosclerotic heart disease, cardiac enlargement, electrolyte abnormalities, and myocardial infarction

2. To assess the status of a patient in a life-threatening situation as a basis for medical or nursing action

3. To provide a visual picture of the heart rhythms, site of the pacemaker, position of the heart, size of ventricles, and presence of injury

II. NURSING PLAN

A. Objectives

1. To act expeditiously in preventing or reversing cardiac arrest

2. To ensure the patient's cooperation and decrease his anxiety by thorough explanation

3. To ensure the patient's safety by continuous monitoring during the Stress Test and Master's ECG

B. Patient Preparation

1. The patient should understand that there is no pain associated with the ECG. He will have to lie still during the actual test. It should be emphasized that there is no danger of electrical shock. The machine measures the electrical impulses emanating from within the patient himself, hence there is no risk or danger involved.

2. There is little actual physical preparation. The technician must have access to the patient's wrists, ankles, and left chest, hence restrictive clothing must be removed.

3. If a Master's ECG or Stress Test is to be done, the patient should be told that he will be expected to participate in somewhat strenuous supervised exercise.

C. Equipment

1. 12-lead ECG machine

2. Two-step platform for Master's ECG

3. Treadmill for Stress ECG

III. IMPLEMENTING NURSING INTERVENTION

A. Therapeutic Aspects

1. The patient should be lying down in a relaxed state. A conductive paste is placed on the parts of the body where the leads are secured to ensure the best graphic picture possible. Leads are strapped to the wrists and ankles, and one lead is moved progressively across the left chest area by means of a suction cup (Fig. 6-1).

2. When the heartbeat wave moves through the heart, it generates a weak but distinct electric current of 1/500 to 1/100 of a volt at the surface of the chest. These impulses are amplified and recorded on the special paper in the ECG machine. The resulting electrocardiogram tracing is interpreted by trained professionals.

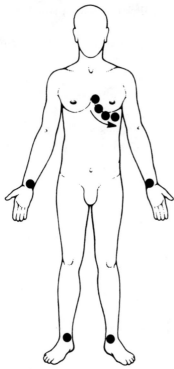

FIGURE 6.1

3. The Master's ECG is used to assess the origin and cause of severe chest pain thought to be angina pectoris. After an ECG is completed with the patient at rest, the patient ascends and descends a two-step platform for the exact number of times specified for a person of his or her age and height. Tracings are made at various intervals to demonstrate the condition of the heart during exercise and recovery. Great care must be taken to ensure that the patient does not overextend himself.

4. The Stress ECG is performed after a period of strenuous supervised exercise. The patient runs on a treadmill set at a certain speed for a predetermined amount of time. ECG tracings are done before running and at intervals afterward.

B. Communicative Aspects

1. *Observations*

   a. The patient must be observed closely during the exercise phase of the Master's and Stress ECG's to ensure that exercise itself does not precipitate a cardiac emergency.

   b. The patient should be observed for compliance with the test.

Movement during the ECG will cause extraneous lines on the graph.

2. *Charting*

DATE	TREATMENT	TIME	OBSERVATION	SIGNATURE
8/6	ECG done at bedside	1400	Pt. relaxed and tol. procedure well. Seems to understand the need for repeat ECG and does not appear anxious.	F. White, R.N.

3. *Referrals*

    a. The American Heart Association may offer its services to the patient.

    b. If cardiac surgery is necessary, there may be local organizations that offer emotional support to the family and patient.

C. Teaching Aspects—Patient and Family

1. The patient and family should understand that subsequent ECG's may be done. An explanation that damage may not show up at first or may be progressive should be given. Prior knowledge of the possibility of the ECG's being repeated may allay a great deal of anxiety.

2. If the patient will have to live with a cardiac abnormality, the nurse should be sure that close family members are familiar with the technique of cardiopulmonary resuscitation (CPR). This should be approached in a matter-of-fact, routine way so that the family will not be alarmed and feel that the situation is worse than they have been led to believe. Knowledge of CPR can save lives, and this is the point that should be stressed.

IV. EVALUATION PROCESS

A. Is the patient less anxious about his general cardiac health after the ECG?

B. Was the patient cooperative during the test?

C. Did the patient understand the physician's interpretation of the ECG?

D. Did the patient withstand the strain of exercise satisfactorily?

E. Did the ECG show abnormalities?

7

Electroencephalogram (EEG)

I. ASSESSMENT OF SITUATION

A. Definition

A graphic record of the electrical activity passing through the surface of the brain

B. Terminology

None

C. Rationale for Actions

1. To detect and determine the location of abnormal electrical activity in the brain, which may indicate such conditions as epilepsy, tumors, or brain damage
2. To assess the presence or absence of electrical activity in determining brain death

II. NURSING PLAN

A. Objectives

1. To prepare the patient adequately by a thorough explanation so that he will not be unduly anxious about the test
2. To elaborate on the physician's interpretation of test results if the patient does not understand
3. To maintain the patient's safety if he is subject to seizures

B. Patient Preparation

1. A thorough explanation of the need for and procedure of electroencephalographic testing is essential. The patient must understand that there is no danger of electrical shock from the electrodes.
2. The patient should avoid the consumption of stimulants (coffee, cola, etc.) and depressants (alcohol) prior to the EEG. Medication will also be withheld unless specified otherwise by the physician.
3. Before the test, the hair and scalp should be shampooed, and no hair preparations should be used after the shampoo.
4. If the physician orders a sleep-deprivation EEG, the patient should not sleep during the 12 hours preceding the test. These are often done early in the morning after the patient has been kept awake all night.

C. Equipment

1. EEG machine and electrodes
2. Conductive paste or jelly

III. IMPLEMENTING NURSING INTERVENTION

A. Therapeutic Aspects

1. The patient is usually reclining or lying down during the EEG. Electrodes are placed at various intervals over the scalp by means of a sticky conductive paste.
2. Tracings are taken over a period of time, during which the patient is relaxed or asleep. He may also be asked to hyperventilate, do simple mental activities, or take certain medications. The entire test may take 45 minutes to 2 hours.
3. The patient should shampoo his hair after the EEG to remove remaining electrode paste.
4. In the comatose patient, absence of brain activity on EEG signifies "brain death" and is utilized in various medicolegal decisions depending upon the laws of the particular state.

B. Communicative Aspects

1. *Observations*

    a. Hyperventilation and sleep deprivation may induce a grand mal seizure in the epileptic patient. However, since measurement of brain conductivity during seizure is desirable, this is not considered a great hazard. Even so, the patient must be protected from injury should a seizure occur.

    b. The patient may be observed for his willingness and ability to follow instructions.

2. *Charting*

DATE	TREATMENT	TIME	OBSERVATION	SIGNATURE
4/7	To x-ray for sleep-deprivation EEG	0730	Pt. has remained awake with some difficulty since 1000 last night. Up in hall most of the night. States he has no reservations about test.	F. White, R.N.

3. *Referrals*

    Not applicable

C. Teaching Aspects—Patient and Family

1. The patient and family should be taught signs of impending seizure (aura) if the patient is diagnosed as epileptic.
2. Management of the epileptic as a functioning participant in modern

society should be emphasized. Unfortunately the stigma attached to "fits" still lingers in some segments of society. If this is the first experience with the reality of epilepsy for the patient, a matter-of-fact, accepting attitude on the part of the nurse can do much to serve as a model for the family to emulate. Emphasizing what the patient can do rather than what he cannot do is very important.

IV. EVALUATION PROCESS

A. Did the patient cooperate during testing?

B. Was the patient able to remain awake all night?

C. Did the patient and family understand the EEG results?

D. Was the EEG normal?

E. Did the patient experience any side effects during EEG?

F. Was there an absence of brain activity?

8

Esophagoscopy, Gastroscopy, Jejunoscopy

I. ASSESSMENT OF SITUATION

A. Definition

1. *Esophagoscopy:* direct visualization of the esophagus by means of a flexible endoscope

2. *Gastroscopy:* direct visualization of the stomach and duodenum by means of a flexible endoscope

3. *Jejunoscopy:* direct visualization of the jejunum by means of a flexible endoscope

B. Terminology

1. *Duodenum:* the first part of the small intestine between the stomach and jejunum

2. *Esophagus:* the tube extending from the pharynx to the stomach

3. *Stomach:* a distensible saclike organ at the end of the esophagus which receives swallowed food, secretes gastric juice, and serves as the organ of digestion

4. *Jejunum:* the second portion of the small intestine between the duodenum and second ileum
5. *Endoscopy:* direct visual examination of certain natural openings or cavities by means of hollow lighted instruments
6. *Eructation:* raising of gas from the stomach; belching

C. Rationale for Actions

1. To detect the presence of pathology
2. To obtain a tissue biopsy
3. To remove a foreign body

II. NURSING PLAN

A. Objectives

1. To prepare the patient adequately and ensure maximum compliance during the procedure
2. To monitor during and after the procedure to detect early signs of complications

B. Patient Preparation

1. These examinations are often done under local anesthetic. A thorough explanation of what to expect and what will be expected of him may help the patient to cooperate more fully (Fig. 8-1).

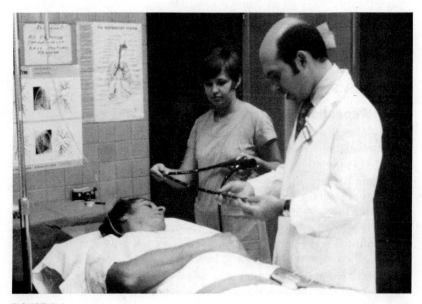

FIGURE 8.1

2. Glands of the mucous membranes lining the GI tract normally produce secretions. When irritated, these glands secrete increased amounts, which may interfere with the endoscopic examination. For this reason, a mucus-inhibiting agent may be administered. Since fluid is essential to the formation of these secretions, fluids are restricted prior to the examination. This also decreases the possiblity of vomiting and aspiration. If the endoscopic examination is done as an emergency measure, aspiration of gastric contents will usually be done first.

3. Suppression of the gag reflex is necessary prior to passage of the endoscope. This is accomplished by general or by local anesthesia. If local anesthesia is selected, the patient should understand that there will be stimulation of the gag reflex during application but that this will pass.

4. Dentures and partial plates should be removed and mouth care given prior to the examination.

C. Equipment

1. Endoscope of appropriate size—setup from surgery
2. Suction pump and tubing
3. Topical anesthetic setup
   a. Agent
   b. Syringe and cannula
   c. Swabs
4. Specimen container or slides and covers
5. Basin with sterile saline solution
6. Emesis basin
7. Tissues

III. IMPLEMENTING NURSING INTERVENTION

A. Therapeutic Aspects

1. Endoscopic examinations depend on illumination of the cavity by an adjacent light source. For this reason, room lights are dimmed. A towel is placed over the patient's eyes.

2. Application of the topical anesthetic must be followed by a brief waiting period while it takes effect. The patient then lies on his left side as the tube is passed (Fig. 8-2). Swallowing by the patient will facilitate tube insertion.

3. Continual reassurance by the nurse during the examination is essential when topical anesthesia is used.

4. A brief cramping sensation may be experienced when the endoscope is passed into the stomach and also when air is pumped in to inflate

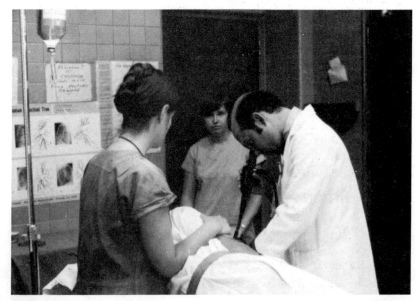

FIGURE 8.2

the stomach for better visualization. The patient should be reassured that this temporary feeling is expected.

5. After endoscopy the patient should be observed for pain, indicating complications. No fluids or food are given until the gag reflex is completely restored.

B. Communicative Aspects

1. *Observations*

   a. Note should be taken of the patient's ability to relax and comply with the tube insertion.

   b. Frequent monitoring of vital signs after gastrointestinal endoscopy will help in early detection of complications. Appropriate monitoring may be every 30 minutes for 3 hours.

2. *Charting*

DATE	TREATMENT	TIME	OBSERVATIONS	SIGNATURE
4/7	Gastro-scopy done in OR Returned to room 650	1115	Gag reflex present. Complains of slight sore throat. No pain. Requesting liquids. B/P 120/78 P 84 R 18	F. White, R.N.

3. *Referrals*

If a carcinogenic lesion is found, referral to the American Cancer Society may be appropriate.

C. Teaching Aspects

1. The patient should be told to report at once any sharp pains in his chest or stomach.

2. A sore throat is not unusual after endoscopy of the GI tract, because of tracheal irritation.

3. The patient should expect to experience increased flatulence or eructation if air is pumped into the stomach during gastroscopy.

IV. EVALUATION PROCESS

A. Was the cooperation of the patient secured before and during the procedure?

B. Does the patient understand possible complications and the need to report them?

C. Did the endoscope pass easily?

D. Are the vital signs within normal limits?

E. Does the patient have a sore throat?

9

Gastric Analysis

I. ASSESSMENT OF SITUATION

A. Definition

Aspiration of the stomach contents through a nasogastric tube for laboratory study

B. Terminology

Urticaria: an inflammatory condition characterized by the eruption of wheals and severe itching; hives

C. Rationale for Actions

1. To determine the presence or absence of acid in the stomach

2. To determine the presence of gastric carcinoma

3. To assess the need for or results of gastric or duodenal surgery

4. To screen the patient for pernicious anemia

II. NURSING PLAN

A. Objectives

1. To allay the fear and anxiety of the patient by adequate preparation

2. To offer reassurance during the course of the procedure

3. To protect the patient from allergic reaction

B. Patient Preparation

1. Because of the duration and unpleasant aspects of the procedure, the patient should know in advance what will happen.

2. Prior to doing the gastric aspiration, a nasogastric tube must be inserted (See Technique 49, Gastric Intubation).

3. To assure that the stomach is empty, the patient will fast for 10 to 12 hours before beginning. Stimulants that might increase gastric secretion must be eliminated; these include smoking, chewing gum, and the consumption of any food or liquids.

C. Equipment

1. See Technique 49, Gastric Intubation

2. Specified stimulant: histamine, caffeine, betazole, alcohol

3. Aspiration syringe

4. Specimen containers and labels

5. Sterile saline solution

III. IMPLEMENTING NURSING INTERVENTION

A. Therapeutic Aspects

1. There are many different methods of obtaining gastric secretions for analysis. The primary concern will be prevention of allergic complications due to the use of certain stimulants. The patient must be NPO for any gastric analysis test.

2. *Twelve-hour secretion test* The nasogastric tube is usually passed in the evening, and the stomach is rinsed with saline solution, which is then drained. The gastric juice collected in the first 15 minutes is usually discarded. The nasogastric tube is then aspirated periodically during the next 12 hours and all gastric contents are saved. The tube may be flushed with sterile saline solution. This long duration test is usually done during the night to minimize the unpleasantness of having the nasogastric tube in place and the withholding of foods and fluids.

3. *Histamine test* Histamine is a strong gastric stimulant but can cause severe allergic reactions. Histalog is often used instead because

it is less likely to cause a reaction. If histamine is used, 0.1 ml is injected intradermally, and if a wheal appears that is greater than 10 mm across, the test is positive and its use is contraindicated. Histamine is never given to patients with a history of asthma, urticaria, or other allergies. If no contraindication is apparent, the nasogastric tube is passed and the gastric contents are aspirated. Histamine 0.01 mg per kg body weight or 0.5 mg Histalog per kg body weight is injected intramuscularly. Gastric content is aspirated at 15 to 20 minute intervals for a prescribed time, usually one hour. The quantity is noted and the specimen is sent to the laboratory.

4. *Caffeine* The nasogastric tube is inserted and gastric contents are aspirated. A solution of 0.5 g caffeine sodium benzoate in 2 dl water is inserted through the tube at the prescribed time. Gastric contents are then aspirated in 30 minutes and every 10 minutes thereafter for 2 hours.

B. Communicative Aspects

1. *Observations*
   a. When histamine is used, the patient must be carefully observed for the following side effects: flushing of the face, headache, hypotension, dizziness, pain at injection site, and nausea.
   b. The amount of gastric secretions should be noted.
   c. The appearance of gastric secretion is significant. If the return is yellowish green (indicating bile), the position of the tube may be in question—it may be in the duodenum. Small streaks of blood may indicate slight trauma during tube insertion. Frank red bleeding indicates a medical emergency, and the physician should be notified at once.

2. *Charting*

DATE	TREATMENT	TIME	OBSERVATION	SIGNATURE
5/7	Histalog gastric analysis begun	0700	No reaction noted to skin test. N-g tube inserted and gastric contents (60 ml) discarded. Histalog given IM. Resting quietly at this time.	G. Ivers, R.N.

3. *Referrals*

Not applicable

C. Teaching Aspects—Patient and Family

1. The patient and family should be warned about signs of allergic reactions that should be reported to the nurse.
2. The effects of certain foods in stimulation of the gastric juices may be discussed if the patient has or suspects that he has an ulcer.

IV. EVALUATION PROCESS

A. Did the patient understand and cooperate during the test?

B. Was the patient offered frequent reassurance during the course of the test?

C. Did the patient manifest any signs of allergic reaction?

D. Was the appearance of the gastric juice normal?

10

Gastrointestinal X-Ray Studies

I. ASSESSMENT OF SITUATION

A. Definition

Radiological study of the gastrointestinal (GI) tract following consumption of a radiopaque substance, also called or including esophagography, barium swallow, upper GI series, small bowel examination

B. Terminology

Gastrointestinal tract: in this instance, the esophagus, stomach, duodenum, and small intestine

C. Rationale for Actions

1. To determine the presence of pathology or abnormalities in the GI tract such as tumors or ulcers

2. To assess the motility and thickness of the gastric wall

3. To determine the presence or absence of right atrial enlargement which will invariably impinge on the esophagus

4. To assess the presence and severity of esophageal varices

II. NURSING PLAN

A. Objectives

1. To explain the procedure thoroughly to the patient

2. To carry out the proper preparations for maximum results

B. Patient Preparation

1. The patient should be told what will happen during the gastrointestinal studies. He should understand that repeated follow-up x-ray

films may be taken as the barium progresses through the GI tract. This may requires several hours, and anxiety is reduced if the patient anticipates the lengthy time requirements.

2. No physical preparation is necessary except withholding food and fluids for 12 hours prior to the test.

C. Equipment

Nonspecific

III. IMPLEMENTING NURSING INTERVENTION

A. Therapeutic Aspects

1. An x-ray is a form of radiant energy that penetrates according to the density of tissue. In order that soft tissues may be visualized, a substance that appears opaque on an x-ray film must be used to fill the organs and cause them to cast an outline shadow on the film. Barium sulfate, a fine, white, odorless, tasteless, bulky powder, that is insoluble in water and impermeable to an x-ray beam, is used to outline the GI tract. In gastrointestinal studies, the patient swallows the "barium milkshake," and the progress of the barium through the GI tract is visualized on the x-ray film. Although the barium is flavored, little can be done to eliminate its chalky taste.

2. The patient stands against a tilting table in the upright position. After the initial swallow he will be secured to the table and tilted at various angles to ensure maximum visualization of all areas. He may be asked to swallow air to add additional contrast. As the barium travels the length of the GI tract, x-ray films will be taken. It can take several hours to complete the x-ray study, and the patient may be allowed to return to his room to wait for the next film. Films may be taken as late as 24 hours after the barium swallow.

3. To ensure adequate spreading of the barium, pressure may be applied manually or with a dome-shaped projection on the x-ray machine. This may be slightly uncomfortable for the patient.

B. Communicative Aspects

1. *Observations*

   a. The patient should be observed during the procedure for faintness or nausea due to the tilting of the table.

   b. The patient's stools should be observed for passage of the barium.

2. *Charting*

DATE	TREATMENT	TIME	OBSERVATION	SIGNATURE
8/15	Returned to room from GI series	1015	Remains NPO. To return to x-ray in 45 min. No c/o discomfort.	F. White, R.N.

3. *Referrals*

Not applicable

C. Teaching Aspects

1. The patient should be prepared for a long wait during the x-ray procedure. He may wish to take reading material or a craft to help pass the time.

2. The patient should be told that he will have chalky stools for several days after the x-ray examination. A laxative, increased intake of high-fiber foods, and large amounts of fluid may help to pass the barium easily.

IV. EVALUATION PROCESS

A. Was the patient adequately prepared for what would happen during the x-ray procedure and for the long waiting periods?

B. Did the patient react calmly to the x-ray experience?

C. Was any abnormality demonstrated on x-ray?

D. Did the patient become nauseated or faint?

11

Glucose and Acetone Testing

I. ASSESSMENT OF SITUATION

A. Definition

Diagnostic tests done on the urine to assess the status of the patient's diabetic condition

B. Terminology

1. *Reagent:* a substance involved in a chemical reaction—often to detect the presence of another substance

2. *Ketosis:* accumulation of ketone bodies

C. Rationale for Actions

1. To determine the presence of glucose in the urine

2. To determine the presence of ketone bodies (acetone) in the urine

3. To provide a guideline upon which to assess the patient's need for insulin

II. NURSING PLAN

A. Objectives

1. To perform the tests correctly
2. To assure the stability and freshness of the reagent tablets
3. To report and take immediate actions when tests indicate glucose or acetone in the urine

B. Patient Preparation

1. In order to perform these tests, a urine specimen is necessary. If the patient understands why the test is being done and the significance of the results in determining his diabetic status, he is much more likely to cooperate. Also, because these tests may be done so frequently, the patient's cooperation is especially vital to the success of diabetic monitoring.

2. In order to have enough urine to produce a specimen when needed, the patient should be adequately hydrated. Fluids should be of the noncaloric type or should be figured into the overall calorie count.

C. Equipment

1. Clean specimen receptacle
2. Reagent materials
3. Test tube and dropper (for Clinitest and Acetest)

III. IMPLEMENTING NURSING INTERVENTION

A. Therapeutic Aspects

1. Diabetic persons suffer from an inadequacy of insulin supply. The body compensates by increasing the blood sugar gradient across the cell walls. When the muscles cannot utilize this oversupply of glucose, the liver forms acidic substances called ketone bodies to supply the needed additional energy to the muscles. This causes ketosis, which is detectable in the urine, and which leads the liver to lose further glycogen. When the blood sugar level reaches 150 to 200 mg/100 ml, the kidney cannot absorb all of the filtered glucose, and glycosuria, the presence of an abnormal amount of glucose in the urine, is a result. Thus a fairly good idea of the patient's systemic diabetic condition can be gained by frequently checking the urine for glucose and ketones (acetone). Since these values must be checked frequently, repetitive withdrawal of blood samples is potentially dangerous and painful to the patient. Monitoring of urinary levels of glucose and acetone is often coordinated with daily blood testing.

2. There are several methods of testing the urine for glucose and acetones:

a. *Clinitest (5-Drop Method)*

(1) The patient voids into a clean container.

(2) The dropper is held vertically, and is filled with urine; 5 drops of the urine are then placed in the test tube.

(3) The dropper is rinsed, and 10 drops of water are added to the test tube.

(4) One Clinitest tablet is dropped into the test tube.

(5) The nurse should observe as the reaction takes place. The test tube should not be shaken during the reaction or for 15 seconds after the reaction has taken place. A pass-through color change can occur if the glucose level is over 2, and the nurse must watch carefully for this change. If the solution passes through orange and dark shades of green-brown, it indicates 4+ (or urine sugar level over 2%), and should be recorded as such.

(6) If no pass-through reaction occurs, the nurse should gently shake the tube after the 15-second waiting period and compare the results with the color scale accompanying the Clinitest set.

b. *Clinitest (2-Drop Method)*

(1) The patient voids into a clean container.

(2) The dropper is held vertically, and is filled with urine; 2 drops of the urine are then placed in a test tube.

(3) The dropper is rinsed, and 10 drops of water are added to the test tube.

(4) One Clinitest tablet is dropped into the test tube.

(5) The nurse should not shake the test tube during the reaction or for 15 seconds after the reaction takes place.

(6) The resulting color is compared with the accompanying chart to determine the approximate percentage of glucose in the urine.

c. *Diastix (glucose)*, *Test-tape (glucose)*, and *Ketostix (acetone)* are strips that are permeated with reagent. They are dipped in the undiluted urine and the results are compared with the color chart.

d. *Acetest tablets* may be used to detect acetone bodies. A tablet is placed on a clean paper towel and one drop of urine is placed directly on the tablet. The results are ascertained by comparison with a color chart.

e. *Keto-Diastix* is a combined ketone-glucose reagent strip that is moistened with urine and compared with a color chart.

3. Urine testing is usually done before meals and at bedtime.

4. All equipment should be rinsed thoroughly after use.

B. Communicative Aspects

1. *Observations*

   a. Careful observation of the chemical reaction during Clinitest is important in detecting pass-through color changes.

   b. Any problems with obtaining the urine specimen should be noted.

   c. The patient should be observed for the following signs of diabetic problems which warrant immediate attention:

   (1) *Insulin shock:* swelling, pallor, tremor, anxiety, tachycardia, palpitation, headache, confusion, emotional changes, slurred speech, incoordination, double vision, drowsiness, convulsions, and coma

   (2) *Diabetic coma:* thirst, anorexia, nausea, vomiting, abdominal pain, headache, drowsiness, weakness, shortness of breath, air hunger, fruity-smelling breath, and coma

2. *Charting*

   On diabetic record

DATE	TIME	CLINITEST	ACETEST	REG. INSULIN	OTHER	SITE
5/14	0700	4+		15 U		L Leg
	1100	2+		5 U		R Leg

3. *Referrals*

   The American Diabetes Association is very active in screening procedures and in the assistance of active diabetics.

C. Teaching Aspects—Patient and Family

1. The patient or a significant family member should be taught to do the urine testing, since this will probably be necessary for the rest of the patient's life.

2. Diabetes is a chronic hereditary disease. For this reason, people with a family history of diabetes should be checked regularly.

IV. EVALUATION PROCESS

A. Does the patient understand and seem eager to learn how to do the urine testing?

B. Does the patient comply with giving the urine specimens on time?

C. Was the test carried out properly?

D. Was the equipment cleaned thoroughly after use so that no residual fluid remains in the test tube or dropper?

12

Intravenous Pyelogram (IVP)

I. ASSESSMENT OF SITUATION

A. Definition

An x-ray study of the kidneys and ureters by means of an injected dye

B. Terminology

1. *Renal calculus* (pl. *calculi*): an abnormal concentration of mineral salts adhering together to form a "stone" somewhere in the urinary system

C. Rationale for Actions

1. To determine abnormalities in the outline of the urinary tract signifying pathology
2. To assess the level of kidney functioning
3. To assess the efficiency of bladder emptying

II. NURSING PLAN

A. Objectives

1. To protect the patient from the threat of allergic reaction
2. To prepare the patient adequately to ensure maximum visualization

B. Patient Preparation

1. A complete assessment of the patient's allergic history is essential prior to the injection of iodine dye.
2. An x-ray is a form of radiant energy which penetrates according to the density of tissue. For this reason, the stomach and bowel should be empty so that they will not interfere with the x-ray visualization of the kidneys, ureters, and bladder, which are close to each other. Food and fluids may be withheld for 12 hours preceding the test. A laxative or enema or both may be used to assure that the bowel is empty in preparation for this x-ray examination.
3. Barium in the GI tract will obscure the urinary tract. If the patient has recently undergone barium studies, a period of about two days should elapse before urologic studies are begun.

C. Equipment
Wheelchair or stretcher for transport to the Radiology Department

III. IMPLEMENTING NURSING INTERVENTION

A. Therapeutic Aspects

1. The patient should be transported to the Radiology Department in a safe manner.

2. In the Radiology Department, the patient will be placed on an x-ray table. An x-ray examination of the KUB (kidneys, ureters, bladder) usually is done first. The dye, which is largely iodine, is then injected by venipuncture. A warm, flushing feeling and an unpleasant taste often accompany injection, but these effects are short-lived. X-ray films are taken at designated intervals. If warranted, a postvoiding film may be taken when the IVP is completed, to determine the efficiency of bladder emptying. The entire x-ray study usually takes an hour.

3. When the patient is returned to his room, the nurse should continue to observe for reaction to the dye.

4. After the x-ray examination, the patient should rest and force fluids in order to flush the dye from his system. Food should also be taken to counteract the effects of dehydration and fasting.

B. Communicative Aspects

1. *Observations*

   a. Observe the patient for any indication of an allergic reaction to the iodine dye.

   b. Note the effect of laxatives or enemas to determine if the colon has been emptied adequately.

2. *Charting*

DATE	TREATMENT	TIME	OBSERVATION	SIGNATURE
7/4	To x-ray for IVP by w/c	0730	States he has no history of any allergies; has used iodine topically. Good results from enema prep. No further c/o right flank pain.	G. Ivers, R.N.

3. *Referrals*

   If abnormalities are found, the National Kidney Foundation may be able to offer services or assistance to the patient.

C. Teaching Aspects

1. The role of adequate hydration in the prevention of renal calculi should be stressed.

2. The inherent safety of x-ray techniques should be emphasized, especially if the patient voices any concern regarding radiation.

IV. EVALUATION PROCESS

A. Did the patient approach the x-ray calmly and did he accept its necessity?

B. Was the patient cooperative throughout the procedure?

C. Did the x-ray film reveal pathology?

D. Did the patient experience any allergic reaction? If so, was it detected early and handled properly?

E. Was visualization obscured by debris in the GI tract?

13

Lumbar Puncture

I. ASSESSMENT OF SITUATION

A. Definition

Insertion of a needle into the lumbar subarachnoid space for the purpose of examining and withdrawing cerebrospinal fluid for diagnostic study or spinal anesthesia. Lumbar puncture is also called spinal tap.

B. Terminology

1. *Subarachnoid space:* space between the pia proper and arachnoid, containing the cerebrospinal fluid

2. *Cervical spine:* the first seven vertebrae

3. *Thoracic spine:* the twelve vertebrae below the cervical spine

4. *Lumbar spine:* the five vertebrae below the thoracic spine

5. *Manometer:* the graduated tube through which fluid flows to determine the pressure of the spinal fluid

6. *Cisternal puncture:* insertion of the needle into the cisterna magna just below the occipital bone in the back of the neck

7. *Queckenstedt test:* compression on one or both of the jugular veins for 10 seconds during lumbar puncture; this should cause a rapid rise in

pressure of the cerebrospinal fluid of healthy persons. The rise in pressure quickly subsides when pressure on the neck is released. When there is a block in the spinal canal, the pressure of the spinal fluid is scarcely affected by this test. This test is contraindicated in the presence of intracranial disease (*i.e.,* hemorrhage or increased intracranial pressure).

8. *Myelogram:* radiologic study of the spinal column using a radiopaque medium

9. *Pneumoencephalogram:* radiologic study of the subarachnoid area of the brain accomplished by injecting gas into the space

C. Rationale for Actions

1. To determine the presence of infection, hemorrhage, increased intracranial pressure, or other pathology

2. To administer spinal anesthesia

3. To inject dyes or gases for the purpose of diagnostic x-ray examination of the spine

II. NURSING PLAN

A. Objectives

1. To prevent contamination and the possibility of infection

2. To minimize the chance of post-lumbar puncture headache

3. To provide adequate explanation, enabling the patient to remain calm and cooperative

4. To secure the patient to assure immobility

5. To send the labeled specimens to the laboratory in an expeditious manner

B. Patient Preparation

1. A thorough explanation should include a description of the spine and spinal cord. It is necessary to emphasize that the cord descends through both the cervical and thoracic spine, to the first or second lumbar vertebra, where it ends. Many patients fear that they will be paralyzed by needle insertion in the spine. The spinal needle is inserted well below the area of the spinal cord, however, usually between the third and fourth lumbar vertebrae. There are many nerve endings in this area, and the needle may encounter one of these. The patient should be reassured that no permanent damage will result, and he should simply tell the physician if he feels a sharp pain in his legs or groin area. Explanation of positioning should also be offered at this time.

2. The possibility of post-spinal headaches should be minimized but not ignored. Many people will have had experiences with those who have greatly exaggerated the likelihood, the duration, and the sever-

ity of these headaches. A positive attitude may do a great deal to prevent the "spinal headache." However, headaches may occur, although the exact cause is uncertain. Many feel that headache is due to leaking of the cerebrospinal fluid, which reduces the fluid's cushioning effect on the brain. When the brain then settles to the base of the skull as the patient assumes the erect position, pain results from pressure on the nerves. The likelihood of headache can be greatly reduced if the patient remains flat in bed for 12 to 24 hours after the lumbar puncture.

3. Since the patient will have to remain in bed for a period of time after the procedure, he should empty his bladder before the procedure is begun.

C. Equipment

1. Spinal tap tray containing syringes and needles for local anesthetic, spinal needle, drapes, test tubes and stoppers, gauze sponges, forceps, and cups for antiseptics
2. Sterile gloves
3. Manometer with three-way stopcock
4. Local anesthetic
5. Topical antiseptic
6. Band-Aid
7. Labels and requisitions

III. IMPLEMENTING NURSING INTERVENTION

A. Therapeutic Aspects

1. Maximum separation of the third and fourth lumbar vertebrae will facilitate needle inservion. This is best accomplished by hyperextension of the spine, which occurs when the patient lies on his side with knees drawn up to the abdomen and the chin displaced downward onto the chest. The nurse may help hold the patient by placing one arm on the back of his neck and the other behind his knees (Fig. 13-1). On occasion, patients may sit on the side of the bed and lean forward onto a table or the nurse. This position is often used for the administration of spinal anesthesia. Spinal pressure readings are inaccurate when the patient is in the sitting position.

2. The normal microorganisms present on the skin may become pathogenic when introduced into the bloodstream or tissues. Penetration of the body's natural defense barrier, the skin, must be preceded by careful cleaning with an antiseptic solution. The site of puncture is then carefully draped to provide a sterile field. The local anesthetic is administered and allowed to take effect.

3. After the physician inserts the spinal needle into the subarachnoid space, the manometer is attached and the fluid is allowed to flow freely into it until it stops. The level at which the fluid stops indicates

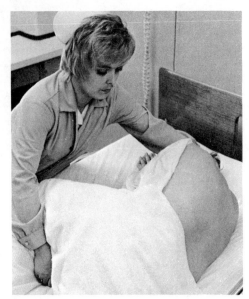

FIGURE 13.1

the spinal pressure. Specimens of the fluid are then placed in test tubes for subsequent laboratory study. The stopcock is turned and the fluid allowed to run or drip into the tubes naturally. Since the rate of flow varies, the patient must be reassured if the length of time begins to seem uncomfortably long. Since some diagnostic tests are done on the first fluid received and some on subsequent samples, the sequence of specimens must be noted and marked on the labels. Likewise, the requisition for the tests should indicate on which specimen they are to be run. Specimens should be sent to the laboratory immediately.

3. After the specimens have been gathered, the needle is removed and direct pressure is applied for a short time. A Band-Aid is then applied, and the patient is placed flat on his back. He should remain flat for 12 to 24 hours. Some physicians allow their patients a small pillow and some allow turning from side to side.

4. When spinal anesthesia is administered, the patient is placed flat on the table and the head of the table is lowered. Progression of anesthesia is assessed by pin sticks on the patient's legs and lower abdomen. When the desired height of anesthesia is reached, the table is leveled or the head slightly elevated, and surgical preparation begins.

B. Communicative Aspects

1. *Observations*

a. The color and appearance of the spinal fluid is significant.

Blood-tinged fluid may indicate a subarachnoid hemorrhage and cloudiness may indicate an infection.

b. The pressure of the cerebrospinal fluid should be noted, as well as the length of time necessary for the fluid specimens to be taken. The normal fluid pressure is 80-200mm of H_2O.

c. In Queckenstedt's test, the pressure variations, as well as the length of time it takes the pressure to normalize, should be noted.

d. Any pain experienced by the patient should be noted. His tolerance during the procedure should be assessed as well.

2. *Charting*

DATE	TREATMENT	TIME	OBSERVATIONS	SIGNATURE
4/9	Lumbar puncture done	0915	Needle insertion accomplished s̄ difficulty. Pressure 100 mm. Fluid appears red tinged— specimens to lab stat. Pt. remains flat in bed and continues to c/o severe headache. Dr. J. notified. B/ P 110/80, P 74, R 22.	G. Ivers, R.N.

3. *Referrals*

Not applicable

C. Teaching Aspects

1. The need for the patient to lie flat for the specified length of time should be explained to enhance cooperation.

2. The subject of post-spinal headaches should be discussed in a matter-of-fact way, so that the patient will not become alarmed if one occurs. However, a positive attitude may greatly reduce the chances of a headache occurring.

3. If spinal anesthesia is administered, the patient must understand that he will regain feeling in his lower body in several hours. Usually, no headache occurs.

IV. EVALUATION PROCESS

A. Did the patient lie still in the proper position?

B. Was his apprehension diminished by adequate preparation?

C. Was the spinal fluid clear?

D. Did the patient experience a post-spinal headache?

E. Was adequate anesthesia produced?

F. Was the fluid labeled correctly and taken to the laboratory quickly?

14

Mammography

I. ASSESSMENT OF SITUATION

A. Definition

X-ray visualization of the breasts to detect the presence of tumors and to determine whether tumors are malignant.

B. Terminology

None

C. Rationale for Actions

1. To determine the presence of tumors of the breasts
2. To determine whether breast tumors are benign or malignant

II. NURSING PLAN

A. Objectives

1. To allay the patient's anxiety about possible breast malignancy
2. To establish a sound diagnostic base upon which to base further action if needed

B. Patient Preparation

1. A patient facing mammography has usually had some basis for suspicion of breast malignancy, such as an unexplained lump or familial history of breast cancer. This may produce a great deal of anxiety as the patient faces the procedure. Reasonable reassurance should be given.
2. An explanation of how the procedure is done and the fact that no pain is involved may reduce the patient's anxiety level. A small amount of discomfort may be experienced if the breasts must be compressed for clearer films.
3. The patient should refrain from the use of deodorants, powders, creams, and other body cosmetics on the day of the procedure.

C. Equipment

In the x-ray department

III. IMPLEMENTING NURSING INTERVENTION

A. Therapeutic Aspects

1. The patient will be asked to remove all clothing above the waist. The x-ray films will be taken with the patient either sitting, standing, or lying.
2. An x-ray is a form of radiant energy that penetrates according to the density of the tissue. The breasts are placed one at a time on the film holder and compressed to try to ensure even density throughout. The films are then taken.
3. Some women may be nervous or embarrassed about exposing their breasts. A female technician may do the x-ray or a female attendant will be present during the examination.

B. Communicative Aspects

1. *Observations*
   a. All female patients should be examined for lumps or irregularities in their breasts during the admission physical examination.
   b. The patient should be observed for undue anxiety about the examination.
2. *Charting*

DATE	TREATMENT	TIME	OBSERVATION	SIGNATURE
11/5	To x-ray for mammography	1015	Examination explained in detail to pt. She seems less nervous p̄ explanation.	F. White, R.N.

3. *Referrals*
   a. The American Cancer Society has booklets explaining Breast Self-Examination, which are free and readily available. If a malignancy is found, the American Cancer Society may also assist by furnishing supplies.
   b. There are local groups, such as "Reach for Recovery," that will assist by counseling and visiting the patient should a malignant tumor be found. These agencies usually seek the permission of the attending physician prior to visiting.

C. Teaching Aspects—Patient and Family

1. The patient and her female family members should be taught how to do self-examination of the breast. They should be encouraged to do this every month, preferably immediately after the menstrual period. After the menopause, the breasts should continue to be checked on a monthly basis.

2. The need for an annual pap smear might also be discussed during the time of teaching about prevention of cancer.

3. Cancer's seven warning signals should be taught to every patient.

IV. EVALUATION PROCESS

A. Was the patient calm and confident before, during, and after the procedure?

B. Does the patient seem to accept the need for regular breast self-examination and yearly pap smears?

C. Did the patient demonstrate an understanding of the correct method of self-examination of the breasts?

D. Was pathology found in the x-ray examination?

15

Myelogram

I. ASSESSMENT OF SITUATION

A. Definition

X-ray visualization of the subarachnoid space around the spinal column by injecting dye

B. Terminology

1. *Lumbar puncture:* insertion of a needle into the subarachnoid space in the area of the third and fourth lumbar vertebrae

2. *Cisternal puncture:* insertion of a needle into the cisterna magna just below the occipital bone in the back of the neck

C. Rationale for Actions

1. To determine the reason for unexplained numbness of legs and arms

2. To rule out pathology of the spinal column such as cysts, herniated discs, or tumors

3. To determine the cause of headaches

II. NURSING PLAN

A. Objectives

1. To allay anxiety and enhance cooperation by thorough explanation
2. To minimize unpleasant side effects

B. Patient Preparation

1. A thorough explanation is essential. The patient should understand what will happen during the myelogram, and should know that removal of the contrast medium after completion of the x-ray examination may cause some pain in the legs or other areas. Making this statement to the patient may reduce the chance the patient's becoming alarmed if pain occurs.
2. Relaxants and tranquilizers may be given as well as antiemetics. Food and fluids are usually withheld prior to the test. As is done for any x-ray study, metal objects and bulky clothing are removed.
3. It is imperative to ascertain that the patient has no allergies to the dye used.

C. Equipment (after return to nursing unit; myelogram is done in the x-ray department)

1. Emesis basin
2. Low pillow

III. IMPLEMENTING NURSING INTERVENTION

A. Therapeutic Aspects

1. Spinal puncture and myelogram are done in the x-ray department. (See Technique 13, Lumbar Puncture.) The nurse should understand what will occur so she can adequately prepare the patient.

    a. Lumbar or cisternal puncture is done. A small amount of spinal fluid is removed, and contrast medium is injected. The patient is strapped to the movable table, which is then tilted to various angles to provide complete visualization. X-ray films are taken at intervals.

    b. After the films are taken, the table is tilted so that the contrast medium collects at the puncture site. It is then withdrawn by a syringe. Failure to withdraw all of the medium may cause inflammation of the subarachnoid space. The needle may be manipulated somewhat in an effort to remove all of the contrast medium. This may cause irritation of the surrounding nerves, resulting in some pain, numbness, and tingling in nearby anatomical structures.

2. After the patient returns from the x-ray department, he is treated as a post-lumbar puncture patient. He is kept flat except for a small pillow (with his physician's permission). Nausea due to motion sick-

ness is a frequent side effect. An emesis basis should be kept close at hand. Fluids should be forced after nausea subsides.

B. Communicative Aspects

1. *Observations*
    a. The patient should be observed closely for any signs of allergy to the contrast medium.
    b. The patient should be observed for headache, nausea, back pain, and stiff neck. A slight fever may occur.
    c. The myelogram procedure and the need to remain flat for a prolonged period may inhibit urination. The patient should be observed closely to make sure that he is voiding a sufficient amount.
    d. Neurological signs should be checked upon return from the x-ray department and periodically for the next 24 hours.

2. *Charting*

DATE	TREATMENT	TIME	OBSERVATIONS	SIGNATURE
3/17	Returned from x-ray after myelogram	1100	Lying flat in bed with small pillow. C/o nausea and sl. headache. Antiemetic given. Neuro signs normal.	F. White, R.N.

3. *Referrals*

Not applicable

C. Teaching Aspects—Patient and Family

1. The patient and family should be told that the procedure will take from 45 minutes to 1½ hours.
2. Proper lifting techniques and body mechanics may be explained to the patient after assessing his readiness and desire to learn.

IV. EVALUATION PROCESS

A. Did the patient understand what would happen during myelogram?
B. Did the patient cooperate by remaining flat for 24 hours?
C. Did the patient experience headache, nausea, or pain?
D. Did the patient void a sufficient quantity during the 24 hours after myelogram?
E. Did the myelogram reveal pathology?

16

Ophthalmoscopic Examination

I. ASSESSMENT OF SITUATION

A. Definition
Examination of the interior of the eye by using a lighted instrument

B. Terminology
1. For anatomical definitions, see Technique 46, Eye, Irrigation of
2. *Strabismus:* eye disorder that occurs when the optic axes cannot be directed to the same object; squint
3. *Nystagmus:* constant involuntary movement of the eyeball

C. Rationale for Actions
1. To examine the inner structures of the eye to determine abnormalities
2. To locate the presence of pathology in the eye

II. NURSING PLAN

A. Objectives
1. To examine thoroughly the inner portion of the eye
2. To minimize the possibility of trauma to the eye and surrounding structures
3. To establish a basis for sound scientific investigation of physiological abnormalities

B. Patient Preparation
1. Because of the proximity of the ophthalmoscope and the examiner to the patient's eye, his cooperation in not moving must be secured prior to beginning. Adequate explanation should serve to secure this cooperation.
2. To ensure maximum visualization and widest possible dilatation of the pupil, room lights are dimmed prior to ophthalmoscopic examination.

C. Equipment
1. Ophthalmoscope
2. Extra batteries

III. IMPLEMENTING NURSING INTERVENTION

A. Therapeutic Aspects

1. Observation is fundamental in all scientific investigations. Observing signs and symptoms of pathology are important functions of the nurse. Using sophisticated equipment such as the ophthalmoscope enables the health care personnel to more accurately determine the patient's health status and plan his care. Therefore, accuracy in observing and reporting is essential.

2. The room lights are dimmed and the scope is turned on. The patient should be told to fix his eyes on a distant object. To examine the right eye, the nurse must have the ophthalmoscope in her right hand in front of the right eye. She uses her left eye and left hand for the patient's left eye. The examiner's head will be very close to the patient's face. The beam is directed onto the patient's eye. A red glow will be present and the examiner should examine the inner aspects of the patient's eye.

3. The closeness of examiner and the ophthalmoscope can cause anxiety in the patient. Reassurance by the nurse can aid compliance and reassure the patient. Because of the possibility of increasing the anxiety level, the examination should not be protracted for an unusually long time.

B. Communicative Aspects

1. *Observations*

    a. Observe for undesirable conditions of the outer eye and surrounding parts

      (1) Eyelids: closure, drooping, swelling, or cysts

      (2) Conjunctiva: inflammation, blood

      (3) Lacrimal ducts: no tears or excessive tears

      (4) Cornea: cloudiness, excessive sensitivity

      (5) Sclera: thinning, bulging, cysts, inflammation

      (6) Anterior chamber: abnormal contents such as blood or pus

      (7) Iris: difference in color, notching, congestion, or infiltration

      (8) Pupil: inequality, dilatation, or constriction

      (9) Extraocular muscles: strabismus, crossed eyes, or nystagmus

    b. Observe the condition of the interior eye

      (1) Retina

      (2) Optic nerve

      (3) Optic disc

      (4) Blood vessels

      (5) Macula lutea and fovea centralis

2. *Charting*

DATE	TREATMENT	TIME	OBSERVATION	SIGNATURE
7/15	Ophthal-moscopic exam of right and left eyes done	0945	No visual abnormalities of the outer eye. Retinal vessels appear abnormal; small amount of intraocular bleeding noted. Dr. Jones notified.	K. Wells, R.N.,

3. *Referrals*

Patients with chronic eye damage may get assistance from the following agencies:
Office of Vocational Rehabilitation American Foundation for the Blind
Braille Institute of America
National Society for the Prevention of Blindness

C. Teaching Aspects

1. The patient should be taught proper eye care and the importance of yearly checkups.

2. Diabetic patients are especially vulnerable to pathology of the eyes. Patients known to have diabetes should be encouraged to have frequent ophthalmoscopic examinations of the eyes.

IV. EVALUATION PROCESS

A. Was the patient cooperative and immobile during the examination?

B. Was the patient anxious about the method of ophthalmoscopic examination or the results of it?

C. Was the inner portion of each eye adequately visualized?

D. Was pathology discovered?

17

Otoscopic Examination

I. ASSESSMENT OF THE SITUATION

A. Definition

Visual examination of the ear using a lighted instrument

B. Terminology

1. *Pinna*: the external ear; auricle
2. *Mastoid process*: the portion of the temporal bone lying behind the pinna; serves for muscle attachment
3. *Tympanic membrane*: membrane separating the external auditory canal from the acoustic cavity

C. Rationale for Actions

1. To determine the condition and the presence of pathology in the external auditory canal
2. To instill medications in the ear
3. To clean the ear and remove wax build-up or foreign bodies

II. NURSING PLAN

A. Objectives

1. To protect the integrity of the lining of the external auditory canal
2. To allay the anxieties of the patient
3. To obtain the patient's cooperation in remaining immobile

B. Patient Preparation

1. Since it is important that the patient remain still during the otoscopic examination, a thorough explanation is necessary to secure his cooperation.
2. Ear treatments often cause anxiety, since the sound produced is exaggerated because of the closeness to the inner ear. Gentleness and efficiency can greatly allay this anxiety.

C. Equipment

1. Otoscope

2. Extra batteries
3. Irrigation syringe or bulb and solution
4. Basin
5. Ear drops

III. IMPLEMENTING NURSING INTERVENTION

A. Therapeutic Aspects

1. The ear has two functions: hearing and balance. The external auditory canal serves to direct sound toward the organs of reception responsible for hearing and to guard against infection. Direct visual examination of this canal using the otoscope can be of great diagnostic value.

2. Handwashing by the examiner must precede the examination. The otoscope should be checked to be sure that the light works. A rounded speculum is placed on the end of the otoscope. The speculum should be the largest which can be inserted into the ear without causing pain or discomfort. Specula are scrupulously cleaned and disinfected after use.

3. During the examination, the speculum is inserted just inside the external opening. The pinna should be pulled upward and backward to enhance visualization of the canal. To visualize the entire canal, the examiner may tilt the otoscope and move his head accordingly. The patient should remain immobile.

4. Minor treatments may be administered through the speculum. Irrigation and application of medications are two treatments for which nurses are often responsible. They may or may not require using the otoscope speculum. Drugs are usually given to soften the skin or wax and to fight infection. Irrigation involves flushing the ear with a fluid such as sterile saline solution to cleanse the canal, soften wax, or remove a foreign body.

B. Communicative Aspects

1. *Observations*

   a. The pinna should be observed for abnormality, fistulas, infection, boils, ulcers, or rash. The condition of the mastoid may be checked by pulling the pinna forward. Swelling or extreme tenderness may signify mastoiditis.

   b. The external auditory canal should be inspected for occlusion, redness, swelling, drainage, foreign body, or tumors.

   c. The tympanic membrane has a dull, bluish, pearly gray, and translucent appearance. It is stretched across and continuous with the auditory canal.

2. *Charting*

DATE	TREATMENT	TIME	OBSERVATIONS	SIGNATURE
4/7	Otoscopic exam complete	0815	Small scratch noted on lower aspect of external auditory canal. Dr. Jones notified. Pt. cautioned about putting sharp objects in his ears.	G. Ivers, R.N.

3. *Referrals*

Persons with severe hearing impairment may be referred to the American Society for the Hard of Hearing.

C. Teaching Aspects

1. The importance of keeping sharp objects out of the ears cannot be overemphasized. Even rubbing or pulling the pinna vigorously can cause ear damage.
2. Foreign objects should be removed only by qualified health care personnel.
3. Ear wax serves the purpose of protecting the inner ear from infectious organisms. It should never be removed by cotton swabs.

IV. EVALUATION PROCESS

A. Did the patient remain immobile during examination?

B. Was the patient's anxiety reduced by prior explanations?

C. Did the patient understand the safety precautions regarding ear care?

D. Were abnormalities or pathology of the ear found?

E. Was wax successfully removed?

F. Was otic medication instillation satisfactorily accomplished?

18
Pneumoencephalogram

I. ASSESSMENT OF SITUATION

A. Definition
X-ray visualization of the ventricles and subarachnoid spaces of the brain following withdrawal of cerebrospinal fluid and injection of air or a gas by way of lumbar puncture.

B. Terminology
Lumbar puncture: insertion of a needle into the subarachnoid space in the area of the third and fourth lumbar vertebrae.

C. Rationale for Actions
1. To locate and determine the size of brain tumors
2. To assess the extent of brain trauma
3. To determine whether cerebrospinal fluid is being blocked

II. NURSING PLAN

A. Objectives
1. To allay anxiety and enhance cooperation by thorough explanation
2. To prepare the patient if there is a possibility of craniotomy
3. To minimize unpleasant side effects

B. Patient Preparation
1. Pneumoencephalogram is a very unpleasant procedure. The ensuing headache is often severe. Nausea and vomiting are frequent side effects. The patient should be thoroughly prepared so that he will not construe these occurrences as a sign that his condition is deteriorating.
2. The night before the x-ray procedure the patient should get a good rest. He will usually be NPO at midnight. Sedatives and analgesics may be given before he goes to the x-ray department. If craniotomy is to be done, the head is shaved. All hairpins and jewelry are removed. Long hair should not be braided, since this could obscure the x-ray film.
3. Some of the films are taken with the patient upside down. He will be securely strapped in a special chair, and there is no danger of falling.

C. Equipment (after return to nursing unit, as pneumoencephalogram is done in the x-ray department)

1. Emesis basin
2. Small pillow

III. IMPLEMENTING NURSING INTERVENTION

A. Therapeutic Aspects

1. Spinal puncture and pneumoencephalogram are done in the x-ray department (see Technique 13, Lumbar Puncture). The nurse should understand what will occur so that she can adequately prepare the patient.

   a. Pneumoencephalography is based on the principle that gas, replacing a fluid within the ventricular and subarachnoid spaces, serves as a contrast medium, since it is less dense than fluid on the x-ray film. Spinal puncture is accomplished, and a small amount of fluid is removed and sent to the lab. An equal amount of air is injected into the subarachnoid space.

   b. The patient is strapped securely in a special chair that rotates slowly to allow the air to travel to the desired location. Some of the films will be taken with the patient upside down.

   c. After the pneumoencephalogram is finished, the chair is placed in an upright position, the needle is removed, and the patient is returned to his room.

2. The bedside care is much the same as that for patients undergoing lumbar puncture. Severe headache and nausea are common. Cold compresses may help relieve the pain. Bent straws will enable the patient to drink without raising his head. A small pillow may be used if it does not cause increased pain.

B. Communicative Aspects

1. *Observations*

   a. The patient is monitored throughout the procedure and should be told to report dizziness, faintness, and difficulty in breathing.

   b. Neurological signs should be monitored every 15 minutes for the first hour, then every half hour for 3 hours. If no problems occur, monitoring every 2 hours for the next 24 hours is appropriate.

   c. Intake and output should be checked for 24 to 48 hours.

2. *Charting*

DATE	TREATMENT	TIME	OBSERVATION	SIGNATURE
4/7	Pneumoencephalogram done in x-ray	1130	Returned to room. C/o severe headache. Flat in bed. Neuro signs stable. Sips of water given c̄ no nausea. Oral med given.	F. White, R.N.

3. *Referrals*

Not applicable

C. Teaching Aspects—Patient and Family

1. The patient and family should be told to keep the staff notified of unusual sensations occurring after the test.

2. During the test, the patient should report unusual pain or problems.

IV. EVALUATION PROCESS

A. Did the patient understand the procedure?

B. Did the patient comply with instructions?

C. Was any pathology found?

D. Did the patient experience any side effects?

E. If the patient experienced headache, was it controlled by drugs and alterations of the environment?

19

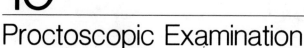

Proctoscopic Examination

I. ASSESSMENT OF SITUATION

A. Definition

Direct visualization of the distal end of the large intestine by use of a lighted tubular instrument

B. Terminology

1. *Anus:* opening of the large intestine to the outside

2. *Rectum:* the terminal six or eight inches of the large intestine

3. *Sigmoid:* the lower part of the descending colon between the iliac crest and the rectum, shaped like the letter "S"

4. *Anoscopy:* visualization of the anus

5. *Sigmoidoscopy:* visualization of the sigmoid colon

6. *Endoscopy:* inspection of cavities by use of an illuminated metal, rubber, or glass tube

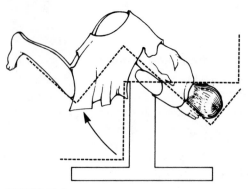

FIGURE 19.1

C. Rationale for Actions

1. To assist in early detection of tumors and other pathology of the large intestine
2. To determine the site of pathology and cauterize to stop rectal bleeding
3. To provide a means for taking a rectal biopsy
4. To remove rectal polyps

II. NURSING PLAN

A. Objectives

1. To allay fear and anxiety by thorough explanation
2. To expedite the procedure by complete preparation and testing of all equipment

B. Patient Preparation

1. A thorough explanation of the procedure should include instructions on the proper position to take during the proctoscopic examination. If the knee-chest position is used, the nurse should show the patient how to assume this position by resting his weight on his legs and chest, not his hands and elbows. Many hospitals have a proctoscopic table that breaks in the middle and tilts to allow the patient to be adequately supported and positioned (Fig. 19-1).
2. The large intestine should be emptied prior to endoscopic examination. This is usually accomplished by a light, low-residue meal the evening before and the administration of a strong laxative such as castor oil. On the morning of the examination, enemas to clear the bowel may be given.

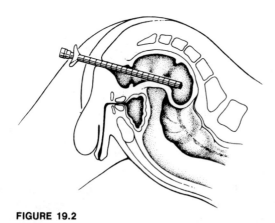

FIGURE 19.2

C. Equipment

1. Appropriate endoscope
2. Suction tips and machine
3. Rectal biopsy forceps and specimen container
4. Sheet for drape
5. Lubricating jelly
6. Rectal swabs

III. IMPLEMENTING NURSING INTERVENTION

A. Therapeutic Aspects

1. The patient should be placed in one of three positions: (1) in bed on his left side with his right leg flexed, (2) on his chest and knees with his buttocks in the air, or (3) on a special proctoscopic table. Continual reassurance throughout the procedure is essential. To avoid embarrassing and exposing the patient unnecessarily, the patient should be adequately draped by using a proctoscopic drape sheet with a circular hole in it. If the drape sheet is not available, use a regular bed sheet and drape the patient according to hospital procedure.

2. Friction, the force opposing motion between two contacting surfaces, can be minimized by lubrication of the scope with a water-soluble jelly.

3. Relaxation of the sphincters guarding the anus will facilitate scope insertion and can be promoted by having the patient take slow, deep breaths. The physician will visualize the bowel as he inserts the scope (Fig. 19-2). If debris is still present, he may elect to use a rectal swab or suction tip.

4. To facilitate visualization between the muscular folds of the rectum, the physician may inflate the lower colon by means of a bulb at-

tached to the scope. Peristaltic action may be stimulated by this distention of the intestinal wall. This will give the patient a full or cramping feeling; slow deep breathing will promote relaxation. Reassurance from the nurse at this time is especially helpful.

5. If a biopsy is taken, the physician will insert the biopsy forceps through the scope and take a small piece of tissue. This may be painful to the patient. The biopsy should be placed in a prepared container that has an appropriate preservative in it and is clearly labeled with the patient's name and the location from which the biopsy was taken.

6. After the scope is removed, the lubricating jelly should be cleaned from the patient's buttocks. If he has been in a position in which his head is lower than his buttocks, he should be slowly raised to a level where head and body are on an even plane and allowed to stabilize for a few minutes. When he no longer feels dizzy or faint, he may be placed in a wheelchair and returned to bed.

7. All equipment used must be cleaned thoroughly or disposed of properly. Specimens should be sent to the laboratory immediately.

B. Communicative Aspects

1. *Observations*

   a. Observe the patient during the procedure for anxiety, cramping, or distress.

   b. If a biopsy is taken, signs of rectal bleeding must be monitored. A small amount of blood-tinged stool may be expected, but bright frank bleeding is an emergency and warrants immediate attention.

2. *Charting*

DATE	TREATMENT	TIME	OBSERVATION	SIGNATURE
10/13	Proctoscopy done	1015	Tol. procedure well. C/o slight abd. cramping. Biopsy taken and sent to lab. Pt. assured nurses he will save his stool for inspection.	F.White, R.N.

3. *Referrals*

   Not applicable

C. Teaching Aspects—Patient and Family

1. The patient should be told that after proctoscopic examination he may have increased flatulence due to inflation of the bowel. Also, if a biopsy is taken, he should be told to report any rectal bleeding.

2. The patient and family should be taught guidelines for proper elimi-

nation habits, judicious use of laxatives, and the effect of diet on elimination.

3. The importance of reporting any rectal bleeding to a physician should be stressed, since this is a warning signal of cancer.

IV. EVALUATION PROCESS

A. Did the patient cooperate during the procedure?

B. Did the patient understand the findings from the examination?

C. Was the bowel adequately prepared for clear visualization?

D. Was the specimen sent to the laboratory promptly?

E. Was the patient returned to his room safely with no dizziness or fainting?

20

Residual Urine

I. ASSESSMENT OF SITUATION

A. Definition

The amount of urine left in the bladder after urination

B. Terminology

1. *Urinary calculus:* an abnormal concentration of mineral salts adhering to form a "stone" somewhere in the urinary system.

2. *B.P.H. (benign prostatic hypertrophy):* an enlargement of the prostate gland often associated with advanced age

C. Rationale for Actions

1. To check for incomplete emptying of the bladder

2. To assess the possibility of enlarged prostate

II. NURSING PLAN

A. Objectives

1. To empty the patient's bladder completely

2. To measure the amount of residual urine in order to assess emptying capability

B. Patient Preparation

1. Explain to the patient why the catheterization must be done and why the bladder must be emptied voluntarily first.
2. Refer to Technique 35, Catheterization, Urethral, for futher preparation steps.

C. Equipment

1. Catheterization equipment (see Technique 35, Catheterization, Urethral)
2. Graduated cylinder for measurement
3. Bedpan, urinal, or commode container

III. IMPLEMENTING NURSING INTERVENTION

A. Therapeutic Aspects

1. The patient should empty his bladder into a container immediately prior to catheterization for residual. This urine must be measured and the amount recorded.
2. The patient is catheterized and the bladder completely emptied. The amount of urine returned is the "residual" amount. This amount must be carefully measured and the amount recorded. Since residual urine is often associated with a partial obstruction of the urethra, such as that caused by an enlarged prostate gland, the resulting stasis of urine in the bladder can lead to infection and calculus. For this reason, complete emptying of the bladder is essential.

B. Communicative Aspects

1. *Observations*
   a. Note the appearance and color of the urine.
   b. Particularly note the amount of residual urine.
2. *Charting*

DATE	TREATMENT	TIME	OBSERVATIONS	SIGNATURE
4/7	Cath'd for residual urine	1015	Pt. voided 350 ml of dark urine. Cath'd with return of 175 ml of residual urine. No c/o discomfort at this time.	B. Smith, R.N.

3. *Referrals*
   Not applicable

C. Teaching Aspects

1. The importance of adequate fluid intake should be emphasized.
2. The male patient over 60 years of age should be told to report a feel-

ing of incomplete emptying and difficulty starting the urinary stream, since these may indicate B.P.H.

IV. EVALUATION PROCESS

A. Did the patient cooperate during the procedure?

B. Was the significance of obtaining residual urine adequately explained?

C. Was any residual urine present?

D. Was sufficient time allowed to completely empty the bladder?

E. Was accurate measurement accomplished?

21

Specific Gravity of Urine

I. ASSESSMENT OF SITUATION

A. Definition

The ratio the weight of a given volume of urine bears to the weight of the same volume of water (normal range 1.010 to 1.025)

B. Terminology

Urinometer: an instrument that contains a mercury bulb attached to a stem with a graduated scale indicating a range of concentration from 1:000 to 1:040

C. Rationale for Actions

1. To test the ability of the kidneys to dilute and concentrate urine

2. To evaluate the extent of kidney damage

II. NURSING PLAN

A. Objectives

1. To allay patient apprehension about diagnostic testing

2. To obtain an adequate amount of urine to assure accurate test results

3. To carry out the specific gravity test in a capable manner

B. Patient Preparation

1. If the test is being done to test the ability of the kidneys to dilute and concentrate urine, the patient may be dehydrated before one specimen and overhydrated before the second specimen.

2. An explanation of what the test is for and the amount of urine needed may encourage the patient to cooperate more fully.

C. Equipment

1. Graduated container holding at least 150 ml

2. Urinometer

III. IMPLEMENTING NURSING INTERVENTION

A. Therapeutic Aspects

1. Urine is formed from the noncolloidal constituents of blood plasma that are filtered by the kidneys and concentrated into urine. The function of the kidneys is to keep the body fluids at their normal composition and volume. Normally, the specific gravity of urine is responsive to the water and electrolyte situation in the body. Profuse perspiration with decreased intake produces a high specific gravity. High fluid intake with no excessive loss will lower the specific gravity. Damaged kidneys cannot adjust to these extremes; and regardless of the degree of hydration, the specific gravity will remain constant, usually between 1.010 and 1.015.

2. At least 20 ml of urine are needed to test specific gravity. The urine is placed in a graduated container and the urinometer is lowered gently into the urine. The specific gravity is the level of the urine on the graduated scale when the urinometer is still. It is read as 00, 01, 02, and so on, through 10, 20, 30, 40, 50, and 60. These are interpreted as: 00 (1.000), 01 (1.001), 10 (1.010), 20 (1.020), and so forth, as measured against the specific gravity of distilled water, which is 1.000. The principle upon which this measurement is based is displacement. This means that the more concentrated the urine, the more the urinometer will be displaced upward and the higher the specific gravity.

3. After the test is completed, all equipment should be thoroughly rinsed and stored properly. Diagnostic testing usually is a cause of apprehension to the patient, hence any possible encouragement should be offered.

B. Communicative Aspects

1. *Observations*

   a. Note the color, odor, and appearance of urine when the specimen is obtained.

   b. Observe the patient's degree of apprehension regarding diagnostic testing.

2. *Charting*

DATE	TREATMENT	TIME	OBSERVATIONS	SIGNATURE
5/4	Sp. gravity of urine 1.015	1400	150 ml of urine obtained for diag. testing. Color yellow clear with no foul odor. Pt. seems very nervous. Readily accepted explanation of purpose of test.	G. Ivers, R.N.

3. *Referrals*

Not applicable

C. Teaching Aspects

1. The influence of adequate hydration on kidney function may be explained.
2. The purpose of the specific gravity test and interpretation of the results should be given to the patient who indicates an interest and desire to know.

IV. EVALUATION PROCESS

A. Did the patient cooperate by providing an adequate specimen?

B. Does the patient seem at ease about the diagnostic testing?

C. Was the specific gravity within normal range?

D. Were the odor and appearance of the urine normal?

22

Urine Examinations

I. ASSESSMENT OF SITUATION

A. Definition

An analysis of the constituents of urine including a description of color

B. Terminology

1. *Clean-catch specimen* (*midstream*): a voided specimen caught in a sterile container after cleansing of the meatus and voiding of a small amount prior to catching the specimen

2. *Catheterized specimen:* insertion of a tube directly into the bladder to obtain a sterile urine specimen

3. *Random specimen:* collection of urine under clean conditions for laboratory study

4. *Timed specimen:* urine collected for a specified period of time, usually 12 or 24 hours

5. *Urinalysis:* analysis of the urine to determine a description of color and degree of cloudiness, pH, specific gravity, presence of protein or glucose, and a microscopic examination of the sediment

C. Rationale for Actions

1. To assess the effectiveness of kidney function
2. To determine the presence of pathology

II. NURSING PLAN

A. Objectives

1. To assist the patient to overcome embarrassment sometimes associated with the eliminative function

2. To collect an adequate amount of urine under clean or sterile conditions

3. For timed specimens, to collect all of the urine excreted during the specified time period

B. Patient Preparation

1. The voluntary process of voiding can be inhibited by feelings of fear, excitement, pressure, and embarrassment. The patient should be given adequate time and privacy to produce the desired specimen.

2. Adequate instructions on the method of specimen collection should be given prior to the request for a specimen.

3. If the specimen is to be gathered over a specified period of time, the patient should understand that *all* urine must be saved and should know the exact amount of time involved.

C. Equipment

1. *Random specimen*
   a. Clean urinal, bedpan, or commode container
   b. Specimen container

2. *Catheterized specimen* (See Technique 35, Catheterization, Urethral)

3. *Clean-catch specimen*
   a. Cotton balls and cleansing solution
   b. Sterile specimen container

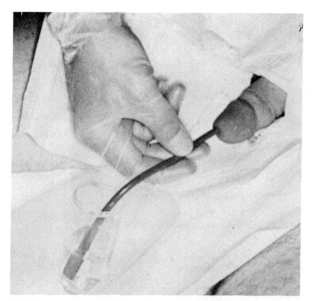

FIGURE 22.1

4. *Timed specimen*
   a. Urinal, bedpan, or commode container
   b. Large specimen bottle with appropriate preservative

III. IMPLEMENTING NURSING INTERVENTION

A. Therapeutic Aspects

1. The time when the urine specimen is collected has a great bearing on the results of the diagnostic tests. Early morning specimens are often desirable for urinalysis because the specimen is more concentrated owing to decreased fluid intake in the hours preceding collection. Tests for certain metabolic disorders may require a specimen collected after a meal.

2. For a random specimen, the patient is asked to void into a clean receptacle (usually a bedpan, urinal, or commode container). The nurse then pours a small amount (usually between 30 to 50 ml) into a labeled specimen container. The specimen container should then be sent to the laboratory with a properly labeled requisition as soon as possible. The remainder of the urine is discarded and the receptacle rinsed thoroughly. This method is usually used for routine urinalysis.

3. For specifics on obtaining a sterile catheterized specimen, refer to Technique 35. Once the catherized specimen has been placed in the container (Fig. 22-1), care must be taken not to contaminate it when replacing the lid. The container should be labeled and sent to the lab-

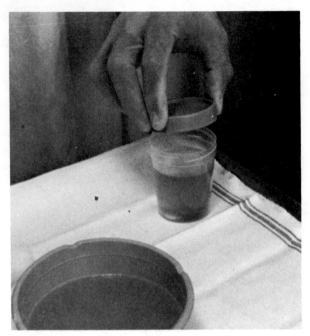

FIGURE 22.2

oratory at once, especially if the specimen is for a culture. A labeled requisition should accompany the specimen.

4. In obtaining a clean-catch specimen (midstream specimen), careful instructions must be given so that the patient does not inadvertently contaminate the specimen. The cap should be removed and replaced with the fingertips on the outside edge to avoid contamination (Fig. 22-2). The cap should be placed top side down on the table while the patient is voiding.

   a. *Women*

   (1) Clean the vulva with an accepted cleansing solution. Emphasis should be placed on cleaning from front to back.

   (2) The labia should be separated during the specimen collection. After passing a small amount of urine, the patient should void directly into the sterile specimen container collecting the midstream portion.

   b. *Men*

   (1) Clean the meatus and surrounding area with cotton balls and a cleansing solution (Fig. 22-3).

   (2) After passing a small amount of urine, the patient should void directly into a sterile container (Figs. 22-4 and 22-5).

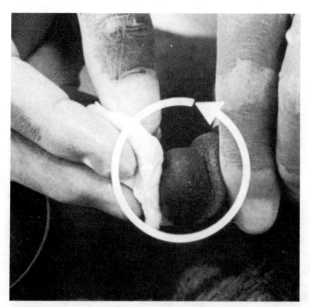

FIGURE 22.3

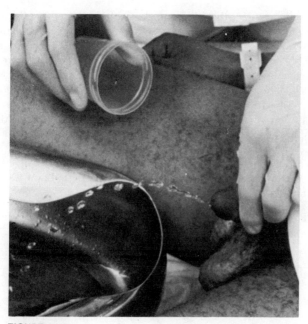

FIGURE 22.4

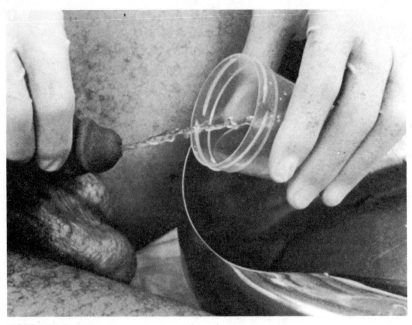

FIGURE 22.5

5. In a timed specimen, the specimen should be collected for the exact amount of time specified. The patient must understand that all of the urine is to be saved. A bottle from the laboratory, with an appropriate preservative, should be labeled and placed in a convenient place where it will not be spilled. It must be kept cold during collection, either by refrigeration or by placing the container in a basin of ice. To begin collection, the patient voids an initial specimen which is discarded. All urine voided after this initial specimen is saved and poured into the collection bottle. At the time the collection is to end, the patient should empty his bladder; this specimen is also saved and poured into the collection bottle. At the end of the specified time, the bottle is taken to the laboratory.

B. Communicative Aspects

1. *Observations*
   a. Note color and appearance of urine.
   b. Note any difficulty in voiding.

2. *Charting*

DATE	TREATMENT	TIME	OBSERVATIONS	SIGNATURE
10/4	24 hour urine specimen begun	0700	Container for urine placed on ice in pt's. bathroom. Complete instructions given to pt., who states he understands and will cooperate.	F. White, R.N.

3. *Referrals*

Not applicable

C. Teaching Aspects

1. Teach the patient the need for adequate hydration for proper kidney function.

2. Caution the patient to collect urine specimens before defecation.

3. Remind the female patients about the importance of cleansing the urinary meatus from front to back.

IV. EVALUATION PROCESS

A. Has the patient cooperated during specimen collection?

B. Did the patient receive full instructions prior to the test?

C. Were the specimens sent to the laboratory expeditiously?

D. Did the patient understand the results?

E. Was the sterility of catheterized and clean-catch specimens maintained?

F. Were the results explained to the patient?

2

Techniques for Adult Patients

23
Admission

I. ASSESSMENT OF SITUATION

A. Definition

The incorporation of a series of activities that occur when the patient enters the hospital

B. Terminology

None

C. Rationale for Actions

1. To give basic, pertinent information to the patient
2. To obtain pertinent information from the patient
3. To make the patient feel comfortable and welcome

II. NURSING PLAN

A. Objectives

1. To make the patient and family feel welcome, and facilitate their adjustment to the hospital environment
2. To observe and evaluate the patient's condition
3. To institute primary diagnostic measures
4. To maintain the individuality of the person being admitted

B. Patient Preparation

1. Greet patient in a courteous manner.
2. Orient patient and family to hospital environment.
3. Explanations concerning hospital regulations for valuables, visiting hours, televisions, telephones, and consent forms, and concerning the operation of equipment (*e.g.,* beds, air conditioner) and the use of side rails should be made. An explanation of hospital routine (*e.g.,* meals, shift changes, doctors' rounds) is also in order. Knowing what to expect reduces unnecessary fear and apprehension, enabling the patient to hear what is said to him. Regardless of the number of details included in admission, each should be explained so that the patient understands that they are in his interest.

C. Equipment

1. Stethoscope and sphygmomanometer

2. Watch with a second hand

3. Hospital gown

4. Portable scale

5. Labeled bedpan and urinal, if needed

6. Admission pack (wash basin, emesis basin, thermometer, hospital lotion, tissues)

7. Admission record

III. IMPLEMENTING NURSING INTERVENTION

A. Therapeutic Aspects

1. Vital signs should be taken when the patient is at rest. Allow him to lie down and relax before beginning this procedure.

2. Vital signs are indicators of the patient's general condition. Temperature, pulse, respiration, and blood pressure should be taken. Weight and height should be recorded as taken or, if necessary, as stated by the patient or family. Physical care procedures also have a secondary purpose of establishing positive interpersonal relations between the patient and his family and the hospital staff.

3. A urine specimen should be obtained from each patient.

4. Adequate patient identification helps prevent errors and cross-contamination. An identification card should be placed on the bed. All personal equipment should be labeled. Allergies should be ascertained and noted on the chart. A patient identification band should be placed on the patient's wrist.

5. The patient should be made comfortable and secure, and the call signal should be left in a convenient place. Valuables and personal clothing may be sent home with the family. The nursing care plan should be initiated on admission.

B. Communicative Aspects

1. *Observations*

   a. The patient and family should be included in all admission explanations. Written instructions may be available for them.

   b. Answer questions readily. Convey confidence by manner and attitude.

2. *Charting*

   a. Record time, date, and mode of admission.

   b. List observations (general appearance and facial expression, pain and type of pain, rashes, bruises, abrasions, drug and food sensitivities, complaints, medications brought by the patient, clothing, valuables, specimens obtained, name of doctor, and timenotified).

   c. The nurse signs the chart.

DATE	TREATMENT	TIME	OBSERVATIONS	SIGNATURE
5/5	Admission	0900	Admitted to room 214 via wheelchair from emergency department. Complaining of nausea, vomiting, and severe pain in right lower quadrant of abdomen. CBC and UA done in E.D. Operative permit for appendectomy signed by patient. Clothes and wristwatch given to husband. Patient states she is allergic to Demerol and tomatoes. Patient states this is her first admission to a hospital. Appears apprehensive. Seems more at ease after being interviewed by head nurse.	
		0910	Dr. A. notified of patient's admission.	F. White, R.N.

3. *Referrals*

Not applicable

C. Teaching Aspects—Patient and Family

1. Explain visiting hours, dining room and snack bar locations and hours, and so forth.
2. If the patient is going to surgery, he and his family should know the approximate time and pertinent details.

IV. EVALUATION PROCESS

A. Have the patient's needs for orientation to his role and his new environment been met?

B. Does the patient perceive the nurse's understanding of his fears?

C. Does the patient understand the functions of the members of the health team?

D. Are the patient's preferences and habit patterns supported whenever possible?

24

Ambulation

I. ASSESSMENT OF SITUATION

A. Definition

The act of walking, with or without assistance, in an attempt to regain normal activity

B. Terminology

None

C. Rationale for Action

1. To build up the physical stamina of the patient in preparation for surgery or treatment
2. To offer a diversion from hospital routine
3. To facilitate wound healing and return of homeostasis
4. To prevent complications, such as pneumonia and contracture

II. NURSING PLAN

A. Objectives

1. To maintain an environment conducive to patient safety
2. To assist with ambulation, as dictated by the patient's condition and progress
3. To offer explanations and reassurance to allay anxieties about ambulation
4. To teach the patient optimal ambulatory techniques and proper posture

B. Patient Preparation

1. Before beginning the ambulation process, the patient should be told exactly what will happen, what will be expected of him, and what limitations, if any, will be placed on his participation (*e.g.*, no weight bearing on right leg, or no extension of affected limb).
2. Assembling all pertinent equipment prior to beginning the procedure will reduce delays and avoid tiring the patient unnecessarily.

C. Equipment

1. Belt (around patient's waist for support)
2. Robe and slippers

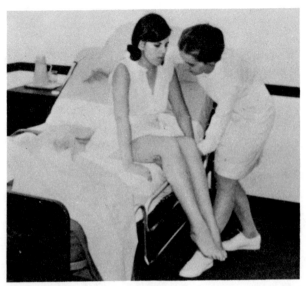

FIGURE 24.1

III. IMPLEMENTING NURSING INTERVENTION

A. Therapeutic Aspects

1. Ambulation helps restore a sense of equilibrium and enhances self-confidence. It should be begun as soon after the surgery or treatment as possible, unless otherwise ordered. Patients in the hospital for studies and examinations should be encouraged to ambulate to preserve muscle tone and encourage a sense of well-being. If activity limitations have been imposed by the physician, the patient should clearly understand the extent of these limitations and the reasons for them.

2. After prolonged inactivity, muscle tone deteriorates, but the patient may feel better than previously and thus overestimate his capabilities. During the first few ambulation periods postoperatively or after severe debilitating illness, two people should accompany the patient. Prevention of injury (*e.g.*, from falls) and complications (*e.g.*, wound dehiscence) should be kept uppermost in mind. A belt may be placed around the patient's waist for the nurse to hold in guiding and supporting him. If there is an abdominal incision, however, a belt is not practical, and an attendant should support each side of the patient.

3. To begin ambulation, the patient should sit on the side of the bed and gain a sense of equilibrium (Fig. 24-1). The bed should be in the low position. He should not attempt to walk until his condition is stable in the sitting position, *i.e.*, no dizziness, nausea. The patient should be discouraged from looking down and encouraged to assume as near

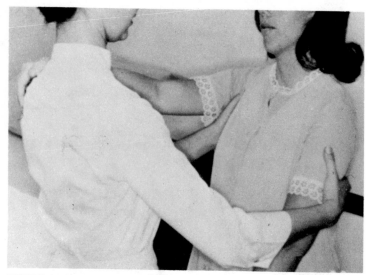

FIGURE 24.2

normal a walking posture as possible. He should begin slowly and deliberately as he is assisted by the nurse, who places one hand under the axilla and the other on the forearm (Fig. 24-2). Standing erect encourages deep breathing and lessens the possibility of wound complications. The patient should then ambulate as ordered or as tolerated.

4. To avoid further fatigue and exertion, the patient's bed may be made while he is up. However, the nurse must remember that ambulation is foremost a form of therapy and is not to be utilized at the patient's expense for her convenience.

5. Special equipment, such as catheters and chest tubes, need not restrict ambulation, provided the physician concurs. If allowed, catheter tubes may be clamped and attached to a drain bag which fastens to the patient's leg, or the regular drain bag may be carried by the nurse. Nasogastric tubes may be clamped, if allowed, and secured to the patient's gown with a pin to prevent pulling. See the appropriate techniques for ambulation with other specialized equipment, such as chest tubes and crutches.

B. Communicative Aspects

1. *Observations*

   a. Observe the patient carefully for readiness to ambulate prior to getting him on his feet. Do not rush him; if he is dizzy or nauseated, let him lie back for a few moments.

    b. After ambulation, observe dressings for more profuse drainage and tubes for changes in drainage.

    c. Observe the patient carefully during ambulation for signs of fatigue, and return him to bed before he becomes overtired.

2. *Charting*

DATE	TREATMENT	TIME	OBSERVATIONS	SIGNATURE
6/1	Amb in room	0800	Amb to door and back. No nausea or dizziness. Some incisional discomfort. Suture integrity maintained. No abnormal drainage.	B. Smith, L.V.N.

3. *Referrals*

    a. If continued assistance and teaching will be needed after dismissal, or if the patient has unusual difficulties in ambulation, referral to a physical therapist may be in order. A physician's concurrence is usually necessary for this.

C. Teaching Aspects—Patient and Family

1. The patient must be told the positive reasons for early postoperative ambulation (*e.g.,* prevention of pneumonia, earlier return to normal activities). He must also be reassured that the suture line will not break open, that he will not damage the operative area, and that he will not cause any complications.

2. Stress the need to stand erect even though the sutures may pull and some discomfort may be present. Walking in a slumped, dependent position inhibits breathing and contributes to complications.

3. Tell the patient that he may feel momentary dizziness on arising but it should pass quickly. Tell him he may feel some pulling sensation in the operative area but it is normal and not an indication of wound breakdown.

4. Stress the importance of not overestimating capabilities. Some patients begin to feel better and try to undertake activities which exceed their stamina. *Moderation* is a key word in ambulation therapy.

5. If the patient is going to require assistance in ambulation after dismissal, the family should be taught proper body mechanics, transfer techniques, and safety precautions.

IV. EVALUATION PROCESS

A. Were accidents prevented by proper attention to safety techniques?

B. Did ambulation therapy progress from dependency to independent activity in reasonable time?

C. Did the patient feel confident about his ambulatory attempts?

D. Has the affected limb healed in correct alignment and normal-position?

E. Have any tubes present remained intact and patent?

F. Did the patient stand erect, breathe deeply, and correctly estimate his abilities?

25

Backrub

I. ASSESSMENT OF SITUATION

A. Definition

The massaging of an individual's back as a therapeutic and comfort measure

B. Terminology

1. *Effleurage:* deep or superficial stroking in massage
2. *Pétrissage:* a kneading movement in massage
3. *Pressure sore (decubitus ulcer):* gangrene of the skin due to pressure; also know as a *bed-sore*
4. *Tapotement:* percussion in massage

C. Rationale for Actions

1. To stimulate circulation and thus increase blood supply to the area
2. To observe the skin for signs of impaired circulation or breakdown (pressure sore)
3. To relieve tension and promote relaxation
4. To convey personal concern for the patient

II. NURSING PLAN

A. Objectives

1. To ensure that the patient has been made as comfortable as possible, especially at bedtime
2. To prevent skin breakdown on the patient who spends a majority of time in bed or is unable to change position easily or often
3. To open and improve lines of communication between the patient and the nurse

B. Patient Preparation

1. Since an important reason for administering a backrub is to relieve tension and promote relaxation, especially at bedtime, the nurse should ensure that the patient is comfortable prior to beginning. General hygiene measures undertaken at bedtime should be completed prior to the backrub. Bed linen should be wrinkle-free and lights lowered appropriately.

C. Equipment

1. Lotion, powder, or alcohol
2. Towel

III. IMPLEMENTING NURSING INTERVENTION

A. Therapeutic Aspects

1. Relaxation promotes rest and sleep. A backrub at the end of the day may alleviate tension and anxiety. The backrub may also be used effectively in establishing or improving communications.
2. Irritation may result if there is friction between the nurse's hand and the patient's back. Lotion or powder reduces friction. The lotion should be warmed in the hand before being applied to avoid stimulation caused by cold lotion.
3. The backrub will be stimulating if it consists of rapid, firm strokes. The pétrissage and tapotement motions are used to achieve this effect (Fig. 25-1).
4. A sedative effect will result if long, slow stroking motions are used, such as the effleurage motion (Fig. 25-2).

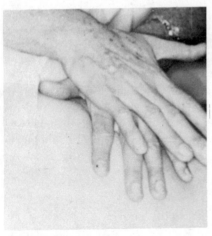

FIGURE 25.1

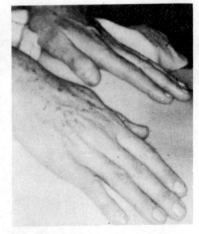

FIGURE 25.2

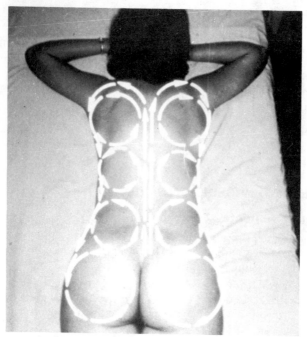

FIGURE 25.3

5. Warmed lotion is applied to the patient's entire back with firm, long strokes. The backrub should begin at the base of the spine and proceed upward to the shoulders. Strokes should begin near the spine and rotate outward to include the entire back (Fig. 25-3). The thumb and first three fingers of one hand may rub the nape of the neck, and the entire process should be continued for 3 to 5 minutes.

6. Body structure will affect the type of stroke selected and the amount of pressure applied to prevent trauma or make the stroke effective. Tapotement should not be used on an emaciated patient. More pressure will have to be applied to the obese or muscular person when using effleurage, or it will affect only the skin itself.

7. Inadequate circulation in bony prominences leads to skin breakdown. Special attention should be given to these areas, especially in patients who are bedfast or have reddened or irritated areas on their backs.

8. To leave the patient comfortable, excess skin moisture should be removed with a towel.

B. Communicative Aspects

1. *Observations*

   a. Note the reaction of the patient to his backrub.

   b. Appearance of back, particularly any areas of discoloration or breakdown or other abnormal findings, should be recorded.

2. *Charting*

DATE	TREATMENT	TIME	OBSERVATIONS	SIGNATURE
5/10	Backrub	2100	Patient appears to enjoy backrub. Skin over back appears pink and healthy.	D. Young, N.T.

3. *Referrals*

Not applicable

C. Teaching Aspects—Patient and Family

1. The family should be taught the backrub technique if the patient will be confined to bed at home.

2. If the patient is confined to bed, he should understand the importance of a backrub in helping to prevent decubitus formation and of ensuring that someone does this for him.

3. The patient should be told the purpose of the backrub (sedation, to help him rest, to prevent pressure, etc.). He should also be told that he will feel pressure and if it is too great, to tell the nurse so she may alter her technique.

IV. EVALUATION PROCESS

A. Was the desired effect achieved (*e.g.*, relaxation, prevention, healing)?

B. Was the nurse–patient relationship enhanced by improved communication?

C. Is the skin on the back in good condition?

D. Has skin breakdown over bony prominences been prevented?

26

Bandaging

I. ASSESSMENT OF SITUATION

A. Definition

The application of a continuous strip of woven material to a body part. Types of bandages are:

1. *Ace*: A commercially prepared bandage of woven elastic material that is capable of giving strong support

2. *Gauze*: A soft, porous, woven cotton of light weight that molds easily to body parts and is used frequently to retain dressings

3. *Kling*: A woven, porous gauze that stretches and molds to body contours and is self-adhesive

B. Terminology

None

C. Rationale for Actions

1. To limit motion of the affected part
2. To secure a dressing
3. To secure splints
4. To provide support
5. To apply pressure
6. To secure traction apparatus
7. To aid the return of venous circulation from the extremities to the heart

II. NURSING PLAN

A. Objectives

1. To allay fear and anxiety
2. To promote physical comfort
3. To maintain body alignment
4. To ensure that the bandage accomplishes its intended purpose (*e.g.*, support or immobilization)
5. To prevent contact of two skin areas by appropriate padding
6. To protect bony prominences by appropriate padding
7. To prevent venous stasis

B. Patient Preparation

1. Microorganisms flourish in warm, moist, contaminated areas. Wounds should be dressed aseptically prior to bandaging (see Technique 44, Dressings, Surgical). A bandage should be applied only over a clean, dry area.

2. Complete assembly of equipment prior to initiating the procedure will reduce the risk of tiring the patient because of unnecessarydelays

C. Equipment

1. Specified bandage
2. Medications, dressings, equipment, as ordered

III. IMPLEMENTING NURSING INTERVENTION

A. Therapeutic Aspects

1. Place the part to be bandaged in normal functioning position to prevent deformity and discomfort and help the circulation of blood in the involved part.

2. Friction and pressure can cause mechanical trauma to the skin. Appropriate padding should be used to separate adjacent skin areas and protect bony prominences.

3. Bandages should be applied from distal to proximal parts, as this aids the return of venous blood to the heart.

4. Uneven pressure can interfere with blood circulation and nourishment of cells, thereby slowing the healing process. When the bandage is applied, care must be taken to ensure even distribution of pressure.

5. Direct visualization of an affected limb is necessary to check circulation. It is best to leave a small area at the end of a bandaged extremity, such as a toe exposed, except when this is the area actually involved in wound healing, such as the stump of an amputated part.

6. Securing the end of the bandage maintains even pressure along the length of the bandage. It may be secured with tape or clips.

7. The basic bandage patterns are:

   a. *Circular*: Each round of bandage overlaps the entire previous round, thus creating a bandage that is the width of the material itself (Fig. 26-1).

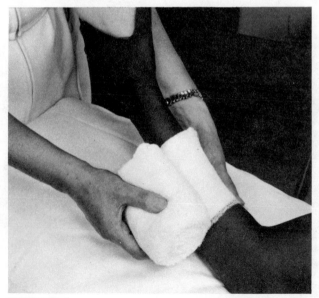

FIGURE 26.1

b. *Spiral*: Each round of bandage slightly overlaps the previous round, to create a progression up the limb (Fig. 26-2).

c. *Spiral reverse*: The bandage is anchored by several rounds of spiral. Then, with each round, the top of the bandage is turned under. Its adaptability to contours makes it excellent for forearm or leg (Fig. 26-3).

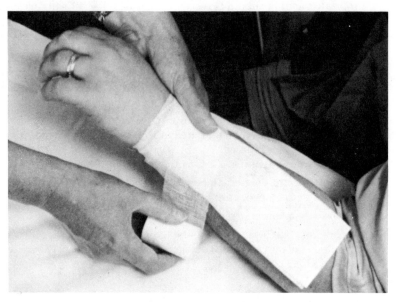

FIGURE 26.2

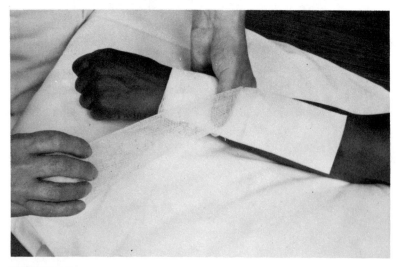

FIGURE 26.3

d. *Figure 8*: This bandage is used for joints. It is anchored with several rounds of spiral bandage below the joint. A round is then made above the joint and alternately below and above until the entire joint is covered (Fig. 26-4).

e. *Spica*: This is the same as a figure 8 bandage, except it usually covers a much larger area, such as the thigh (Fig. 26-5).

f. *Recurrent*: This bandage is used for anchoring a dressing on the head, a stump or a finger. The bandage is first postioned by two circular turns. The roll is then turned perpendicular to the circular turns and passed back to front and front to back, overlapping each time until the area is covered. It is secured by making two circular turns over the circular initial turns (Fig. 26-6).

B. Communicative Aspects

1. *Observations*

   a. Signs of restricted circulation must be observed frequently by checking for:

   (1) Blanching

   (2) Erythema (redness)

   (3) Cyanosis

   (4) Tingling sensation

   (5) Edema

   (6) Coldness of the tissues

   b. Unusual drainage or odor may indicate a pressure area or- infection.

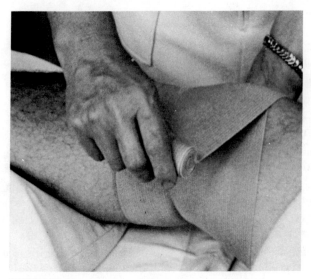

FIGURE 26.4

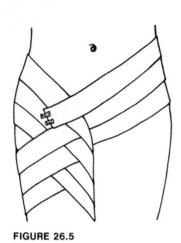

FIGURE 26.5

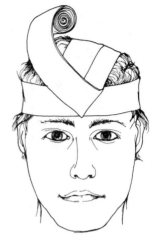

FIGURE 26.6

2. *Charting*

DATE	TREATMENT	TIME	OBSERVATIONS	SIGNATURE
5/19	Ace bandage	1500	Ace bandage applied to both legs, from toe to groin. Rt foot very edematous. States, "I had phlebitis in my rt leg before."	B. Smith, L.V.N.
		1515	Toes blanch. States, "My leg doesn't tingle and feels warmer."	B. Smith, L.V.N.

3. *Referrals*

The patient and family should be told where they may purchase bandages and the type of bandage they should buy.

C. Teaching Aspects—Patient and Family

1. Instruct patient and family how to hold and apply bandages if patient is to be dismissed with them.

2. Inform patient and family where to purchase bandages and how to wash them, if washable. (Wash in mild detergent and drip dry.)

3. Instruct patient to elevate body part if signs of impaired circulation are present.

4. Instruct patient to report changes in appearance of the affected part to the physician.

5. Tell the patient that the bandage will be snug; however, if the bandaged part becomes numb, loses sensation or becomes painful, he should notify the nurse at once.

IV. EVALUATION PROCESS

A. Is the patient at ease and comfortable?

B. Has the patient accepted and cooperated with activity limitations imposed by the presence of the bandage?

C. Is the body in proper alignment?

D. Has the bandage accomplished its intended purpose (*e.g.*, support, immobilization)?

E. Are adjacent skin areas separated?

F. Are bony prominences protected?

G. Is adequate circulation being maintained?

27

Baths, Cleansing

I. ASSESSMENT OF SITUATION

A. Definition

The medium and method of cleansing the body. Types are:

1. *Complete bed bath:* The entire body of the patient is washed at the bedside by the nurse.

2. *Abbreviated bed bath:* Only the parts of the patient's body that might cause illness, odor or discomfort, if neglected, are washed. This includes face, axillae, genitalia, anal region, back, and hands.

3. *Partial bath:* Complete or partial bathing of the patient's body at the sink or tub or in the shower.

B. Terminology

None

C. Rationale for Actions

1. To cleanse the skin to remove accumulated perspiration, secretions, microorganisms and debris. Removing these accumulations, which act as culture media for pathogens, prevents infection and preserves the healthy, unbroken condition of the skin.

2. To provide comfort and relaxation to a tired, restless patient

3. To stimulate circulation, both systemically and locally

4. To promote muscle tone by active or passive exercise

5. To promote elimination from the skin

6. To prevent lung congestion by stimulating respiration through change of position

7. To improve the patient's self-esteem through improved appearance, which leads to increased interaction with others

II. NURSING PLAN

A. Objectives

1. To promote hygiene and comfort for the patient

2. To observe the patient's skin condition

3. To assess the patient's range of motion

4. To encourage the patient to be as independent as possible or allowed

5. To assess the patient's physical and mental status

6. To establish a communication pattern between patient and nurse that promotes health teaching and expression of patient concerns

B. Patient Preparation

1. If the patient understands what will happen, he will be more at ease and more likely to cooperate.

2. All necessary equipment should be gathered prior to beginning the procedure to avoid chilling the patient with unnecessary delays.

3. In a bed bath, the top bed linen should be removed and replaced with a bath blanket, which provides warmth, absorbs moisture, and is less cumbersome.

C. Equipment

1. Bath towel

2. Washcloth

3. Soap

4. Lotion

5. Powder, if desired

6. Bath basin for bed bath

7. Toilet articles

III. IMPLEMENTING NURSING INTERVENTION

A. Therapeutic Aspects

1. *Bed bath*

   a. Warm water (110° to 115° F.) tends to relax muscles and increase circulation by dilatation of the blood vessels. Excessive heat should be avoided, however, as it may cause burns or diversion of blood from the vital centers of the brain, resulting in syncope (fainting). The water may be changed as often as necessary to maintain warmth.

b. Soap decreases surface tension of water, which aids in more efficient cleaning. It is, however, an irritant to certain delicate tissues, such as the eyes. Soap should not be used if the patient objects, is allergic to it, or has excessively dry skin.

c. The dangling ends of the washcloth are annoying to a patient. The washcloth should be folded around the hand to prevent dangling and to keep it warm longer. This may be done by laying the open hand palm side up on the cloth and folding each side over and the top down. The top may be tucked under the palm side to secure it (Figs. 27-1, 27-2, 27-3, 27-4, and 27-5).

d. Using firm, gentle strokes in bathing the patient tends to stimulate muscles and aid circulation (Fig. 27-6).

e. Cleansing contaminated areas last will reduce the chance of spreading microorganisms. The suggested sequence is:

(1) Face

(2) Arms, hands, axillae

(3) Chest and abdomen

(4) Legs and feet

(5) Back

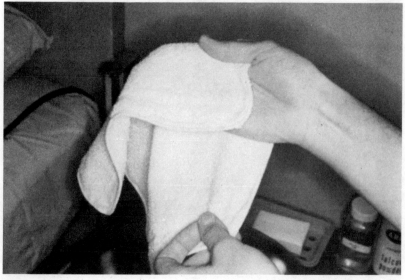

FIGURE 27.1

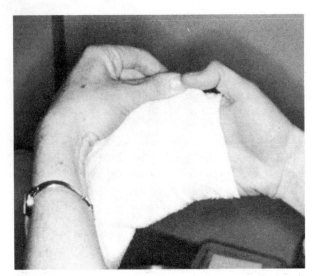

FIGURE 27.2

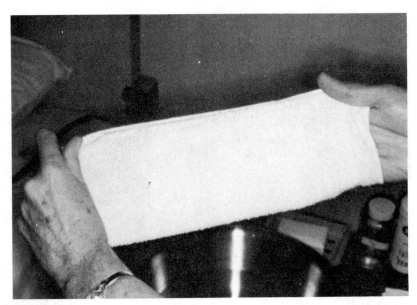

FIGURE 27.3

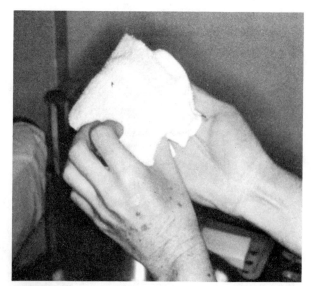

FIGURE 27.4

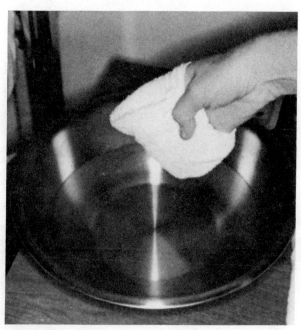

FIGURE 27.5

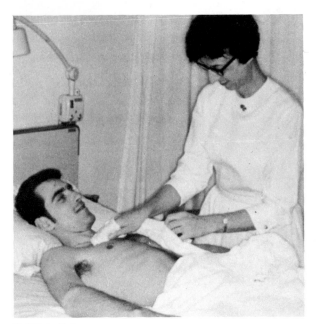

FIGURE 27.6

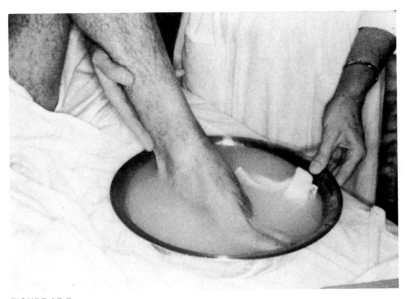

FIGURE 27.7

(6) Perineum

(7) Anal region

f. Immersion of accessible body parts, such as hands and feet, in the basin of water will aid in dissolving contaminants, removing debris, softening nails, as well as refreshing the patient (Fig. 27-7).

g. All body parts should be moved through their full range of motion during the bath, unless medically contraindicated. Active or passive exercises prevent contractures and improve circulation (Figs. 27-8, 27-9).

h. When in contact with the skin for a prolonged period of time, soap is drying and can cause itching. The soap should be rinsed off quickly and thoroughly.

i. Keeping the skin dry aids in the prevention of pressure sores (decubiti) and discourages bacterial growth.

j. Care should be taken to avoid scratching the patient with sharp fingernails or jewelry.

k. Lotion may be applied to soften the skin and prevent drying and cracking.

2. *Partial bath*

The same principles apply as for the bed bath. Additional safety measures include:

a. Assisting the patient to and from the bathing area

b. Remaining with the patient during the bath if necessary or carefully instructing him in use of the signal light in case he needs help

c. Providing a chair or stool for debilitated patients

d. Instructing the patient in the use of the handrail

e. Remaining within easy call of the patient

B. Communicative Aspects

1. *Observations*

a. Observe patient's activity, responses, mood, and general appearance.

b. Note skin changes, such as rash, discoloration, or other unusual characteristics.

c. Check progress of healing wounds.

d. Observe areas around bony prominences, where the hazard of skin breakdown may develop from constant pressure or friction.

e. Observe patient's physical condition and evaluate the amount of exercise the patient can tolerate without undue fatigue; weakness of any particular part of the body is easily detected at this time.

f. Opportunity for conversation affords opportunity to assess the

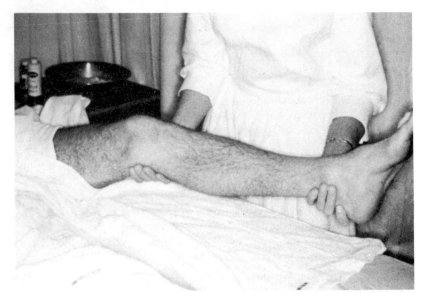

FIGURE 27.8

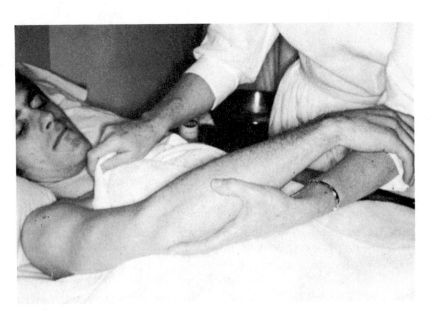

FIGURE 27.9

patient's general frame of mind or mood; he may reflect feelings about his illness.

   g. Observations of general hygiene help to identify the need for health teaching.

  2. *Charting*

DATE	TREATMENT	TIME	OBSERVATIONS	SIGNATURE
7/31	Complete bed bath	0815	Reddened area observed over coccyx during bath. Area massaged gently. Skin is dry, with poor turgor. Lotion applied. States concern about surgery tomorrow. Explanation and information given about surgery procedure.	F. White, R.N.

  3. *Referrals*

   Not applicable

C. Teaching Aspects—Patient and Family

1. If observation indicates inappropriate attention to hygiene, patient or family should be instructed in cleanliness.
2. If patient indicates concern about his condition, the bath may afford an opportunity for appropriate teaching.
3. If the patient has a physical disability, instruction should be given to patient or family concerning exercise and range of motion.

IV. EVALUATION PROCESS

A. Was the patient allowed and encouraged to assist according to his capabilities?

B. Is the nurse aware of the patient's physical and emotional status?

C. Was the patient able to verbalize his feelings?

D. Is the patient clean and comfortable?

E. Has the patient's skin condition been evaluated?

F. Does the patient have full range of motion?

G. Was the patient allowed to assist according to his capabilities?

28
Baths, Therapeutic

I. ASSESSMENT OF SITUATION

A. Definition

The medium and method of treating the body therapeutically by immersing the body or body parts in water of varying temperatures or in water with emollients added. Types of therapeutic baths are:

1. *Sitz bath:* The immersion of the body from mid-thigh to iliac crest in water of a temperature from 110° to 115°F

2. *Emollient bath:* The immersion of the body in a regular bathtub of water at 95° to 100° F., containing one of the following:

    a. Three cups of oatmeal

    b. One pound of cornstarch

    c. Eight ounces of sodium bicarbonate

    d. Medication as ordered by the physician

B. Terminology

Emollient: a soothing and softening agent, applied locally

C. Rationale for Actions

1. *Sitz bath*

    a. To promote phagocytosis through increased peripheral vasodilatation

    b. To stimulate formation of new tissue through increased blood supply

    c. To relieve pain by relieving pressure on nerve endings caused by deep congestion of blood

    d. To promote relaxation of local muscles

    e. To promote suppuration

2. *Emollient bath*

    a. To soften and remove dermatologic crusts

    b. To relieve pruritus by protecting irritated skin from air currents or by coating skin with the palliative substance

    c. To apply medication to a large area of skin

    d. To protect skin lesions

II. NURSING PLAN

A. Objectives

1. To promote healing
2. To relieve pain or pruritus
3. To promote relaxation
4. To promote psychological comfort by soothing irritation
5. To promote normal body functions, such as defecation or micturition, through relief of pain and relaxation
6. To provide for cleanliness

B. Patient Preparation

1. Explanations of the reasons for the bath and the actual procedure to be followed will help put the patient at ease and may increase his cooperation.
2. All necessary equipment should be assembled prior to taking the patient to the bath area.
3. Soiled dressings are contaminated. They should be removed in the patient's room if possible and disposed of properly. If an inner dressing adheres to the wound, it may be soaked off in the tub.

C. Equipment

1. Bath tub, sitz tub, or portable sitz tub
2. Water of indicated temperature
3. Medication, as ordered
4. Rubber or plastic ring for sitz bath, if indicated
5. Washcloths and towels

III. IMPLEMENTING NURSING INTERVENTION

A. Therapeutic Aspects

1. *Sitz bath*

   a. Water temperature of 100° to 115° F. promotes peripheral vasodilatation but will not burn the patient. The sitz bath may be given in a regular bathtub, filled approximately one sixth full. There are specially designed sitz tubs that allow the patient to sit comfortably with hips and buttocks immersed in water. A portable sitz basin is available for use in commodes, chairs or even in bed. If nothing else is available, a large basin may be used.

   b. Sitting the patient on a rubber or plastic ring will relieve pressure and discomfort if he has rectal or perineal sutures or pain.

   c. Various aspects of the hospital regimen may cause weakness or fainting. These include surgical procedures, pain, tension, anxiety, and the medical treatments. The nurse should provide adequate patient assistance to, during, and from the bath.

d. Local vasodilatation of the lower extremities will draw blood away from the perineal area. If possible, the feet and legs should not be immersed in the water; thus seating a patient in a basin is more desirable than seating him in a bathtub.

e. Fluctuations in water temperature can cause cardiovascular stress. A constant water temperature can be maintained by adding warm water as needed.

f. Maximum benefit is obtained within the first 10 to 20 minutes. Prolonging the procedure tires the patient and increases the chances of cardiovascular stress.

g. Avoid patient chilling, as this causes vasoconstriction. A bath blanket may be placed around the patient's shoulders while he is in the tub.

h. Irregular or accelerated pulse may indicate cardiovascular stress. Pulse should be checked periodically during the bath. If irregularity occurs, the patient should be returned to bed immediately.

2. *Emollient bath*

a. An emollient bath should be given at 95° to 100° F., as this will prevent vasodilatation, which may increase pruritus.

b. Unpleasant skin conditions create fear of disfigurement and rejection by others; the nurse must demonstrate her acceptance of the patient.

(1) Avoid staring or showing signs of revulsion.

(2) Look at the person rather than the lesion or affected area.

(3) Allow the patient to verbalize feelings about his disfigurement.

c. Rubbing increases irritation. Light, gentle strokes of a washcloth will apply solution to body parts not immersed in the tub. The skin should be patted dry, not rubbed.

d. A bath lasting 20 to 30 minutes provides adequate time for the emollient to coat the skin.

e. The patient with a skin problem should be protected from drafts, as he is prone to chilling.

B. Communicative Aspects

1. *Observations*

a. Note appearance of area treated.

b. Record amount and character of drainage.

c. Observe patient's reaction to the procedure, including tolerance of it and results obtained (*e.g.,* relief of pain or pruritus).

2. *Charting*

DATE	TREATMENT	TIME	OBSERVATIONS	SIGNATURE
9/21	Sitz bath	0900	Sitz bath to perineal region at 115° F for 20 minutes. No change in pulse noted. Incision appears clean, with no drainage. Patient experienced relief of pain following bath.	D. Young, N.T.
10/2	Corn starch bath	0930	Cornstarch bath at 98° F for 30 minutes. Bathing removed crusts and exudate from abdomen. Extremities appear reddened and weeping. Patient experienced moderate relief of pruritus.	D. Young, N.T.

3. *Referrals*

   Not applicable

C. Teaching Aspects—Patient and Family

1. *Sitz bath*

   a. Instruct patient to keep fingers away from wounds.

   b. Instruct patient to take a sitz bath after every bowel movement and as needed for relief of pain after rectal surgery.

   c. Emphasize the importance of correct water temperature.

   d. The patient should be told to expect that the initial sensation in the wound area will be unpleasant, due to the tenderness already present. However, this soon subsides, and the sitz bath provides an excellent means of relief from pain and discomfort.

2. *Emollient bath*

   a. Discourage patient from scratching affected areas.

   b. Instruct patient to avoid temperature extremes and tight clothing.

   c. Reinforce physician's instructions concerning diet and allergies, if appropriate.

   d. Tell the patient he may expect an unpleasant sensation on entrance into the water. This is due to the already irritated condition of his skin. However, the tub bath should relieve his itching and discomfort and promote relaxation.

IV. EVALUATION PROCESS

A. Does the patient appear mentally and physically relaxed?

B. Is the patient using proper body mechanics in entering and leaving the tub?

C. Is the patient able to decrease the amount of scratching?

D. Does the treated area appear to be improving?

E. Was the pain or pruritis decreased?

F. Is the patient regaining normal body functions?

G. Does the treated area appear clean?

29

Bedmaking

I. ASSESSMENT OF SITUATION

A. Definition

The process of applying or changing bed linens. Types are:

1. *Open bed:* the bedmaking process when the bed is unoccupied or when the occupant is able to be up while the bed is made

2. *Occupied bed:* the bedmaking process in which the bed is made while the patient is in it

3. *Surgical bed:* the bedmaking process in which the bed is prepared to receive a patient with a minimum of disturbance after his return from the recovery room

B. Terminology

1. *Draw sheet:* a shortened sheet placed across the bed over the bottom sheet. It covers the area between the chest and knees and is stretched tightly and tucked under each side of the bed. The draw sheet protects the mattress and lower sheet and helps keep the patient dry and comfortable.

2. *Mitered corner:* a means of anchoring sheets on a mattress. It is accomplished on the bottom sheet by placing the end of the sheet evenly under the mattress (Fig. 29-1). The side edge of the sheet is then raised onto the bed (Figs. 29-2 and 29-3), and the remaining portion is tucked under the mattress edge (Figs. 29-4, 29-5, 29-6). The entire side section is then folded under the side of the mattress. To miter the foot section of the top sheet, the raised side edge is lowered to the side of the bed rather than tucked under, making a neat and serviceable corner.

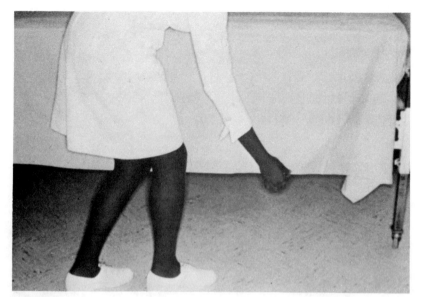

FIGURE 29.1

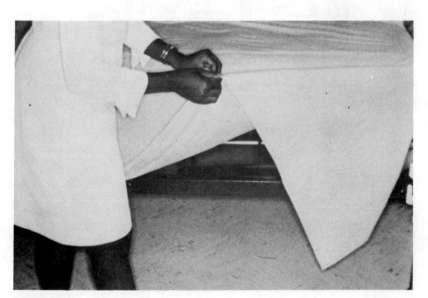

FIGURE 29.2

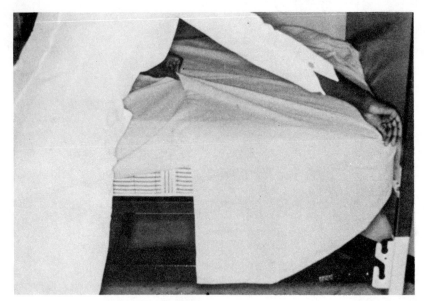

FIGURE 29.3

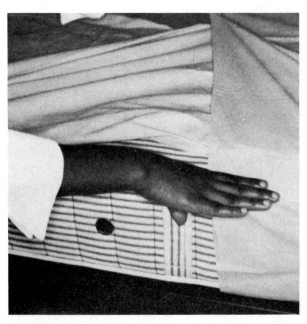

FIGURE 29.4

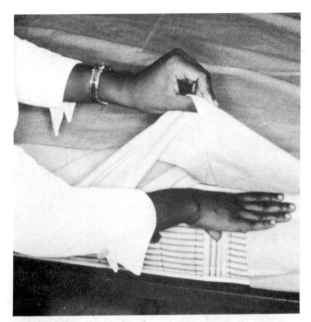

FIGURE 29.5

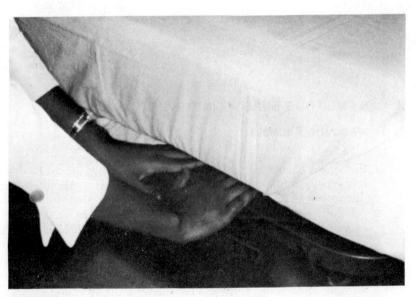

FIGURE 29.6

C. Rationale for Actions

1. To provide a suitable environment in which the patient will be able to carry on normal body activities 24 hours a day when he cannot be out of bed

2. To provide a suitable environment for comfort and rest for the patient who is able to be out of bed for periods of time

II. NURSING PLAN

A. Objectives

1. To provide a clean environment
2. To promote physical comfort
3. To promote psychological comfort by providing a neat environment in which the patient can receive visitors
4. To prevent cross-contamination
5. To prevent undue strain for patient and nurse

B. Patient Preparation

1. The patient should be bathed before the occupied bed is made.
2. The nurse should explain what actions will be expected from the patient to facilitate the bedmaking process. Having all equipment at hand prior to beginning will reduce unnecessary delays.

C. Equipment

1. Contour sheet or flat sheet
2. Top sheet
3. Pillowcase(s), as needed
4. Draw sheet, if needed
5. Spread, if needed

III. IMPLEMENTING NURSING INTERVENTION

A. Therapeutic Aspects

1. *Open bed*

    a. Bed linens harbor microorganisms that can be transferred by direct contact to the nurse's hands and uniform. In order to avoid the spread of such microorganisms, the nurse should utilize a scrupulous handwashing technique before and after making the bed. She should also avoid contact of the linens and her uniform.

    b. Fanning soiled linens can spread microorganisms through the air. The linens should be stripped from the bed, formed into a compact bundle, and placed in a hamper or pillowcase. Contact with the floor is unsightly and conducive to the spread of microorganisms.

c. Completing one side of the bed before moving to the other side saves the nurse's time and energy. The bed should be raised to its highest position to avoid unnecessary stooping. The bottom sheet should be placed with its center fold in the center of the mattress. If it is a contour sheet, the top and bottom corners on the side nearest the nurse are placed over the mattress corners. If it is a flat sheet, the end may be even with the foot of the mattress and the top corner nearest the nurse secured with a mitered corner. Both head and foot portions may be secured with mitered corners, if desired. The center fold of the draw sheet should be placed in the center of the bed, and the entire edge nearest the nurse tucked securely under the mattress. The top sheet is placed with the center fold in the center of the bed, and the top edge even with the top of the mattress. It then is tucked in at the bottom on the side nearest the nurse and secured with a mitered corner. The spread is applied in the same way as the top sheet. The nurse then moves to the other side of the bed and repeats the entire process in the same sequence.

d. A taut, wrinkle-free foundation lessens discomfort and pressure on the patient. The bottom sheet and draw sheet should be pulled firmly and tucked securely.

e. Using one's weight to counteract resistance from the sheet lessens effort and strain on the nurse. The back should be kept straight to lessen the strain on the smaller, weaker back muscles. Tightening of the bedding should be accomplished using the weight of the body applied through the large muscles of the legs and gluteals.

f. The top linens should not be tight, as this can exert pressure on the lower extremities of the patient, resulting in discomfort and tissue breakdown. The bed should be finished by forming a cuff with the top sheet over the spread and a toe pleat at the foot of the bed before tucking in the top linens.

g. The top bedding should be fanfolded to the foot of the bed to facilitate the patient's return to the bed.

2. *Surgical bed*

a. The surgical bed is prepared in the same fashion as the open bed, with the following exception.

b. The top linen is not tucked in at the foot. It is fanfolded to the side of the bed away from the door (Fig. 29-7), to facilitate transfer of the returning patient from the stretcher to the bed without undue exposure and strain.

3. *Occupied bed*

a. Since rolling requires less strain on both the nurse and the patient than pushing, the patient should be rolled to the far side of the bed, while he helps himself if possible by holding onto the raised side rail.

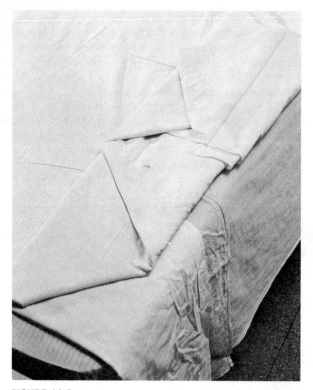

FIGURE 29.7

b. The fewer position changes required, the less strain and fatigue will be felt by patient and nurse. The soiled linen on the vacated side of the bed is loosened and tucked under the patient (Fig. 29-8). The clean bottom linen is placed and fanfolded to the center of the bed (Fig. 29-9). In one movement, the patient is rolled over the soiled and fanfolded linen to the clean side of the bed, with the rail up (Fig. 29-10). The nurse then moves to the other side of the bed, removes the soiled linen and finishes foundation and top linens as for an open bed (Fig. 29-11).

c. Protect the patient's modesty by ensuring adequate draping during bedmaking.

B. Communicative Aspects

1. *Observations*

   a. Observe the condition of the patient's skin.

   b. Observe any limitations or problems with range of motion.

2. *Charting*

   Chart anything unusual about the patient.

3. *Referrals*

If the patient will need a hospital bed at home, he should be referred to a hospital supply house where such beds may be rented or purchased.

C. Teaching Aspects—Patient and Family

1. Demonstrate the technique of bedmaking to the family if the patient will require such services after dismissal.

2. This is an excellent opportunity to teach proper body mechanics to the patient and family, if appropriate.

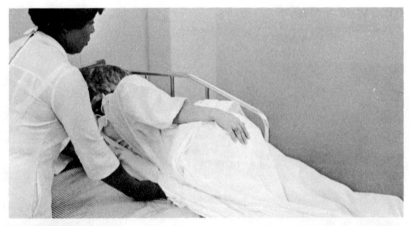

FIGURE 29.8

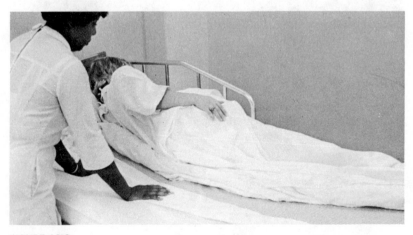

FIGURE 29.9

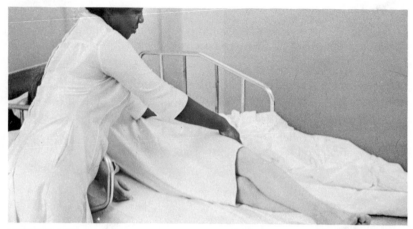

FIGURE 29.10

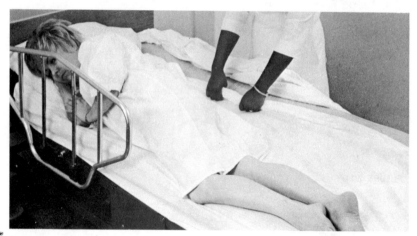

FIGURE 29.11

IV. EVALUATION PROCESS

A. Is the environment clean?

B. Were proper body mechanics used throughout the procedure?

30

Binders, Application of

I. ASSESSMENT OF SITUATION

A. Definition
A broad bandage encircling the abdomen or chest. There are 4 types:
1. Straight abdominal binder
2. Scultetus (many-tailed) binder
3. Breast binder
4. T-binder

B. Terminology
None

C. Rationale for Actions
1. To retain dressings
2. To provide abdominal support
3. To prevent tension on sutures and wounds
4. To prevent irritation when patient is allergic to adhesive
5. To reduce breast engorgement for a non-nursing parturient

II. NURSING PLAN

A. Objectives
1. To reduce patient's fears about tension on sutures and wounds
2. To offer an alternative to tape for an allergic patient
3. To relieve the postpartum patient of the discomfort of breast engorgement
4. To bring the presenting part of the fetus into proper alignment in the maternal pelvis

B. Patient Preparation
1. The expected effects of the binder application should be explained to the patient so that he will understand why the binder is being applied.
2. Equipment should be gathered before beginning. It might be helpful

to show the patient what the binder looks like and how it will be applied so that he will know how best to cooperate.

C. Equipment

1. Binders of appropriate type
2. Safety pins

III. IMPLEMENTING NURSING INTERVENTION

A. Therapeutic Aspects

1. *Straight abdominal binder* (*Fig. 30-1*)

   a. Maximum support is provided when pressure is equally distributed. The binder should be placed under the patient, with the lower border well down under the hips and fastened firmly to avoid friction, which causes irritation.

   b. Support from below reduces tension on the wound and adjacent parts. In surgical application, the nurse should begin fastening binders at the bottom.

   c. For obstetrical application, the nurse should observe these principles:

      (1) Applying downward pressure will direct the uterus intothe pelvis, so the binder should be fastened from the top downward.

      (2) Lack of abdominal muscle strength reduces the support of the uterus, resulting in poor alignment of the uterus, poor contractions and slow cervical dilation. After the binder is applied, the patient must be observed closely for precipitate delivery.

   d. A tight binder may reduce chest expansion during respirations. The nurse should make darts where necessary so the binder will fit snugly but allow adequate room for breathing. If the binder extends above the waistline, loosen it slightly to avoid interfering with respirations.

2. *Scultetus* (*many-tailed*) *binder* (*Fig. 30-2*)

   a. The binder should be placed well under the hips, with no wrinkles. The two innermost straps are brought straight across the body and tucked at the opposite side. The remaining straps are brought across the center one by one, alternating sides and slanting to achieve a fishtail effect. The final two straps come straight across the body, as the first two, and the top strap is secured with two safety pins placed horizontally.

   b. On obstetrical patients, fasten the last two straps on *both* sides. If the patient is extremely large, it may be necessary to secure *each* strap with a safety pin.

   c. Examine for compression of tubes and drains.

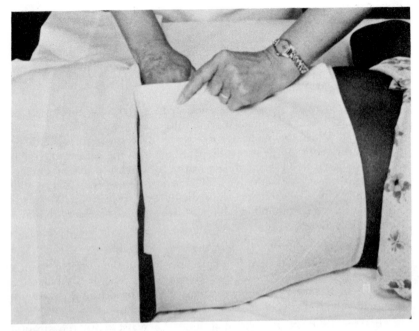

FIGURE 30.1

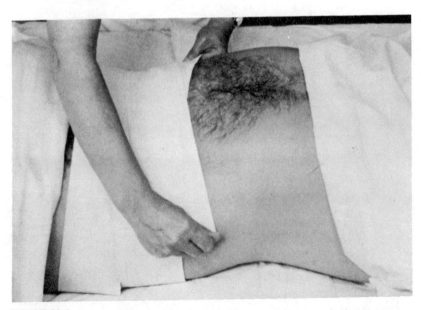

FIGURE 30.2

3. *Breast binder (Fig. 30-3)*

    a. Lactiferous structures in the breast may become engorged during the early puerperium. The breast binder is designed to reduce engorgement. The binder should be spread on the bed, and the patient should lie supine on it. The arm openings must be adjusted so that the material will not chafe.

    b. Alignment of glands and ducts reduces tension. Involution of breast tissue is promoted when alignment and support are applied. When the binder is correctly in place, the nipples should be in the center of the breast tissue. Starting at the bottom, the binder should be fastened snugly at the front with at least six safety pins placed horizontally. Make darts if necessary to assure adequate fit. The shoulder straps should be fastened to fit. Allow the patient to sit up and check for fit. Reapply as necessary to maintain snugness.

4. *T-binder (Fig. 30-4)*

    a. The T-binder is used to secure dressings in the perineal area. A single T-binder is used for women and a double T-binder for men. If surgery has been extensive and the dressing is large, a double T-binder may be used on a woman.

    b. The T-binder is secured around the waist, with the strap(s) brought up between the legs and secured to the waistband.

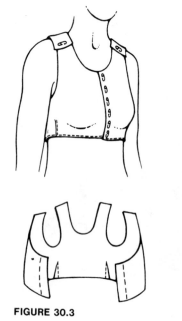

FIGURE 30.3

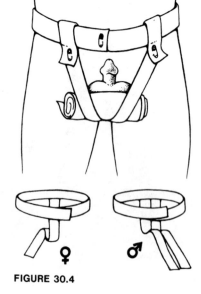

FIGURE 30.4

B. Communicative Aspects

1. *Observations*

    a. Check for drainage under the binder, both amount and characteristics.

    b. Appearance of sanguineous drainage calls for close observations and appropriate measures to prevent extensive blood loss.

    c. Observe for any strong or foul odor, which indicates drainage from an infected wound.

    d. Observe the binder during patient activity for fit and effect.

2. *Charting*

DATE	TREATMENT	TIME	OBSERVATIONS	SIGNATURE
4/29	Binder applied	0930	Scultetus binder applied to retain dressing on surgical wound. Patient reassured that binder is secured so that it will not be uncomfortable and that it will be reapplied as it becomes loose. Patient states she feels more comfortable about moving.	B. Smith, L.V.N.

3. *Referrals*

    a. If the patient will need a binder after dismissal, he should be told where replacements may be purchased.

    b. The American Cancer Society will provide equipment such as binders to cancer patients.

C. Teaching Aspects—Patient and Family

1. Instruct the patient that if the binder is loose or uncomfortable in any way, he should ask for it to be reapplied.

2. Inform the patient of the reason for the binder. Tell him that after a period of time, the binder may begin to cause irritation; he should report this to the nurse. Tell him the binder may feel constricting and uncomfortable at first, but this should subside. If it does not, he should inform the nurse.

IV. EVALUATION PROCESS

A. Can the patient maintain normal body alignment and correct posture after the application of the binder?

B. Is the patient comfortable and able to move about freely?

C. Is the dressing held securely in the proper place?

D. Is the breast engorgement discomfort reduced or relieved by application of the breast binder?

31

Bladder Irrigations

I. ASSESSMENT OF SITUATION

A. Definition

The process of introducing a stream of solution into the bladder via catheter and draining it by natural or artificial means

B. Terminology

1. *Bladder:* the vesicle which acts as reservoir for urine
2. *Catheter:* a tube for evacuating or instilling fluids
3. *Plain irrigation:* a single process of introducing and emptying solution from the bladder
4. *Intermittent irrigation:* the process of introducing and emptying solution from the bladder through a closed system at designated intervals
5. *Tidal (thru-and-thru) irrigation:* an automatic continuous process of introducing and emptying solution from the bladder through a closed system

C. Rationale for Actions

1. To relieve inflammation of the bladder wall
2. To prevent or treat infection
3. To minimize formation of blood clots
4. To maintain patency of urinary drainage system

II. NURSING PLAN

A. Objectives

1. To provide mental comfort to patient
2. To maintain a sterile bladder drainage system
3. To preserve patency of bladder drainage system
4. To observe characteristics of urinary drainage
5. To instruct patient and family in the indicated method of irrigation

B. Patient Preparation

1. When hand irrigation of a catheter is needed, the patient should be told that he may feel a sensation of fullness and perhaps cold.
2. Occasionally a clot may stop up a three-way catheter, which will cause distention and spasms of the bladder if not relieved. If the pa-

tient begins to feel excessive fullness or pain during tidal irrigation, he should notify the nurse at once. If he is told to watch for these symptoms during the preparation period, complications may be avoided.

3. Application of a pad beneath the patient's hips may prevent the bed linen from becoming wet owing to leakage or spills during manual irrigation.

C. Equipment

1. *Plain irrigation*

   a. Disposable irrigation set or 50 ml irrigating syringes and sterile basin

   b. Sterile solution, as ordered

   c. Emesis basin

   d. Bed protector (disposable or reusable hip pad)

2. *Intermittent irrigation*

   a. Intermittent bladder irrigation setup

   b. Heavy IV standard

   c. Sterile solution, as ordered (2,000-ml bags)

   d. Catheterization tray with 3-way catheter (if not already in place)

3. *Tidal (thru-and-thru) irrigation*

   a. Tidal irrigation setup

   b. Heavy IV standard

   c. Sterile solution, as ordered (2,000-ml bags)

   d. Drainage bottles (3)

   e. Large basin

III. IMPLEMENTING NURSING INTERVENTION

A. Therapeutic Aspects

1. *Plain irrigation (Fig. 31-1)*

   a. Aseptic technique must be employed owing to the susceptibility of bladder tissue to injury and infection. The urinary tract offers a favorable location for the multiplication of microorganisms, because it is dark, warm, and moist. When disconnecting the drainage tubing to irrigate the catheter, the nurse should avoid contaminating the ends of either the catheter tubing or the drainage system. A sterile drainage tube protector should be placed over the end to prevent contamination.

   b. To prevent dilution of the blood as a result of reabsorption of the irrigating fluids, sterile normal saline is preferred for irrigation, unless otherwise ordered. The irrigating solution is poured into a sterile basin and drawn into the sterile syringe.

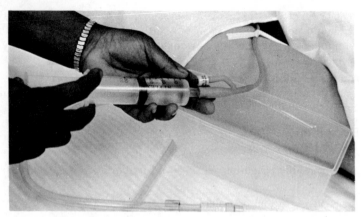

FIGURE 31.1

c. Increase in pressure on any portion of a confined liquid is transmitted undiminished to all parts of the liquid. As the volume of urine rises to about 250 ml, the pressure in the bladder becomes 130 mm, which is sufficient to initiate nerve pulses that can produce pain or the desire to void. Unless otherwise ordered, instill a total of 100 ml of solution in 30-ml amounts, being careful not to contaminate the tip of the syringe.

d. Siphonage is produced when the free surface of the liquid in one vessel is lower than the free surface of the liquid in the other, causing a difference in pressure. The fluid in the bladder should be allowed to return by gravity. This is effected by holding the catheter over a basin below bladder level. If no return is obtained, the syringe may be used to initiate or complete gentle withdrawal of irrigation fluid.

e. Leave the patient in a clean, comfortable environment.

2. *Intermittent irrigation (Fig. 31-2)*

a. Maintaining a closed system decreases the chance of contaminating the urinary system. The intermittent irrigation system is used when frequent irrigation is needed and it is undesirable to open the system frequently for plain irrigation. To initiate the intermittent irrigation, remove the covering from the large 2,000-ml bag and attach the drip chamber of the tubing to the insert opening labeled "outlet."

b. The pressure of water in a container for irrigation has been established as approximately ½ pound for every foot of elevation. Low pressure is utilized for bladder treatments, because of the bladder's musculature and ability to expand. The bag should be hung on a standard and adjusted to place the drip chamber 2½ to 3 feet above bed level.

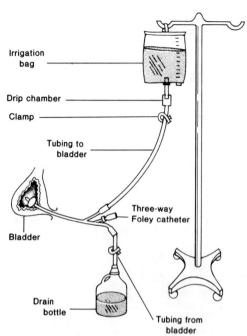

Irrigation bag

Drip chamber

Clamp

Tubing to bladder

Three-way Foley catheter

Bladder

Drain bottle

Tubing from bladder

FIGURE 31.2

c. Instillation of air into the bladder may cause painful distention. Flush the tubing with solution, close the clamp below the drip chamber, and attach the tubing to the inlet of a 3-way catheter. Connect the drainage system to the catheter outlet, and attach the tubing to the bed to facilitate free drainage. Close the clamp on the drainage tubing.

d. To irrigate the bladder, open the tubing to the bladder and allow 100 ml of solution to flow into the bladder by gravity. Close the clamp, and allow the solution to remain in the bladder 15 to 20 minutes, or as ordered. After the specified time, open the drainage clamp, and allow the irrigating solution to drain. The clamp on the drain tube should be left open.

e. Leave the patient in a clean, comfortable environment.

3. *Tidal (thru-and-thru) irrigation (Fig. 31-3)*

a. Maintaining a closed system decreases the chance of contaminating the urinary system. Continuous tidal irrigation is used when a constant bathing of the inner aspects of the bladder is necessary. To initiate tidal irrigation, remove the covers from two 2,000-ml bags. Insert the drip chamber of tubing into the large hole on one bag labeled "outlet." Place one end of the tandem tubing in the inlet of bag 1 and the other end in the outlet of bag 2. The vacu-

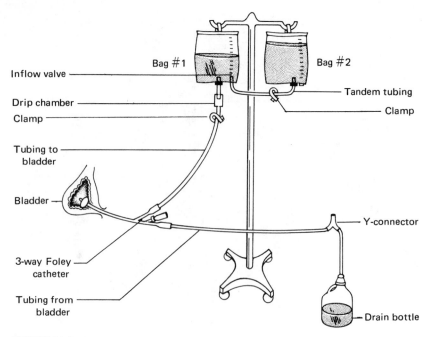

Inflow valve

Drip chamber

Clamp

Tubing to bladder

Bladder

3-way Foley catheter

Tubing from bladder

Bag #1

Bag #2

Tandem tubing

Clamp

Y-connector

Drain bottle

FIGURE 31.3

um from bag 1 will draw the water from bag 2 and prevent air from running into the bladder. Close the clamps before hanging the bags on a standard adjusted to place the drip chamber 2½ to 3 feet above bed level.

b. Air in the bladder can cause distention. If this happens, open the clamps and flush the tubings. After reclamping, attach the distal end of the tubing to the inlet of the patient's 3-way catheter. A glass or plastic connector may be inserted into the outlet and fastened to the drain tube so that the appearance of irrigation fluid can be noted as it leaves the bladder.

c. Pressure within the bladder will not exceed that amount exerted by the air vent or the Y-connector, which should be fastened to the foot of the bed at bladder level. This produces an anti-gravity flow, to allow the gradual decompression of normal bladder tissue. The Y-connector connects drain tubing with final tubing, the distal end of which should be placed in a drainage bottle. Open all clamps, and regulate flow by adjusting the clamp on the tubing that leads into the bladder.

d. The patient should be left in a clean and safe environment. Tubing should be adequately secured to prevent accidental pulling or jerking yet should allow as much freedom of movement as possible. Drainage bottles should be placed in a large basin to prevent accidental overflow on the floor.

B. Communicative Aspects

1. *Observations*

   a. Observe color, appearance, and amount of urinary drainage.

   b. Check tubings frequently to assure patency of drainage system (*e.g.,* no kinks, twists, loops below bed level).

   c. All tubes leading from the bladder should be below bladder level.

   d. Observe that all solution going in the bladder is returning and that the bladder is not overly distended.

   e. Observe the patient for any great discomfort, and be sure the catheter is draining adequately before giving any pain medication.

2. *Charting*

   Record intake and output measurements on an I&O form.

DATE	TREATMENT	TIME	OBSERVATIONS	SIGNATURE
4/9	Foley cath irrigated with 30 ml sterile D/W at room temp	0900	30 ml solution returned by gravity. Light yellow in color, with no sediment. Patient expressed no discomfort or pain.	C. Allen, L.V.N.
4/10	Bladder irrigated with 100 ml room temp $KMnO_4$ 1:10,000 qh 1000 to 1400	1015	Irrigation solution withdrawn by gravity after 14 minutes. Solution contained numerous solid particles. Patient expressed slight senstion of pressure during procedure.	C. Allen, L.V.N.
4/11	Cont thru-and-thru bladder irrigation started	0600	4,000 ml room temp D/W hung and dripping slowly. Returning slowly. Light red in color. Patient states he is more comfortable; seems to be resting. Instructed to drink more liquids and not disconnect the tubing.	C. Allen, L.V.N.

3. *Referrals*

If bladder irrigation is to be done at home, a public health or visiting nurse referral may be needed.

C. Teaching Aspects—Patient and Family

1. Instruct the patient that tubing should be free of kinks, twists, bends, and pressure from body parts, as urine drains by gravity.

2. Instruct the patient never to disconnect tubing, as touching could contaminate the drainage system.

3. Instruct concerning adequate fluid intake if the patient's condition permits.

4. If bladder irrigation is to be done at home, the patient or family will need specific instructions and demonstrations. A public health referral may be needed.

5. Preoperatively, the patient should have been prepared for an indwelling catheter. He should know that the feeling of urgency and desire to void is expected during the first postoperative hours. He should be told that straining and trying to void around the catheter will only increase tissue irritation and cause fatigue.

6. Prior to plain or intermittent irrigation, the patient should be told that he will have a feeling of fullness and desire to void when the fluid is instilled. Deep breaths may help him relax and overcome this feeling. During continuous irrigation, the patient should be told to expect a feeling of slight fullness. However, should pain or spasm occur, he should call the nurse at once, as a clot may be blocking the catheter or the tubing may be kinked. An overly distended bladder is very undesirable in patients with recent urologic surgery.

IV. EVALUATION PROCESS

A. Were sufficient explanation and preparation given to the patient to allay his anxiety and elicit his cooperation?

B. Has the family been included in the treatment regime?

C. Has the patient (or significant other person) demonstrated his willingness and capabilities in learning to do his own (or the patient's) irrigations, if indicated?

D. Are physical and psychological support and comfort being maintained?

E. Is the drainage system being kept patent?

F. Does the intake and output record reflect adequate hydration and elimination?

G. Has the family been included in the treatment regimen?

32
Body Mechanics

I. ASSESSMENT OF SITUATION

A. Definition

The efficient use of the body as a machine and as a means of locomotion

B. Terminology

1. *Tonus*: the normal status of a healthy muscle consisting of a partial steady state of contraction while awake
2. *Contracture*: a permanent contraction state of a muscle
3. *Atony*: decrease or absence of normal tonus
4. *Atrophy*: decrease in size and loss of normal function of a muscle
5. *Posture*: body alignment
6. *Fulcrum*: the fixed portion of a lever which allows movement
7. *Center of gravity*: the point at which the mass of an object is centered

C. Rationale for Actions

1. To avoid unnecessary muscle strain and possible injury
2. To assist in locomotion of the patient in and out of bed with minimal strain for nurses and patient
3. To perform everyday activities safely and properly by utilizing correct principles of body mechanics

II. NURSING PLAN

A. Objectives

1. To teach the patient, his family, and co-workers the proper use of the body as a machine of activity, utilizing proper principles to prevent injury
2. To recognize and change incorrect habits of body mechanics, substituting proper activities in their place
3. To reinforce correct behavior

B. Patient Preparation

Patient preparation for proper body alignment and body mechanics is brought out in each individual technique.

C. Equipment

Not applicable

III. IMPLEMENTING NURSING INTERVENTION

A. Principles of Body Mechanics

1. The center of gravity is the point at which the whole weight of the body may be considered to be concentrated. In humans, the center of gravity is considered to be in the center of the pelvis at the level of the second sacral vertebra. The feet form the supporting area of the body. The greater the supporting area and the lower the center of gravity, the more stable the body will be. Therefore, a more stable base of support can be achieved by separating the feet.

2. Good posture is the key to body mechanics and involves more than just standing erect. It keeps the center of gravity as nearly as possible in the same vertical line when standing, sitting, or squatting (Fig. 32-1). Good posture contributes to a pleasing appearance and also provides for correct functioning of the weight-bearing joints.

3. When a force acting on the body tends to rotate the body in one direction or another, the principle involved is called torque. The direction of torque is either clockwise or counterclockwise. For the body to be in equilibrium and not rotate, a force of equal resistance in the opposite direction must be applied. The major factor in determining torque deals with the distance between the center of gravity and the object causing resistance. This explains why some positions are better

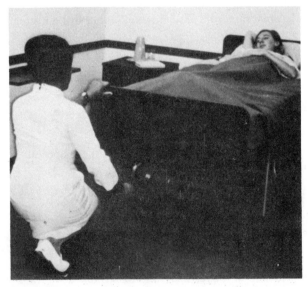

FIGURE 32.1

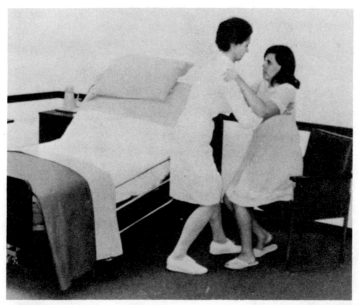

FIGURE 32.2

than others for work activities—namely, those which require less energy and cause less strain. For example, in lifting an object from the floor, stooping requires greater strain because the distance from the center of gravity to the object is greater than that required by bending at the knees and picking up the object.

4. Laws that govern balance in the standing position also apply when the body is in motion. To prevent strain, proper contraction of the muscles to counteract gravitational resistance is necessary. For example, carrying a heavy object at arm's length produces far greater strain than carrying it close to the body, which allows correct body alignment. Lifting a patient by bending forward at the waist produces unnatural body alignment and will likely result in back strain. Lifting by flexing the hips and knees, placing one foot forward (broadens base of support), and keeping shoulders in the same plane as the pelvis reduces the amount of energy necessary to accomplish the task with much less strain on the body muscles (Fig. 32-2).

5. Many simple laws of physics can lighten the nurse's workload. It is easier to slide an object than lift it (Fig. 32-3). Sliding on an even surface requires less energy than moving the object on an incline. Friction increases the amount of energy required to accomplish a task. Friction can be reduced by application of an intermediate object such as a draw sheet on a bed (Fig. 32-4). When lifting, face the work situation and avoid rotary movements of the spine. Utilizing

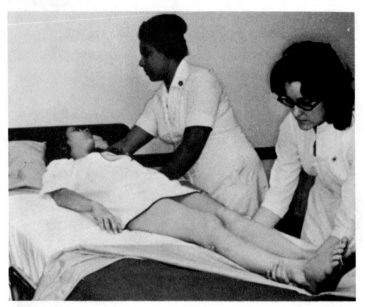

FIGURE 32.3

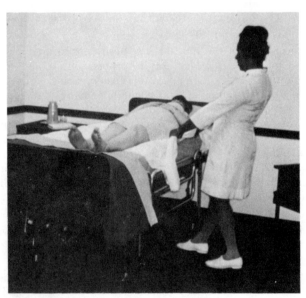

FIGURE 32.4

smooth, continuous movements requires less energy than continually stopping and starting movement.

B. Communicative Aspects

1. *Observations*

    a. Notes should be made about the patient's posture.

    b. All patients, but especially those with orthopedic problems, should be observed for proper knowledge and application of correct body mechanics.

2. *Charting*

    Not applicable

3. *Referrals*

    Not applicable

C. Teaching Aspects—Patient and Family

1. All patients should be taught proper posture and body mechanics. The best method is the nurse's good example as she carries out her daily tasks.

2. When the family will care for a bedridden patient at home, the nurse should explain and demonstrate the principles of proper body mechanics in turning and lifting a patient and should allow the family member to demonstrate understanding of these before the patient is dismissed.

IV. EVALUATION PROCESS

A. Does the patient cooperate during moving and lifting procedures?

B. Do nurses understand the need for proper body mechanics and seem eager to demonstrate them to others?

C. Do nurses, family, and patients utilize principles of proper body mechanics?

33
Cast Care

I. ASSESSMENT OF SITUATION

A. Definition

Observations and nursing interventions which prevent or alleviate complications resulting from the application of a cast.

B. Terminology

1. *Blanching:* a method of pressing the nailbed to ascertain circulatory impairment. The nail should whiten momentarily, then quickly return to normal pink color
2. *Full-leg cast:* a cast extending from mid-thigh to toes
3. *Hanging cast:* a cast extending from axilla to fingers, usually with a bend in the elbow
4. *Plaster of Paris:* quick-drying cast material, used in rolls
5. *Short-leg cast:* a cast extending from below the knee to the toes
6. *Spica cast:* a cast involving a great portion of the main trunk of the body, front and back, and possibly one or more extremities
7. *Spreaders:* an instrument used to spread or loosen a cast which is too tight
8. *Stockinette:* a soft, cloth-like material used under the cast, next to the skin, to protect delicate tissues

C. Rationale for Actions

1. To maintain desired anatomical position
2. To provide traction for reduction of a fracture
3. To prevent or correct contractures

II. NURSING PLAN

A. Objectives

1. To ensure immobilization and desired anatomic position
2. To prevent impairment of circulation
3. To prevent pressure areas under cast
4. To prevent pressure on nerves
5. To record observations of extremities in a cast

6. To teach the patient and family observations that should be made while in the hospital and following discharge

B. Patient Preparation

1. On admission to the unit, minimal handling of the affected extremity will prevent further trauma. Clothing should be removed from injured limbs first.

2. Firmness and support keep the cast in correct conformity until drying is complete. Preparation of the bed should include bedboards, if indicated, to prevent sagging, and enough plastic-covered pillows to support the base in the desired anatomical position.

3. Tell the patient that the affected limb will feel warm immediately after cast application, because the plaster is dipped in warm water to make it usable. Emphasize the need for him to lie still until the cast dries to prevent misshaping the new plaster and possibly causing pressure areas. The patient should expect some discomfort, but pain or continuous localized pressure should be reported. When getting up with a cast, the patient should expect to have to compensate for the alteration in his center of gravity due to the added weight. He might be told to expect pressure from the hanging cast when he stands erect, and soreness due to reduced mobility of the affected part.

C. Equipment

1. Cast cart, including bucket for water, stockinette and plaster in all sizes, and any other supplies used in cast application

III. IMPLEMENTING NURSING INTERVENTION

A. Therapeutic Aspects

1. Firmness and support keep the cast in correct conformity until drying is complete. It usually requires at least 24 hours for the cast to dry completely. Bed covers should be kept away until drying is complete. Uneven pressure should be avoided until cast is dry. If the cast must be lifted, the palms should be used, rather than the fingertips (Figs. 33-1, 33-2). Exposing the cast to circulating air (using a blow drier for instance) will hasten drying. An extremity cast should be turned every 2 hours, to ensure even drying. Four people are needed to turn a patient in a drying spica cast, to prevent cracking. The cast is completely dry when it no longer feels damp or slightly soft to the touch.

2. The rough edges of a plaster cast may traumatize the skin, especially in children. The pressure of the rim of the cast may also cause bruises. Extra padding, such as moleskin, over the edges may prevent skin irritation.

3. A plaster cast is porous and will absorb water and urine. Every effort should be made to keep the cast dry.

4. Poor venous return is common in an injured part. Cold applications constrict blood vessels, anesthetize nerve endings, and aid in blood co-

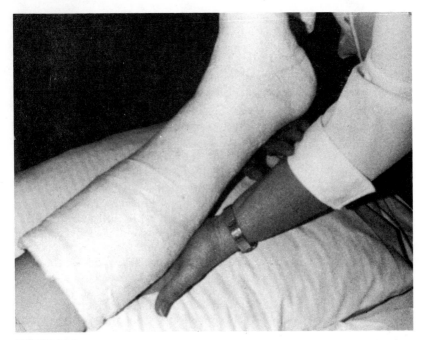

FIGURE 33.1

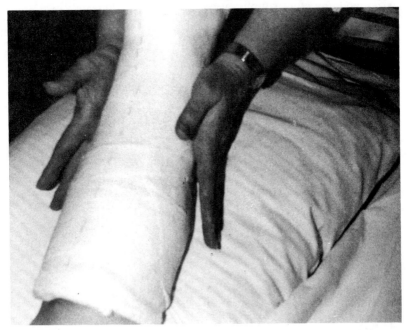

FIGURE 33.2

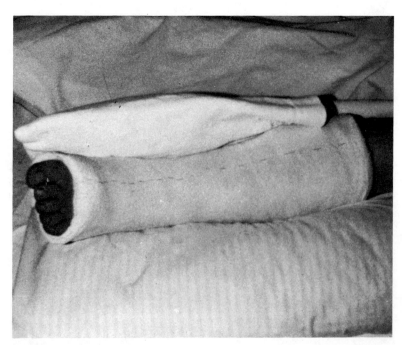

FIGURE 33.3

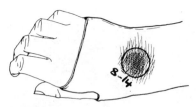

FIGURE 33.4

agulation. Casted extremities should be elevated, with all contours supported to prevent cracking. Ice may reduce edema (Fig. 33-3).

5. A plaster cast is not flexible and tends to shrink as it dries; it thus can inhibit circulation, and swelling often occurs in the fracture area. Especially during the first 24 hours, the fingers or toes must be checked frequently for early signs of circulatory embarrassment. The signs include numbness and tingling, unusual color (pale or cyanotic), skin warm to touch, obvious edema, and blanching of nailbeds. Any seepage of blood through the cast should be circled at its exact perimeter and dated, so that further seepage can be evaluated (Fig. 33-4). Any such drainage and its progression should be noted in the nurses' notes and called to the physician's attention.

6. Proper body alignment and positioning are extremely important to a patient in a cast, because:

   a. Pinching of skin and formation of pressure areas on bony protrusions must be avoided.

   b. Maximum chest expansion for respiration must be facilitated.

   c. Maximum comfort must be provided. To avoid complications, frequent position changes are mandatory.

7. Elimination usually presents problems to the patient in a hip spica, as it is difficult to use the bedpan. Steps should be taken from the start to prevent soiling the cast. Sheets of plastic around the open perineal edges of the cast will help prevent soiling. For female patients, an emesis basin may be the best receptacle in which to urinate.

8. Foreign particles under the cast will precipitate skin irritations and infections. Devices for scratching under the cast must be well-padded and used with extreme care. Scratches under the cast can easily become infected, due to the warm, dark, moist environment. A musty odor coming from under the cast may indicate pus formation.

9. Exudates and secretions should be removed carefully, gently, and by means appropriate to preventing skin trauma. Following cast removal, the skin will be flaky, the muscles and joints sore and stiff. The skin should be washed gently with mild soap and warm water.

B. Communicative Aspects

1. *Observations*

   a. Symptoms of nerve or circulatory impairments should be made hourly until all symptoms are negative. Check toes and/or fingers for:

      (1) Color (blanching sign)

      (2) Sensation (numbness or tingling)

      (3) Edema

      (4) Temperature

      (5) Mobility

      (6) Pain

      (7) Skin irritations at the edge of the cast

   b. Bleeding may occur if there is a wound. Observations for bleeding should be made at frequent intervals and charted as indicated with time.

   c. Bony prominences, such as the heels, ankles, wrists, elbows, and feet, may develop pressure areas if allowed to remain on the bed. Check frequently and relieve pressure areas.

   d. Detection of a foul odor or a hot spot on the cast may indicate an infectious area beneath.

2. *Charting*

   a. Circulation sheet

DATE	HOUR	COLOR	SWELLING	TEMPERA-TURE	MOBILITY	SENSATION
4/2	0700	Pink	None	Warm	Good	Good
	0800	White	Slight	Cool	Decreased	Tingling
	0900	Cyanotic	Moderate	Cold	None	Numbness

   b. Nurses' notes

DATE	TREATMENT	TIME	OBSERVATIONS	SIGNATURE
4/2	Short-leg boot cast applied to rt leg by Dr. D.	0800	Toes of rt foot appear slightly edematous, white, cool; decreased movement; complaining of tingling. Dr. D. notified.	G. Ivers, R.N.
		0900	Dr. D. here. Toes of rt foot appear moderately edematous, slightly cyanotic; loss of mobility; cold and complaining of numbness. Dr. D. split cast.	G. Ivers, R.N.

3. *Referrals*

   a. The patient should be given the name(s) of available orthopedic appliance suppliers in case he needs to replace such items as slings, crutch pads, or traction equipment he might need after dismissal.

C. Teaching Aspects—Patient and Family

1. Instruct patient and family to observe for symptoms of nerve and/or circulatory impairment.

2. Instruct patient and family to observe for possible pressure areas under the cast.

3. Instruct patient and family on the importance of exercising unaffected extremities to prevent atrophy.

4. Instruct patient of the importance of isometric execise of the extremity in a cast, to maintain muscle tone.

5. Instruct patient concerning support that will be used following the removal of cast.

IV. EVALUATION PROCESS

A. Has the patient learned maximum self-care and function to the fullest extent possible in view of limitations caused by the cast?

B. Do the patient and his family understand what symptoms to watch for that might indicate complications?

C. Is the cast intact?

D. Did the cast dry evenly and completely?

E. Has trauma to the skin around the cast edges been prevented?

F. Have padding and preventive efforts kept the cast clean and free of waste contamination?

G. Have complications been prevented?

H. Have proper observations of extremities and cast been made and recorded?

34

Catheter (Foley), Care of

I. ASSESSMENT OF SITUATION

A. Definition

Cleansing of the indwelling catheter and meatus to prevent urethral irritation and inflammation

B. Terminology

See Technique 35, Catheterization, Urethral.

C. Rationale for Actions

To prevent infection or inflammation of perineal area, meatus, or urethra

II. NURSING PLAN

A. Objectives

1. To provide mental and physical comfort to the patient
2. To control introduction or presence of microorganisms
3. To instruct patient and family on care of catheter system, if the catheter must remain indwelling after dismissal from hospital
4. To observe characteristics of perineal care

B. Patient Preparation

1. Thorough handwashing by the person performing this procedure is essential.
2. The patient should be told the reason for cleaning the catheter.
3. Adequate screening or drapes should be available prior to beginning the procedure.

C. Equipment

1. Container of cotton balls with antibacterial cleansing agent
2. Washbasin with water
3. Soap
4. Hand towel and washcloth

III. IMPLEMENTING NURSING INTERVENTION

A. Therapeutic Aspects

1. The skin and mucosa harbor pathogenic microorganisms. The urinary tract offers a favorable location for the multiplication of such organisms, which can fulminate into urinary pathology, especially in the presence of an indwelling (Foley) catheter. Perineal care may be given with soap and warm water. To give catheter care, two cotton sponges saturated with cleaning solution are needed.
2. Indwelling catheters are usually one of two types. The single-lumen tube (2-way Foley) has an inflation tube as well as a tube that allows irrigation fluid to be inserted and urine to drain from the same lumen (Fig. 34-1). The double lumen tube (3-way Foley) has an inflation tube and two other tubes—one to insert irrigation fluid and the other to allow the simultaneous drainage of urine (Fig. 34-2).
3. Pressure on the urethral-vesicle area, caused by pulling the urethral catheter, will overstimulate neural bladder control, causing bladder spasms and pain. The catheter should be held taut but not pulled.
4. For catheter care in the male, the penis is raised and the foreskin retracted approximately ½ to 1 inch. The mucous membranes should be kept clean and free from possibly infective exudate and excretions. The urinary meatus is cleansed with one cotton ball, the Foley is cleansed from the point of insertion outward (Fig. 34-3). Care should be taken not to bring contamination from the anus forward. The cleansing procedure should be repeated until all secretions and crusts are removed. A fresh cotton ball should be used each time.
5. In the female, the perineal area should be kept free from secretions, feces, and menstrual flow. Discharge which coats the catheter at the meatus soon becomes colonized with bacteria. In the female patient, separate the vulva by placing the thumb and first forefinger between the labia minora. The urethral meatus is cleansed with cotton balls. With fresh cotton balls, the perineum is cleansed from the meatus

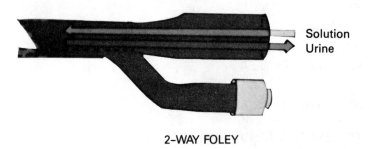

2–WAY FOLEY

FIGURE 34.1

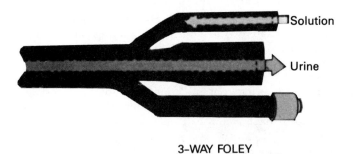

3–WAY FOLEY

FIGURE 34.2

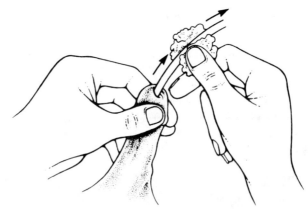

FIGURE 34.3

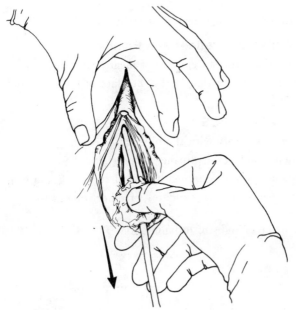

FIGURE 34.4

downward and outward, using a fresh cotton ball for each stroke (Fig. 34-4).

6. The patient should be left comfortable. The drainage tube should be pinned to the sheets, with no tension or unnecessary pull. The tubing should be kept free of kinking or twisting.

7. Catheter care is performed b.i.d. and p.r.n.

B. Communicative Aspects

1. *Observations*

   a. Observe skin and meatus. Be certain there is no redness, skin eruption or swelling at the insertion site or surrounding area.

   b. Inspect proximal end of the catheter and meatus and keep it free of dried crusts and blood.

   c. In the perineal area, observe for signs of inflammation and accumulation of discharge.

2. *Charting*

DATE	TREATMENT	TIME	OBSERVATIONS	SIGNATURE
9/30	Foley	0800	Catheter cleansed with Zephiran chloride sponges. No redness or swelling noted.	D. Young, N.T.

3. *Referrals*

   (See Technique 35, Catheterization, Urethral.)

C. Teaching Aspects—Patient and Family

1. Instruct concerning proper cleansing of meatus and catheter.

2. Instruct regarding observation of skin at place of insertion and surrounding area.

IV. EVALUATION PROCESS

A. Did the patient cooperate with the nurse?

B. Was the patient comfortable during the procedure?

C. Was the patient's privacy guarded by use of screening and drapes?

D. Is the catheter free of crusts, exudates, or other undesirable materials?

E. Is the meatus free of signs of inflammation?

35

Catheterization, Urethral

I. ASSESSMENT OF SITUATION

A. Definition

Insertion of a catheter into the urinary bladder. Types are (See Fig. 35-1.):

1. *Nonretention:* plain or straight catheter, for temporary intubation
2. *Retention:* Foley catheter, for prolonged intubation and continuous free drainage

B. Terminology

1. *Bladder:* the vesicle that acts as a receptacle for urine
2. *Catheter:* tube for evacuating or injecting fluids
3. *Clitoris:* The female erectile structure, located beneath the anterior labia, partially hidden by the labia minora
4. *Foley catheter:* a self-retaining catheter that is held in place in the bladder by an inflatable balloon

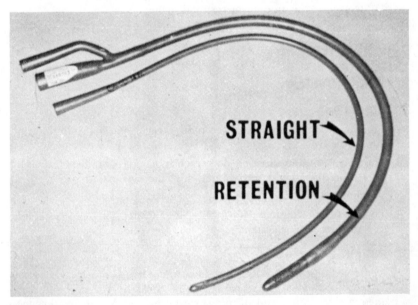

FIGURE 35.1

5. *Labia majora:* two folds of cellular adipose tissue, lying on either side of the vaginal opening and forming lateral borders of the vulva

6. *Labia minora:* two thin folds of tissue that lie within the labia majora and enclose the vestibule

7. *Meatus:* external opening of the urethra

8. *Pathogenic organisms:* microorganisms capable of causing disease

9. *Penis:* male organ of copulation and urinary excretion

10. *Perineum:* that mass of skin, muscle, and fascia located between the vagina and rectum in the female and between the meatus and rectum in the male

11. *Residual urine:* urine that remains in the bladder after voiding

12. *Suppression:* complete failure of the natural excretion of urine

13. *Urethra:* canal for discharge of urine, extending from the bladder to the external meatus

14. *Vulva:* the external female genitalia

C. Rationale for Actions

1. To facilitate the evacuation of urine

2. To obtain a sterile urine specimen

3. To control urine flow

4. To irrigate the bladder

5. To instill medications

6. To determine the amount of residual urine

7. To prevent strain on pelvis or abdominal wounds from distended bladder

II. NURSING PLAN

A. Objectives

1. To allay fear and anxiety of the patient regarding his condition and the procedure

2. To control the introduction or presence of microorganisms, thereby preventing infection or inflammation of the perineal area

3. To minimize trauma to the urinary tract

4. To instruct the patient and family, if indicated, on reason for and care of the catheter system

B. Patient Preparation

1. Explain the procedure to the patient and elicit as much cooperation as possible. Since this procedure can be embarrassing to the patient, adequate screening and draping are necessary. A sign on the door will help ensure that there are no interruptions

2. If the catheterization is to determine the amount of residual urine, the patient should void prior to catheter insertion

3. If the purpose is to obtain a sterile specimen, the patient should not have voided for 30 minutes prior to the procedure.

C. Equipment

1. Catheterization tray, including sterile gloves, specimen container, lubricant, cleansing solution, and cotton balls

2. Appropriate catheter

3. Appropriate drainage system (for retention types)

4. Bath blanket

5. Sterile perineal pad (if needed)

6. Gooseneck lamp

7. Forceps

III. IMPLEMENTING NURSING INTERVENTION

A. Therapeutic Aspects

1. The patient should be positioned as follows, depending on ability: a woman, recumbent with knees flexed and separated; a man, supine. Relaxation of the abdominal and perineal muscles during insertion of the catheter greatly enhances the patient's comfort during this procedure. The lamp should be placed in such a position as to ensure maximum visual assistance without danger of burning the patient or contaminating the sterile field.

2. The human skin and mucosa harbor pathogenic microorganisms. The urinary tract offers a favorable location for multiplication of such organisms, which can proliferate into urinary pathology. In a postpartum patient or any patient with vaginal or meatal discharge, the perineal pad should be removed and disposed of and routine perineal care given before beginning the procedure. The nurse should wash her hands thoroughly before beginning catheterization. A sterile field should be established by opening the catheterization setup, maintaining inner sterility of the wrapper, and donning sterile gloves (Fig. 35-2). Lubrication decreases friction between the catheter and the urethral tract, minimizing mechanical injury to tissue, which would predispose to urinary tract infection and inflammatory processes. A sterile lubricant, such as K-Y jelly, may be applied to the distal 3 inches of the catheter (Fig. 35-3). The container to receive the urine is also prepared at this time, and drapes are applied under the buttocks and over the perineum (Fig. 35-4). If a Foley catheter is being used, a syringe with the proper amount of water for balloon inflation should be ready, also. To cleanse the involved area in the female, separate the vulva by placing thumb and index finger between the labia minora, and clean the urinary meatus with a single downward motion (Fig. 35-5). Repeat several times, using a fresh applica-

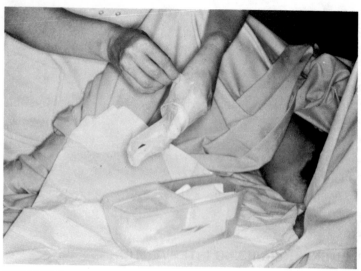

FIGURE 35.2

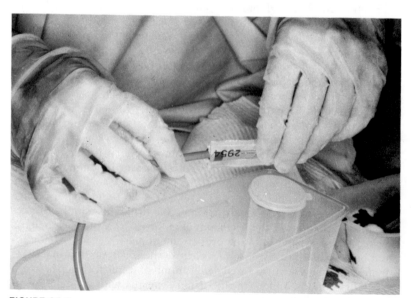

FIGURE 35.3

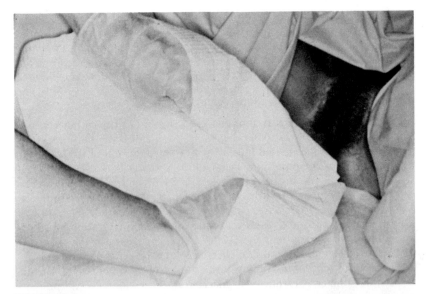

FIGURE 35.4

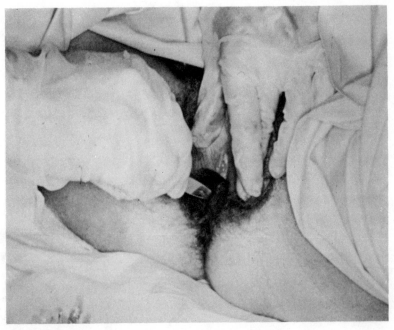

FIGURE 35.5

tor each time. The urinary meatus should be indentified (Fig. 35-6). The urethra of a postpartum patient is edematous, and the entire perineal area is tender; therefore, great care and gentleness should be used in cleansing and catheterizing. In the male patient, raise the penis to a 60° to 90° angle with one hand. This will reduce the angle of catheter entry. Retract the foreskin and cleanse the meatus, using single circular outward motions (Fig. 35-7).

3. Maintenance of sterility must be kept in mind as the catheterization procedure progresses. After cleansing the meatus, the hand touching the skin is contaminated and must not be reintroduced to the sterile field. The sterile hand now removes the catheter from the tray, leaving the drain end in the receptacle to prevent spillage. After reidentifying the urinary meatus, the catheter is slowly inserted into the bladder (Figs. 35-8, 35-9, 35-10). A degree of voluntary relaxation of the urinary sphincter can be produced by deep inspiration and slow exhalation. The patient should be instructed to breathe deeply as the catheter is gently inserted. Never force a catheter; if difficulty or obstruction is encountered, notify the nurse in charge or the physician. If the catheter is erroneously inserted into the vagina, it is contaminated, and a new catheter must be used. If a sterile specimen is needed, place the open end of the catheter in a sterile collection container. Sterile specimens should be taken to the laboratory as soon as possible.

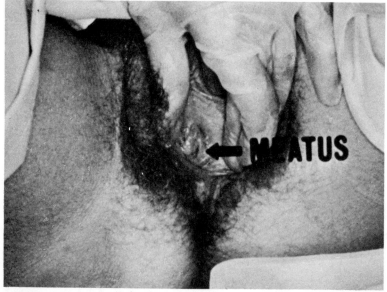

FIGURE 35.6

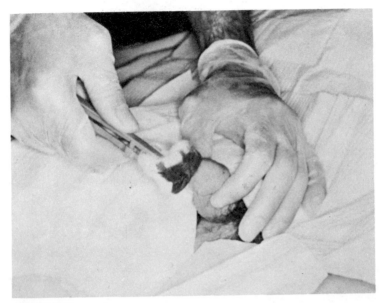

FIGURE 35.7

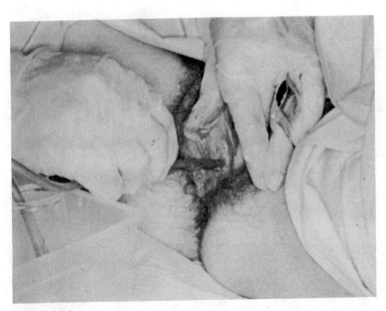

FIGURE 35.8

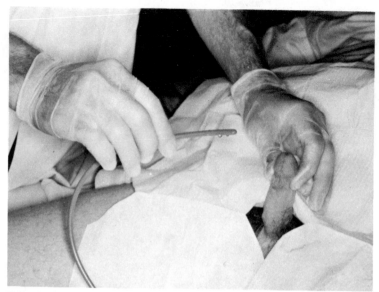

FIGURE 35.9

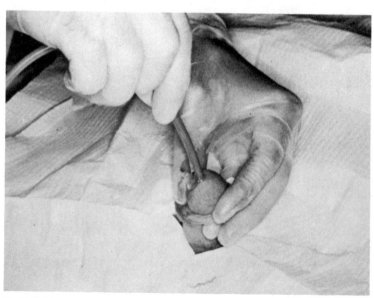

FIGURE 35.10

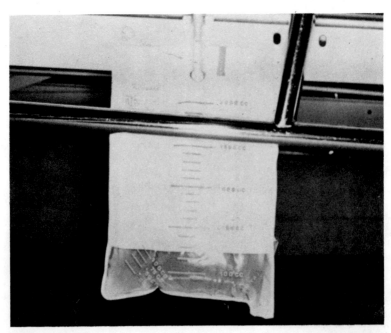

FIGURE 35.11

4. The important aspect of catheter drainage is maintenance of sterility and patency. Various types of drainage apparatus are described below.

   a. The drainage bag is connected by a long, plastic-type tubing, inserted into the catheter tube drainage opening. This method works by gravity; for this reason, the bag must be kept at a level below the bladder (Fig. 35-11). If the bag is raised, it can cause urine to flow back into the bladder and might cause infection. Care must be taken to avoid pinching or kinking the tubing, thus causing urinary retention and stasis in the bladder. The drainage bag is emptied by draining it into a graduated container for accurate measurement (Fig. 35-12).

   b. A leg urinal is a small plastic bag with a short tubing, which fastens to the catheter. It has two flexible straps, which fasten around the leg and hold the bag in place. It may be worn under trousers, skirts, or robes and cannot be seen. It must be emptied periodically by means of a release valve on the bottom of the bag. If worn over a long period of time, it must be cleaned each day, using a bacteriostatic solution.

   c. An hourly container is a small, graduated tube used to measure hourly urine output. It depends on gravitational flow and is usually emptied by means of a stopcock on the bottom side.

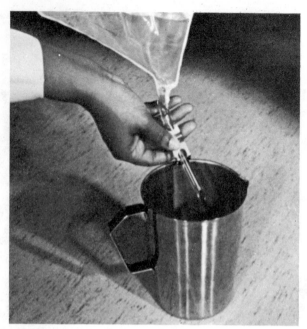

FIGURE 35.12

5. Decompression of an overly distended bladder may cause shock or hemorrhage from rupture of vessels due to rapid change in intravesical pressure. It is suggested that no more than 1,000 to 1,500 ml of urine be taken at one time. In the postpartum patient, however, the bladder should be completely emptied before removing the catheter.

6. Remove the nonretention catheter by pinching tubing and withdrawing gently; pressure on the urethral-vesicle area caused by pulling the catheter will overstimulate neural bladder control, causing bladder spasms and pain. With the retention-type catheter, instill the proper amount of sterile water to inflate the retention balloon (Fig. 35-13). Overinflation may cause the balloon to burst (Fig. 35-14). The open end of the catheter should be attached to the appropriate drainage system. The tubing should be taped to the leg, with some ease between meatus and tape to prevent pulling. The drain tubing is then secured to the bed sheet in such a way that the force of gravity causes the urine to flow downward into drain bag, and the chance of someone snagging extra tubing and pulling the catheter are minimized. In postpartum patients, a perineal pad may be applied gently over the catheter in a manner most comfortable to the patient. (For correct positioning of the catheter, see Figs. 35-15 and 35-16.)

7. After the procedure, the patient should be left in a clean, comfortable environment. Situate the bedside table to facilitate easy reach of needed articles. Reassure the patient that he may move about within

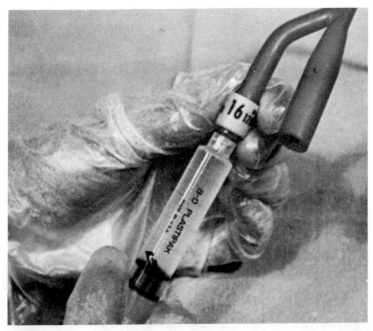

FIGURE 35.13

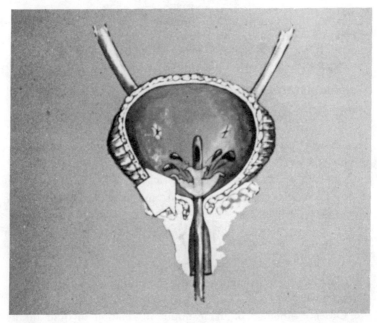

FIGURE 35.14

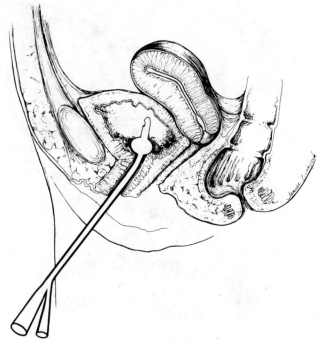

FIGURE 35.15

the extent of his medical limitations without fear of dislodging the catheter. The initial burning sensation and discomfort will subside shortly. Record the amount of urine on the bedside intake and output record and on the chart. Label and send specimen to lab, if needed.

B. Communicative Aspects

1. *Observations*

   a. Note color, appearance, and amount of urine removed.

   b. Observe for unusual discomfort of patient while inserting or removing the catheter.

   c. Observe for efficient drainage system:

      (1) Tubing is free of kinks, twists, and pressure fom resting body parts.

      (2) Tubing is below the bladder level to facilitate gravitational flow.

      (3) End of tubing is above the urine receptacle level.

   d. Note signs of inflammation or accumulation of discharges in perineal area.

   e. Observe amounts of urine ouput in relation to fluid intake to evaluate adequate kidney function.

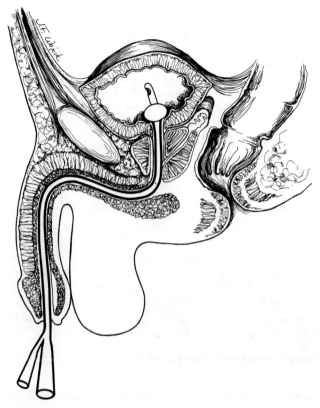

FIGURE 35.16

2. *Charting*

    a. Accurate urinary output and fluid intake should be measured on the patient's intake and output (I&O) forms.

    b. Nonretention catheterization

DATE	TREATMENT	TIME	OBSERVATIONS	SIGNATURE
5/3	#14 French cath inserted to obtain sterile urine specimen for culture	1400	650 ml cloudy, dark amber urine obtained. Patient tolerated procedure with minimal fatigue and discomfort. Full explanation given prior to and during procedure. Spec and req to lab.	F. White, R.N.

c. Retention catheterization

DATE	TREATMENT	TIME	OBSERVATIONS	SIGNATURE
5/3	#16 Foley cath inserted and connected to gravity drainage system	1400	500 ml clear, pinkish yellow urine obtained. Explanation and reason given prior to and during procedure. Patient stated, "Another tube won't tie me down." Instructed concerning ambulating with a Foley. Keeping I&O record. Keeping tubing patent. Left in Fowler's position, reading. Sterile U.A. spec to lab for culture.	F. White, R.N.

3. *Referrals*

   a. If the catheter must remain in place after the patient is discharged from the hospital, the patient should be referred to a visiting nurses' association for follow-up to assure that the catheter is kept clean and changed as indicated.

   b. If the patient will need catheter equipment at home, the family should be instructed on where and what to purchase.

C. Teaching Aspects—Patient and Family

1. Nonretention catheterization

   a. Instruct patient or parents to report any difficulty or change in voiding after catheterization.

   b. Instruct in importance of increased fluid intake to assist in production of urine for a least 8 hours after catheterization.

2. Retention catheterization

   a. Instruct concerning maintenance of system while ambulatory and in bed.

   b. Instruct concerning importance of adequate fluid intake.

   c. If physician wishes, teach technique for irrigation and replacement of catheter system to parents or other family member.

3. For both retention and nonretention catheterizations, tell the patient to relax as much as possible during insertion but to expect a burning sensation. The burning and discomfort may continue for several minutes but will gradually subside. If the catheter is to remain in the patient, reassure him that he will no longer feel it in an hour or two.

IV. EVALUATION PROCESS

A. Was the patient's privacy guarded?

B. Was sterility maintained?

C. Was the patient adequately instructed on what to expect after catheterization?

D. Was infection prevented?

E. Was the tubing adequately secured to prevent trauma to the bladder from accidental pulling?

F. Was adequate bladder drainage achieved?

36

Charting Abbreviations

I. RULES GOVERNING INITIALS AND ABBREVIATIONS FOR CHARTING

A. Abbreviations should be used consistently. Imaginative abbreviations that mean something to only a few persons have no place on the patient record.

B. The proper place for initials and abbreviations is in the portions of the chart that are least likely to be utilized for legal purposes.

C. Abbreviations are utilized to save time and space; however, if there is any question, the word should be written out in its entirety.

II. ACCEPTABLE INITIALS AND ABBREVIATIONS FOR CHARTING

A. General Terms

abd	abdomen
a.c.	before meals
AC	alternating current
accom	accommodation
ACTH	adrenocorticotropic hormone
ad	to, up to
ad. lib.	as desired
adm	admission
AK	above knee
alb	albumin
alk	alkaline
A.M.	morning

amb ambulate
amp ampule
amt amount
anes anesthesia, anesthetic
ant anterior
A-P anterior-posterior
APC aspirin, phenacetin, caffeine
approx approximately
ASA acetylsalicylic acid (aspirin)
ASHD arteriosclerotic heart disease
A.V. node atrioventricular node

BCG bacillus Calmette-Guerin (vaccine for tuberculosis)
b.i.d. twice a day
bisp bispinous or interspinous diameter (pelvic measurement)
BK below knee
B.M. bowel movement
BMR basal metabolic rate
B.P. blood pressure
BPH benign prostatic hyperplasia
BRP bathroom privileges

C centigrade
$\bar{c}$ with
C_1, C_2 (etc.) first cervical vertebra, second cervical vertebra (etc.)
Ca calcium
CA cancer; carcinoma
cap capsule
cath catheter; catheterized
C.C. chief complaint
cc cubic centimeter
CCU coronary care unit
CHF congestive heart failure
CHO or carbo carbohydrate
Cl chloride
cm centimeter
CNS central nervous system
CO_2 carbon dioxide
c/o complains of
COLD chronic obstructive lung disease
comp compound
cont continued; continuous
CPR cardiopulmonary resuscitation
C.S. central service; cesarean section
CSF cerebrospinal fluid

CVA	cerebrovascular accident
CVP	central venous pressure
cysto	cystoscope; cystoscopy
DC	discontinue; direct current
D.C.	diagonal conjugate (pelvic measurement)
D&C	dilatation and curettage
diab	diabetic
diag	diagnosis
diam	diameter
disc	discontinue
DNS	Director of Nursing Service
DOA	dead on arrival
Dr.	doctor
dr	dram
D.T.s	delirium tremens
D/W	distilled water
Dx	diagnosis
EDC	expected date of confinement
EENT	eye, ear, nose and throat
elix	elixir
EOM	extraocular movement
epith	epithelial
E.R.	emergency room
et	and
etc.	and so on
exam	examination
exp. lap.	exploratory laparotomy
expir	expiration; expiratory
ext	extract; external
F	Fahrenheit
F. cath.	Foley catheter
F.H.	family history
FHS	fetal heart sound
fl, fld	fluid
fract	fracture
ft	feet
G in W *or* glyc. in W	glycerin in water
gal	gallon
G.B.	gallbladder
G.C.	gonorrhea
GI	gastrointestinal
Gm	gram
gr	grain
Grav. I, Grav. II (*etc.*)	primigravida, secundigravida (etc.)

gt	drop
G.U.	genitourinary
gyn	gynecology

H *or* (H)	hypodermic
h	hour
H et H *or* H&H	hemoglobin and hematocrit
H&P	history and physical
Hb *or* Hgb	hemoglobin
HC	head circumference
HCl	hydrochloric acid
Hct	hematocrit
Hg	mercury
H_2O	water
H_2O_2	hydrogen peroxide
HOB	head of bed
hosp	hospital
hr	hour
h.s.	hour of sleep; bedtime
ht	height

I	iodine
ICU	intensive care unit
I&D	incision and drainage
IICU	infant intensive care unit
I.M.	intramuscular
inspir	inspiration; inspiratory
inter	between
I&O	intake and output
IPPB	intermittent positive pressure breathing
iss	one and one-half
I.T.	inhalation therapy; intertuberous (pelvic measurement)
IV	intravenous

K	potassium
Kg	kilogram
$KMnO_4$	potassium permanganate

L	liter
L *or* lt	left
L_1, L_2, L_3 (*etc.*)	first lumbar vertebra, second lumbar vertebra, third lumbar vertebra (etc.)
lab	laboratory
lap	laparotomy
lat	lateral
lb	pound
lg	large

liq	liquid
LLL	left lower lobe (lung)
LMP	last menstrual period
L.P.	lumbar puncture
L.R.	lactated Ringer's (IV solution)
LUL	left upper lobe (lung)
L&W	living and well

M	male; meter
m	minum; meter
max	maximum
mcg	microgram
med	medicine
mEq	milliequivalent
Mg	magnesium
mg, mgm	milligram
M.I.	myocardial infarction
min	minute; minimum
ml	milliliter
mm	millimeter
Mn	manganese
mo	month
M.S.	morphine sulphate; multiple sclerosis

N	normal; nitrogen
Na	sodium
N.B.	newborn
neg	negative
neuro	neurology; neurological
no.	number
noct	nocturnal (night)
non. rep.	do not repeat
NPO	nothing by mouth
N.S.	neurosurgery
N/S	normal saline
N&V	nausea and vomiting

'o'	orally
O_2	oxygen
O_2 cap	oxygen capacity
O_2 sat	oxygen saturation
obs or OB	obstetrics
O.C.	obstetrical conjugate (pelvic measurement)
occ	occasional
occ. th.	occupational therapy
o.d.	daily
O.D.	right eye
OFC	occipital frontal circumference

oint	ointment
op	operation
ophth	ophthalmology
o. pt.	outpatient
opt	optimal
O.R.	operating room
ortho	orthopedic
O.S.	left eye
O.T.	occupational therapy
oto	otology
O.U.	both eyes
oz	ounce
P	pulse
p̄	after or post
P-A	posterior-anterior
palp	palpable
PAR	post anesthesia recovery
Para I, Para II (*etc.*)	primipara, secundipara (etc.)
paracent	paracentesis
path	pathology
p.c.	after meals
P.E.	physical education
ped	pediatrics
percuss. & ausc.	percussion and ascultation
PKU	phenylketonuria
P.H.	past history
pH	hydrogen concentration
P.I.	present illness
PID	pelvic inflammatory disease
P.M.	afternoon
PMP	previous menstrual period
PNP	pediatric nurse practitioner
P.O.	phone order
p.o.	per os (by mouth)
poplit	popliteal
pos	positive
post-op	postoperative
prep	preparation
pre-op	preoperative
PRN	whenever necessary
prog	prognosis
prot	protein
pt	patient; pint
P.T.	physical therapy
pulv	powder
PVC	premature ventricular contraction
PZI	protamine zinc insulin

q	every
q.i.d.	four times a day
qh	every hour
q2h, q3h (*etc.*)	every 2 hours, every 3 hours (etc.)
q.o.d.	every other day
q.n.	every night
q.n.s.	quantity not sufficient
q.s.	quantity sufficient
qt	quart
quant	quantity; quantitative
resp	respiratory; respiration
req	request; requisition
RHF	right heart failure
RLL	right lower lobe (lung)
RLQ	right lower quadrant (abdomen)
RML	right middle lobe (lung)
ROM	range of motion
rt	right
rt'd	returned
RUL	right upper lobe (lung)
RUQ	right upper quadrant
Rx	therapy; treatment
s̄	without
SAD	sugar and acetone determination
S.A. node	sinus atrial node
S.C.	subcutaneous
SCIV	subclavian intravenous
S.H.	social history
sig	write or label
sm	small
SMR	submucous resection
sod. bicarb.	sodium bicarbonate
sol	solution
SOS	may be repeated once if urgently required
spec	specimen
sp. fl.	spinal fluid
sp. gr.	specific gravity
s. s. enema	soap suds enema
Staph	Staphylococcus
stat	immediately, once only
stillb	stillbirth
Strep	Streptococcus
subcu	subcutaneous
subling	sublingual (under the tongue)
surg	surgery, surgical
sympt	symptom

syr   syrup

T   temperature
T&A   tonsillectomy and adenoidectomy
tab   tablet
TAT   tetanus antitoxin
Tb   tubercle bacillus
Tbc   tuberculosis
tbsp   tablespoon
temp   temperature
t.i.d.   three times a day
tinct   tincture
T.L.   tubal ligation
TLC   tender loving care; total lung capacity
TLV   total lung volume
TPR   temperature, pulse, respiration
tr   tincture
trach   tracheostomy
tsp   teaspoon
TUR   transurethral resection

U   unit
U.A.   urinalysis
ung   ointment
URI   upper respiratory infection
UTI   urinary tract infection
urol   urology; urological

vag   vaginal
V.C.   vital capacity
V.D.   venereal disease
V.I.   volume index
vit   vitamin
vit. cap.   vital capacity
V.O.   verbal orders
vol   volume
V.S.   vital signs

WBC   white blood cells
wd   well-developed
wn   well-nourished
wt   weight

B. X-ray Abbreviations

A-P   anterior-posterior
A-P & Lat   anterior-posterior and lateral
Au^{198} radioactive gold

Ba enema   barium enema
Ba swallow   barium swallow

Co   Cobalt

ECG (EKG)   electrocardiogram
echo   echo encephalogram
EEG   electroencephalogram
EMG   electromyograph; electromyogram

G.B. series   gallbladder series
G.I. series   gastronintestinal series

I^{131} radioactive iodine
IV cholangiogram   intravenous cholangiogram
IVP   intravenous pyelogram

KUB   kidney, ureters, bladder

MFT   muscle function test

UGI   upper gastrointestinal series

C. Laboratory Abbreviations

acid p'tase   acid phosphatase
AFB   acid fast bacillus
A-G   albumin-globulin ratio
alk   alkaline
alk p'tase   alkaline phosphatase
ANA   antinuclear antibody (test for lupus erythe-
matosus)
ASO *or* ASTO   antistreptolysin

baso   basophile
bili   bilirubin
bl. cult.   blood culture
Bl. time   bleeding time
Br   bromide
BSP   bromosulphalein
BUN   blood urea nitrogen

C   carbon
Ca   calcium
CBC   complete blood count
ceph. floc.   cephalin flocculation test
chol   cholesterol
chol. est.   cholesterol ester

CI	color index
Cl	chloride
CPK	creative phosphokinase
CO_2	carbon dioxide
coag. time	coagulation time
creat	creatinine
CRPA	C-reactive protein antiserum
diff	differential count
eos	eosinophils
FBS	fasting blood sugar
Fe	iron
fib	fibrinogen
glob	globulin
gluc	glucose
Gm %	grams per hundred milliliters of serum or blood
Hct	hematocrit
Hgb *or* Hb	hemoglobin
h.p.f.	per high powered field (used only in describing urine sediments)
I	iodine
ict. ind.	icterus index
LDH	lactic dehydrogenase
L.E. cell	lupus erythematosus cell
lymph	lymphocytes
MCH	mean corpuscular hemoglobin
MCV	mean corpuscular volume
mg %	milligrams per hundred milliliters of serum or blood
mono	monocytes
NH_3N	ammonia nitrogen
NPN	nonprotein nitrogen
PBI	protein-bound iodine
pCO_2	partial pressure of carbon dioxide
pH	hydrogen concentration
PKU	phenylketonuria
PO_4	inorganic phosphorus
polys	polymorphonuclear leukocytes

pro. time	prothrombin time
PSP	phenolsulfonphthalein
RBC	red blood count
sed. rate	sedimentation rate
SGOT	serum glutamic oxaloacetic transaminase
SGPT	serum glutamic pyruvic transaminase
SMAC	sequential multiple analyzer with computer
SMA-12	sequential multiple analysis of 12 chemistry constituents
STS	serologic test for syphilis
T_3 test	triiodothyronine test
TGR	thromboplastin generation time
TPI	*Treponema pallidum* immobilization test
U.A.	urinalysis
VDRL	flocculation test for venereal disease
WBC	white blood count
Zn	zinc

37

Charting Guidelines

I. DEFINITION

The chart is a written record of the care administered by hospital personnel to a patient. The record is to include:

A. The health history of the patient

B. Observations and symptoms of the patient

C. The nursing care administered

D. Therapy and response

II. PURPOSE

The patient's record is kept to provide:

A. A means of communication
B. A basis on which medical therapy is prescribed
C. An aid to the physician in diagnosis
D. Evidence of continuance
E. Material for research and education
F. A legal document, admissible in courts as evidence

III. GENERAL GUIDELINES

A. All entries on the chart must be accurate and factual. Exactness is essential in charting times, effects and results of treatments and procedures. Full dates, including the year, should be used; the year is omitted from dates in charts in this text.

B. Entries may be printed or in script but must be legible and in ink.

C. Each entry must be followed by the writer's first initial, last name, and title, *e.g.*, J. Doe, R.N. All last names, including physicians, hospital staff, patients, and relatives, should be spelled in full. Such names are initialed in the charts of this text only to avoid associations with living people.

D. Ditto marks and erasures are not acceptable. They may lead to legal questions, should the chart be used in court proceedings. Errors are corrected by drawing a single line through the incorrect material and writing "error" above it, as illustrated:

error
~~1000 Amb. in hallway.~~

1000 Amb. in room.

E. Descriptions are essential when charting about drainage, stools, vomitus, pain, and so forth.

F. Lines should never be left completely or partially blank. If a line is skipped or not completely used, a single line should be drawn through it to prevent charting by someone else.

G. The time should be recorded on all entries.

H. Only abbreviations listed in Technique 36, Charting Abbreviations are to be used.

I. Each page must be stamped with the correct addressograph plate.

IV. SPECIFIC GUIDELINES

A. Physician's Orders

1. Each order should have the date and time that it was written.

2. Some system of indicating which orders have been transcribed or carried out is necessary.

3. The licensed person who assumes responsibility for noting the orders must sign the time and her name and title to verify she has noted them.

B. Graphic Records and Treatment and Procedure Sheets

1. Graphic records for temperature and pulse must reflect accurately the patient's actual vital signs.

2. Discrepancies, such as elevated temperature or abnormally depressed pulse, should be reported to the charge nurse.

3. All treatments and procedures must have the time that they occurred. There must also be a place to chart patient response, untoward side effects, and outcome.

C. Patient Progress Notes (Nurses' Notes)

1. These must reflect the ongoing care and response of the patient. They should be patient-oriented and comprehensive.

2. All entries should be meaningful and pertinent. Meaningless phrases, such as "a good 8 hrs.," should be avoided

3. Some specific situations follow (for others, see the particular technique):

   a. *Dressings:* Chart amount and appearance of drainage, appearance of wound, type of dressing applied, and patient's response.

   b. *Hot and cold applications:* Chart where and how long applied, appearance of skin, and patient's response.

   c. *General care:* Back care, decubitus care (size and appearance, drainage, type of care given), positioning, and so forth, should be charted.

   d. *Diagnostic tests:* Time, type of test, side effects, outcome and response, and patient's response are to be charted.

   e. *Admission:* Complete description of patient, method and time of arrival, and patient's response are charted.

   f. *Dismissal:* Chart method and time of departure, instructions and equipment given to patient, who accompanied patient, and patient's response.

   g. The nurses' notes should reflect the nursing process as related to the following legal function of nurses:

   (1) Application and execution of physician's legal orders

   (2) Observations of symptoms and reactions

   (3) Supervision of patient

   (4) Supervision of those participating in care (except physician)

   (5) Reporting and recording

(6) Application and execution of nursing procedures and techniques

(7) Promotion of physical and emotional health by direction and teaching

38

Colostomy Care

I. ASSESSMENT OF SITUATION

A. Definition

The diversion of waste products through an artificial opening on the abdominal surface; specifically, care of an opening of the colon

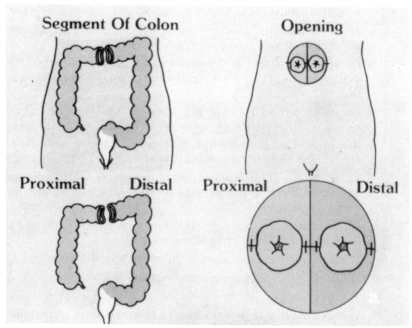

FIGURE 38.1

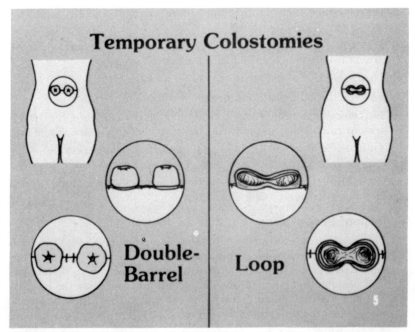

FIGURE 38.2

through the abdominal wall. (See Figs. 38-1 and 38-2.) Types are:

1. *Temporary orifice:* an opening formed in transverse segments of the colon to permit the escape of feces, known as a transverse loop or double-barrel colostomy

2. *Permanent orifice:* the rectum or lower sigmoid portion of the large intestine is excised, and an artificial orifice is created from the remaining or proximal end of the bowel

B. Terminology

None

C. Rationale for Actions

1. To establish regularity in the emptying of the colon of gas, mucus and feces, so the patient can go about his social and business activities without fear of fecal drainage.

2. To prevent excoriation by maintenance of clean, dry skin

3. To cleanse the intestinal tract and prevent obstruction

II. NURSING PLAN

A. Nursing Objectives

1. To know the patient as an individual

2. To encourage early participation by the patient and his family in care of the colostomy

3. To maintain an attitude of patience, concern, and support while the patient learns to accept and care for his colostomy

4. To observe the stoma for discoloration and stenosis

5. To keep the skin clean and prevent excoriation

6. To demonstrate colostomy irrigation and be available for return demonstrations and to teach use and care of the irrigation appliance

7. To assist in establishing a regular pattern of evacuation by seeing that irrigation is carried out at the same time each day

8. To teach the patient and family the importance of resuming normal diet and activities as soon as possible

B. Patient Preparation

1. Preparation for a colostomy should begin well in advance of the actual procedure, if possible. This drastic alteration to his physical appearance is a dreaded and frightening experience. With a little encouragement and opportunity, the patient may verbalize the hostility and fear he feels. A willingness to listen and answer questions is the nurse's best tool in helping the patient cope with this difficult period.

2. A presurgical and a postsurgical visit by a capable ostomy volunteer may be an excellent psychological lift for the patient. The physician should be consulted prior to initiating this action.

3. The patient with a colostomy faces a tremendous threat to his body image. He will need time to adjust to his altered physical and emotional situation. He should not be pushed faster than he is able to develop. A positive and patient attitude on the part of the nursing staff can help the new colostomy patient face the reality of his situation. He should become involved in his care early and begin doing the colostomy care himself as soon as possible.

C. Equipment

1. Irrigating appliance (various commercial ones available)
2. Irrigating solution:
   a. Tapwater
   b. Saline solution
   c. Soap solution
3. Bedpan or commode
4. Stand to hold irrigating solution
5. Protective pad for bed
6. Towels and washcloths
7. Clean colostomy bag or dressing
8. Paper bag

9. Water-soluble lubricant

III. IMPLEMENTING NURSING INTERVENTION

A. Therapeutic Aspects

1. *Irrigation*

   a. Normal body position for bowel evacuation provides psychological comfort and well-being. If the patient is physically able, the irrigation should be done in the bathroom, in a sitting position (Fig 38-3). However, if he is unable to sit up, turn him to the side on which the colostomy is located and elevate his head slightly. The equipment should be completely assembled and conveniently arranged. A full explanation of what is done and why will enhance cooperation.

   b. The temperature of the solution should be 105° F. If it is too cool, it may cause cramping, and if too warm, it may injure the mucous lining. The irrigation bag is filled with the type and amount of solution prescribed by the physician. The flow control clamp must be closed at this time. For the first irrigation, only 250 ml is usually given. This may be increased daily up to 1,500 ml. There should be a stoma guard on the colon tube below the flow control clamp. The nurse should remove or assist in the removal of the bag or dressing, which is disposed of in a paper bag. The stoma and surrounding tissue should be thoroughly cleansed.

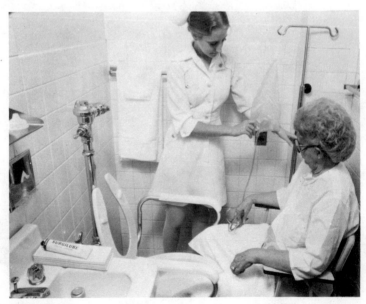

FIGURE 38.3

c. The type of irrigation appliance may vary. The most common type consists of a gasket held over the stoma by a belt around the patient's waist (Fig. 38-4). The gasket opens into a long plastic bag open at both ends. The irrigation tubing is inserted through the upper opening of the bag, and the lower opening is allowed to fall into the bedpan or commode (Fig. 38-5). The belt is fastened to the gasket on one side and, with the gasket securely over the stoma, is passed around the patient's waist and fastened to the other side of the gasket. The belt should fit snugly to prevent leakage. Place the guard over the tube. (Fig. 38-6).

d. Air introduced into the colon only adds to distention and discomfort. Fill the tubing with solution and expel the air. Then the distal tip of the tube should be lubricated with a water-soluble lubricant, such as K-Y jelly (Fig. 38-7).

e. Introduce the colon tube through the guard into the stoma, 2 to 3 inches or as ordered by the physician (Figs. 38-8, 38-9). Never use force on inserting the tube, because the bowel may be perforated. If resistance is met, pull the tube out slightly, release a small amount of solution, pause a minute, and again gently attempt insertion. If resistance cannot be overcome without force, notify the physician. When the tubing is properly inserted, open the clamp and allow water to flow into the colon. Hang irrigation bag on an IV standard, rack, or hook at shoulder level.

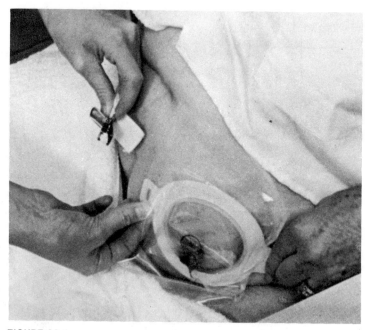

FIGURE 38.4

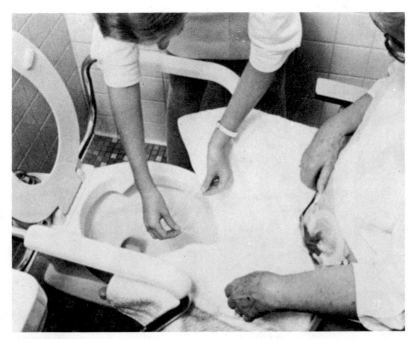

FIGURE 38.5

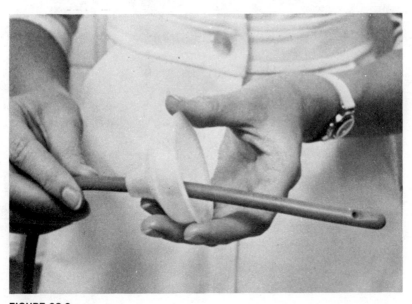

FIGURE 38.6

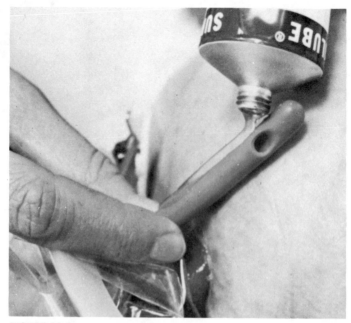

FIGURE 38.7

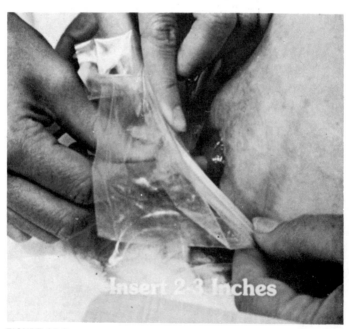

FIGURE 38.8

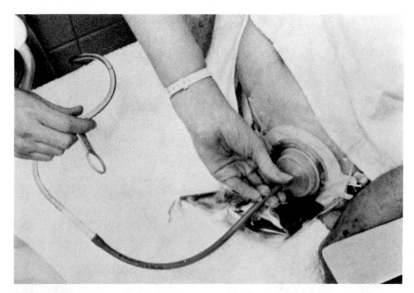

FIGURE 38.9

    f. The amount of pressure on the flowing water is determined by the height of the bag. If the patient complains of cramping, lower the container, clamp the tubing, and allow the patient to rest before resuming irrigation at a slower rate.

    g. Solution should remain in the colon 5 to 15 minutes. Remove tube and clamp top of bag. The bowel contents can usually be evacuated in 30 minutes. The patient will learn the physical signs or feelings that indicate evacuation is complete. After evacuation, assist the patient to clean the stoma and surrounding tissue with soap and warm water and dry it *completely* (Figs. 38-10, 38-11). A clean bag or dressing should be applied (Fig 38-12). The patient and nurse should both wash their hands well.

    h. For the emotional health and well-being of the patient, leave him clean and comfortable; wash, dry, and store the irrigation equipment properly. Praise and encouragement will do much to help the patient gain the confidence and self-assurance he will need to deal with his colostomy in the future.

2. *Dressing change*

    a. Preventing excoriation and irritation of skin is vital to a colostomy patient. Skin breakdown can delay the fitting and wearing of a permanent bag. The skin should be cleaned with soap and water each time the dressing is changed. Medicated ointments may be ordered.

    b. Stoma dressings are intended to absorb the liquid part of the stool

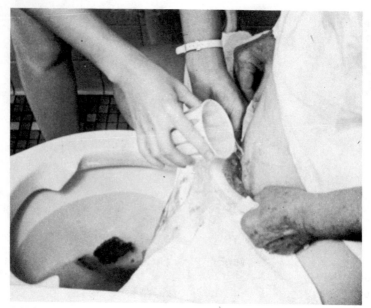

FIGURE 38.10

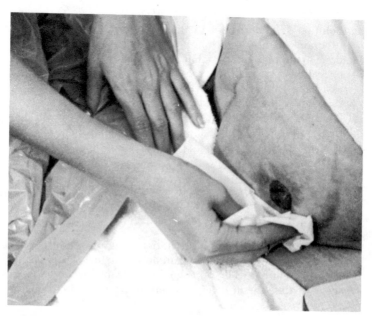

FIGURE 38.11

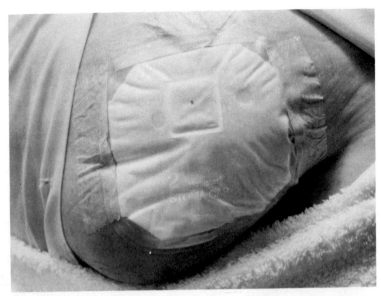

FIGURE 38.12

and to prevent soiling clothes and bed linens. Gauze pads may be placed over stoma with a larger dressing over them. The dressings may be held in place with Montgomery strips to prevent skin irritation due to frequent changes of adhesive tape. Ostomy bags may be applied as soon as ordered.

c. Stoma bags are available for the patient to wear and may be held in place by a belt or may be self-adhering to the skin. It is very important that the skin around the stoma be kept clean and dry. As soon as the colostomy is working, a bag should be applied and instructions given to the patient about care of his colostomy appliance. The common colostomy bag has a round opening in the upper portion which fits over the stoma. Thus, the evacuated contents are allowed to fall into the bag. The bags should be changed as needed. The irrigation bag can be rinsed with warm soapy water and then with clear water and left to dry. The belt may also be washed in warm soapy water and should be rinsed thoroughly and allowed to dry before reapplication.

B. Communicative Aspects

1. *Observations*

   a. Observe the patient and his environment to determine how he sees himself, particularly in relation to his illness. Observe for expressions of self-doubt, self-assurance, autonomy, orientation toward family and friends, and adaptive ability.

   b. Observe the fecal return for appearance, color, and consistency.

c. Observe the skin around the colostomy for signs of redness or excoriation.

d. Observe the colostomy for any change in appearance.

e. Observe for signs and symptoms of fluid and electrolyte imbalance.

f. Observe the patient for signs of acceptance or rejection of the altered body image.

2. *Charting*

DATE	TREATMENT	TIME	OBSERVATIONS	SIGNATURE
5/15	Colostomy irrigated with 500 ml tap water	0830	No difficulty inserting tube. Returned dark brown, formed material. Stoma appears pink; patient looked at stoma for first time and asked questions about irrigation. Appears to be ready for teaching. Dressing applied.	F. White, R.N.

3. *Referrals:*

a. *Ostomy therapist:* if an ostomy therapist is available, he can be a valuable resource to facilitate a smooth transition from hospital to home.

b. *Ostomy club:* many cities have clubs composed of ostomy patients who meet regularly to discuss mutual problems.

C. Teaching Aspects—Patient and Family

1. The nurse should be familiar with the following information to assist the patient to maximum rehabilitation potential.

a. How soon after surgery is the colostomy irrigated?

b. How often and when should the irrigation take place?

c. What constitutes adequate nutrition for the colostomy patient?

d. What effect does dehydration have on proper colostomy function?

e. How often and what kind of bowel movements should be expected?

f. What is the best and most economical irrigating device for this particular patient?

g. How and where will irrigation be done at home?

h. How is equipment kept clean and odor-free?

i. How and where is new equipment obtained when needed?

j. What other family member can be taught colostomy care to ensure proper care if the patient cannot do it himself?

k. Why are periodic follow-up visits essential?

l. What unusual signs should be called to the physician's attention immediately?

m. What community resources are available?

2. The following information should be given to the patient and his family.

a. Before the operation, the patient should understand what is involved in the surgery and how it will affect his normal life. However, overpreparation may serve to frighten or upset him. Teaching should be geared toward his response and acceptance, which are measured by questions and degree of interest. In teaching, stress should be placed on the function remaining rather than on the function which will be lost.

b. After surgery, the patient should be encouraged to look at his stoma and to participate in his care. However, if he seems resistant or hesitant, he should not be pushed but allowed to progress at his own pace.

c. He should be told that the large size of the stoma may diminish in time.

d. The low-residue diet is usually followed for several weeks with progression to a normal diet. The patient should be advised to chew all food thoroughly. Some foods which may need to be avoided are onions, beans, cabbage, and nuts, which are known to cause gas; spicy or irritating foods, which may cause diarrhea; and certain drugs, such as antibiotics. The patient may be instructed to keep some type of antidiarrhea medication on hand.

e. The patient should be cautioned against overrestricting himself in such ways as severe dietary restrictions, never going out socially, not traveling, taking excessive supplies or clothing along when going out, etc. Once regulated, he will probably be able to resume most of his normal activities.

f. The patient should be told to return as requested by his physician for regular medical examinations.

IV. EVALUATION PROCESS

A. Is the patient showing signs of accepting his colostomy?

B. Is the patient participating in the colostomy irrigation process?

C. Will the patient look at his colostomy?

D. Does the patient know how to care for and replace the colostomy equipment?

E. Is the colostomy irrigation being done at the same time each day?

F. Is the irrigation achieving adequate colonic evacuation?

G. Has a successful irrigation posture and routine been achieved?

H. Is the skin around the colostomy healthy and intact?

39

Contact Lens, Removal of

I. ASSESSMENT OF SITUATION

A. Definition

Removal by the nurse of corneal or scleral lenses of a patient who is incapacitated or injured and cannot remove the lenses himself; corrective lenses that fit either the cornea or sclera of the eye for correction of refractive errors

B. Terminology

1. *Corneal lenses:* the most widely used type of lens, which is so small that it covers only the cornea
2. *Scleral lenses:* a larger lens which covers both the sclera and cornea and is the size of a quarter

C. Rationale for Actions

To remove the lens from the eye without trauma

II. NURSING PLAN

A. Objectives

1. To prevent injury to the eyes
2. To avoid loss or damage to the lenses

B. Patient Preparation

1. If the patient is conscious but incapacitated, it should be explained to him that his lenses will be gently removed by the nurse.
2. If the patient is unconscious, he will probably be in a recumbent position and the nurse can accomplish the removal of his lenses in this position.

C. Equipment

1. Suction cup for removing contact lenses
2. Case for storage of contact lenses

III. IMPLEMENTING NURSING INTERVENTION

A. Therapeutic Aspects

1. Method used for either scleral or corneal lens removal with rubber suction holder:

a. The surface of the suction cup must be free from dirt and grease.

b. The lower lid of the patient's eye should be pulled down gently. Too much pulling lowers the upper lid at the same time, which is not desirable. Too much suction cannot be produced at this time.

c. The suction should be placed on the center of the lens. Care must be taken that force is applied to the lens rather than the eye. All edges of the suction cup should be in contact with the lens.

d. The nurse then releases the pressure of the suction on the lens.

e. The lens should be pulled from the bottom in a rocking motion to break the suction at the lower scleral portion. Care is taken to avoid pulling the entire globe from the socket by remembering that suction must be broken before pulling the lens forward.

f. The lens is pulled out and down from the eye.

g. Measures to take if there is difficulty in breaking the suction from the bottom portion of the lens:

  (1) Attach the suction cup to the lens.

  (2) Raise the upper eyelid of the patient.

  (3) Break the suction from the upper scleral portion.

  (4) Remove lens from under lower lid, pulling outward and upward.

2. Manual Removal—use with corneal lens:

a. The nurse places the tip of the forefinger of one hand horizontally on the lower lid below its margin.

b. Next, she places the top of the forefinger of the other hand on the upper lid above its margin and observes to determine if the lens is visible.

c. The nurse then manipulates the two lids against each other in scissors motion while the patient closes, opens, and rolls his eyes. The lens should slide out between the lids.

B. Communicative Aspects

1. *Observations*

a. If the contact lens cannot be removed with ease, removal efforts should be discontinued and an ophthalmologist should be called.

b. Note and record the condition of the eyes before and after removal of the lens.

2. *Charting*

a. Time

b. Removal procedure

c. Storage of lens

d. Response of patient

DATE	TREATMENT	TIME	OBSERVATIONS	SIGNATURE
4/18	Removal of both corneal lenses	0900	Both corneal lenses removed from patient with casts on both arms. Contact lenses placed in contact lens case and placed in locked storage compartment in room.	J. Day, R.N.

3. *Referrals*

If the patient is having difficulty with the lenses, he should make an appointment with an optometrist or ophthalmologist.

C. Teaching Aspects—Patient

1. Since the patient has had the lenses prior to coming to the hospital, he should know all of the aspects of the care and wearing of contact lenses. However, review of any aspect may be needed with emphasis on proper storage when not in use.

IV. EVALUATION PROCESS

A. Was the removal of the lenses conducted without injury or discomfort to the patient?

B. Was the patient given a thorough explanation of what was going to be done?

C. Were the lenses properly stored with proper labels for each eye?

40

Crutchwalking

I. ASSESSMENT OF SITUATION

A. Definition

Aiding the disabled person in increasing stability and reducing body weight on one or both of the lower extremities. Types of crutchwalking are:

1. *Four-point gait:* Weight-bearing is permitted on both legs, and the pattern is as follows: right crutch, left foot; left crutch, right foot (Fig. 40-1). It is the normal reciprocal walking pattern, with crutches.

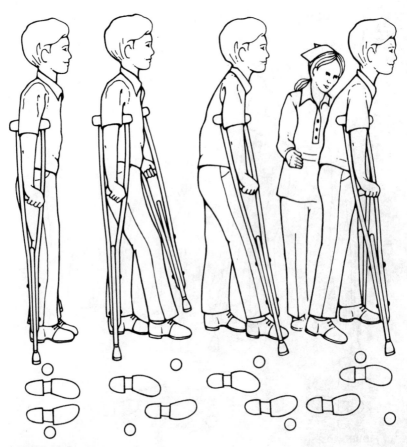

FIGURE 40.1

2. *Two-point gait:* Weight-bearing is permitted on both legs, and the pattern is a speed-up of the 4-point gait: right crutch and left foot forward at the same time; left crutch and right foot forward at the same time (Fig. 40-2).

3. *Three-point gait:* Weight-bearing is permitted on only one leg; the other leg cannot bear weight, but it acts as a balance in the process. This gait is also used when partial weight-bearing is allowed on the affected extremity. The pattern is as follows: both crutches and the nonsupportive leg go forward; then the good leg follows through as weight is borne on the palms. The crutches and impaired leg are brought forward immediately, and the pattern is repeated (Fig. 40-3).

4. *Swing-through gait, swing-to gait, tripod gait:* The body is supported on the hands and the crutches, and the body is then brought through the crutches in a swinging motion. Advance both crutches simultaneously while bearing body weight on both legs. Lean forward,

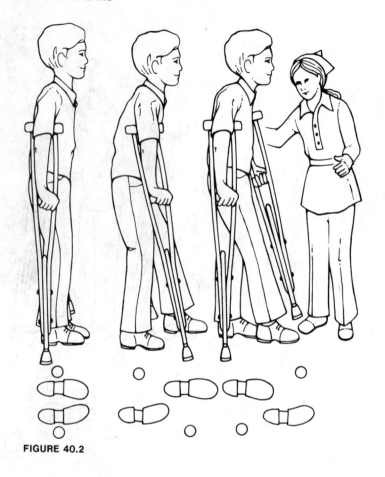

FIGURE 40.2

transferring the body weight onto the extended crutches. Swing the legs up to the crutches or beyond the crutches (Fig. 40-4). This gait is used by paraplegics and those with braces on both legs.

B. Terminology

None

C. Rationale for Actions

1. To promote mobilization
2. To promote patient independence through ambulation
3. To prevent injury to affected limb

II. NURSING PLAN

A. Objectives

1. To teach patient crutchwalking

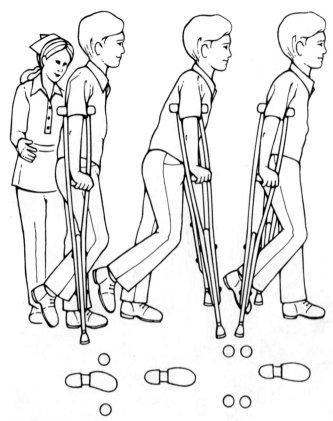

FIGURE 40.3

2. To alleviate fear and anxiety of the patient in crutchwalking

3. To prevent development of faulty habits in crutchwalking

4. To record daily progress of crutchwalking

B. Patient Preparation

1. Due to the dependent nature of the patient's condition, the nurse must ensure patient safety and prevent further injury due to falls or incorrect use of crutches. A safety belt should be used until the patient gains stability. Adequate instruction should be given prior to any attempts at crutchwalking. A nurse or therapist must be with the patient during his early crutchwalking periods.

2. Exercise is the foundation of preparation for ambulation. Preconditioning exercises that the nurse can teach and supervise are as follows: quadriceps sitting, gluteal sitting, sit-ups, push-ups, raising arms and pull-ups. The exercises will strengthen the muscles of the shoulders, chest, arms, hands, and back.

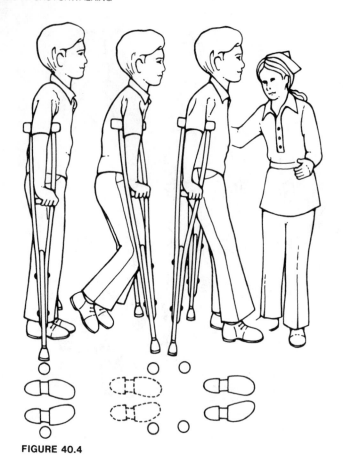

FIGURE 40.4

C. Equipment

1. Adjustable crutches
2. Rubber crutch tips
3. Axillary arm pads
4. Safety waist belt
5. Tape measure

III. IMPLEMENTING NURSING INTERVENTION

A. Therapeutic Aspects

1. Adjustable crutches are practical, as the disease may cause changes in the muscles and the joints, or the patient may improve and progress to a different crutch base and gait. To measure a standing patient for crutches, measure 1½ to 2 inches from the axillary fold to a position

on the floor 4 inches in front of the patient and 6 inches to the side of his toes. Allow a 2-finger width insertion between the axillary fold and the arm piece. If the patient must be measured lying down, measure from 2 inches below the axilla to 4 to 6 inches out from the sole of the foot.

2. In order to give the patient a feeling of security and as an added safety measure, the patient should learn from the first day the proper way to balance on crutches. The starting position is a tripod, formed by the patient's body and the two crutches.

3. Correct standing position is essential for maintaining balance. The patient stands with his feet slightly apart, and the crutches are placed forward and out from the body in such a fashion that a line drawn between them would form the base of a triangle, whose apex would be the patient's feet.

4. Pressure on the brachial plexus will cause temporary or permanent paralysis of the arm. The patient should be taught to extend and stiffen his elbow and to place the weight of his body on his palms.

5. The type of disability determines the crutchwalking gait. In general, the following will apply to most orthopedic patients:

   a. When a patient may bear partial weight on each limb, teach the 4-point or 2-point gait.

   b. When the patient may bear only a little or no weight on one extremity, teach the 3-point gait.

   c. When paralysis of hips and legs is complete, teach the swing-through gait.

B. Communicative Aspects

1. *Observations*

   a. Anxiety and fear experienced by the patient may interfere with ability to learn to walk on crutches.

   b. Correct balance, posture and gait should be observed to prevent complications.

   c. Physical tolerance should be observed in relation to the crutchwalking program.

2. *Charting*

DATE	TREATMENT	TIME	OBSERVATIONS	SIGNATURE
5/25	Crutch training	0900	Patient ambulated with crutches for first time, using 2-point gait. Is using poor posture at this time but appears excited about starting to walk. Correct posture demonstrated.	C. Allen, L.V.N.

3. *Referrals*

The patient or family should be told where orthopedic supplies may be purchased after dismissal so that such items as crutch tips, crutch pads, may be replaced as needed.

C. Teaching Aspects—Patient and Family

1. Instruct the patient in the crutch gait to be used.
2. Instruct the patient in the importance of good posture in crutch-walking.
3. Instruct both patient and family in safety measures: no wet spots, loose rugs or other obstacles in the way when patient is crutch-walking.
4. Inform the patient that crutch tips must be intact and should be replaced when there is any sign of thinness in the rubber.

IV. EVALUATION PROCESS

A. Were fear and anxiety identified and alleviated early in treatment?

B. Were faulty crutchwalking habits prevented?

C. Does the patient exhibit proper body posture during crutchwalking?

D. Have physical limitations and restrictions been considered in adopting a crutchwalking gait?

41

Dentures, Care of

I. ASSESSMENT OF SITUATION

A. Definition

Cleaning the false teeth of an individual

B. Terminology

1. *Dentifrice:* a preparation intended to clean and polish the teeth
2. *Stomatitis:* inflammation of the mouth
3. *Vulcanite:* porous material used in making dentures

C. Rationale for Actions

1. To maintain cleanliness and comfort

2. To prevent infection of the mouth

3. To prevent bacteria from traveling to the digestive tract

II. NURSING PLAN

A. Objectives

1. To teach the proper care of dentures to the patient

2. To prevent complications associated with inadequate cleaning of the mouth and teeth

3. To handle dentures with care to prevent breakage

B. Patient Preparation

1. If the patient is alert and able to care for his own dentures, the proper equipment should be brought to the patient's bedside for his own use.

2. If the patient is unable to care for his dentures, the nurse can clean his dentures as part of the hygienic care given to the mouth.

3. If the patient is unconscious, the dentures should be removed from his mouth and placed in a labeled dental container in water or normal saline solution to keep the dentures moist.

4. To give mouth care, the head of the bed should be raised to Fowler's position unless contraindicated. If the patient is unable to sit up and care for his mouth and dentures, he can be turned to the side facing the individual giving the care.

C. Equipment

1. Denture brush or toothbrush

2. Container for dentures

3. Denture cleaner

4. 4×4 if needed to clean the mouth of the patient

5. Towel and curved basin to give mouth care

III. IMPLEMENTING NURSING INTERVENTION

A. Therapeutic Aspects

1. The dentures should always be cleaned when giving mouth care to the patient. The mucous membrane lining of the mouth should be kept clean, as well as the patient's dentures. Hot water should never be used to rinse dentures, since it will damage the denture material.

2. If a patient cannot remove his dentures, they may be removed in the following manner:

   a. The upper denture, which is held in place in the mouth by a vacuum, can be grasped with the thumb and index finger on each hand (Fig. 41-1). The upper denture is then moved up and down

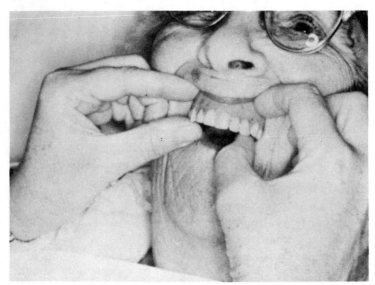

FIGURE 41.1

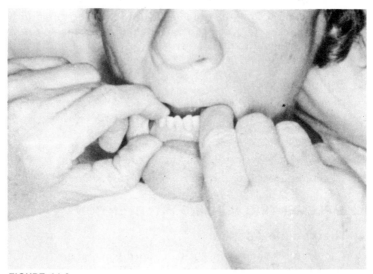

FIGURE 41.2

gently to break the seal of the vacuum. Once this seal is broken, the upper denture can be slipped gently out of the mouth.

b. The lower denture is not held in place by a vacuum, and may be removed by taking a firm grasp with the thumb and index finger of each hand and lifting it gently out of the mouth (Fig. 41-2).

During the removal, care must be taken to turn the lower dentures slightly to prevent stretching the patient's lips.

c. Once the dentures have been removed, they should be placed in a basin. The basin then may be taken to the sink to wash (Fig.41-3).

d. A toothbrush and denture powder are used to clean the dentures by the application of brushing motions. The upper dentures are brushed in a downward motion, whereas the brush is moved in an upward motion on the lower dentures. When the dentures are cleaned, they must be held over the basin of water or over a soft towel.

e. The dentures are rinsed with running warm (not hot) water. Care must be taken not to drop the dentures while cleaning them. If the dentures are cleaned over a basin filled with water, there is less likelihood of damage to dentures if they are dropped (Fig. 41-4).

f. After the dentures have been cleaned, they should be replaced in the patient's mouth unless contraindicated. The upper lip can be elevated with one hand while the upper denture is inserted with the other hand (Fig. 41-5). Once the dentures are in place, the nurse should press gently on the upper denture to ensure that they are securely in place (Fig. 41-6). The same procedure is followed with the lower denture, with pressure applied in a downward motion (Fig. 41-7).

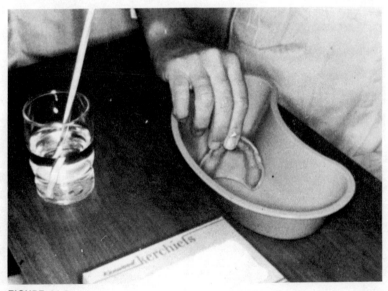

FIGURE 41.3

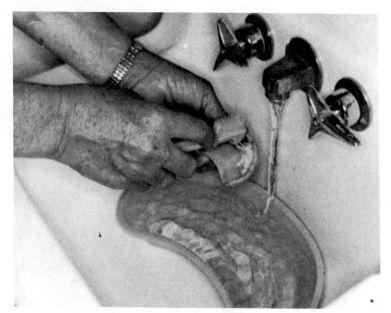

FIGURE 41.4

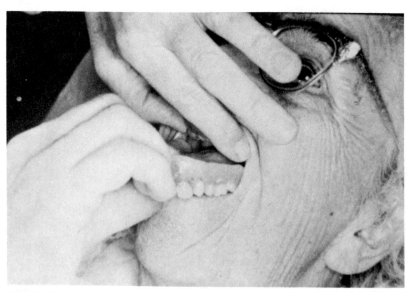

FIGURE 41.5

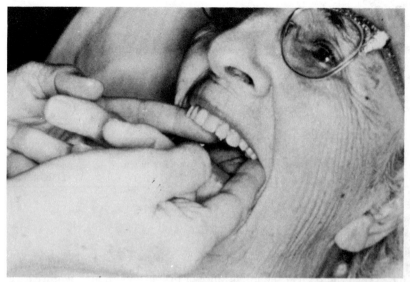

FIGURE 41.6

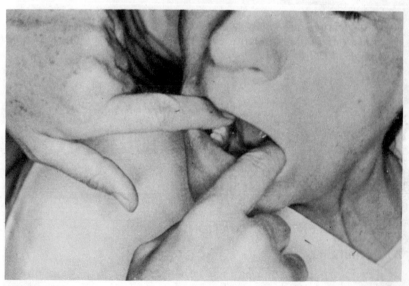

FIGURE 41.7

B. Communicative Aspects

1. *Observations*

   a. Carefully observe the condition of the mouth.

   b. Be sure that the dentures fit properly.

   c. Note the condition of the dentures.

2. *Charting*

DATE	TREATMENT	TIME	OBSERVATION	SIGNATURE
5/1	Dental care	0830	Mouth is in good condition. Lower denture does not fit well in mouth.	M. Doe, R.N.

3. *Referrals*

   Not applicable

C. Teaching Aspects—Patient

1. Teach the patient the importance of proper mouth and denture care.

2. Stress the importance of dentures fitting properly in mouth. A patient should be taught that when he keeps dentures out of his mouth for long periods, the gum line will change, increasing the chances for improperly fitting dentures.

IV. EVALUATION PROCESS

A. Were all the food particles removed from the dentures?

B. Did the patient appear to be comfortable after the dentures were cleaned?

C. If the dentures are not to be kept in the mouth, is there a labeled container for the dentures in a storage area where they will not be in danger of falling to the floor?

42

Discharge Planning

I. ASSESSMENT OF SITUATION

A. Definition

The incorporation of a series of activities leading to the departure of the patient from the hospital

B. Terminology

None

C. Rationale for Actions

1. To facilitate departure under optimal conditions
2. To teach the patient special procedures
3. To interpret the physician's orders
4. To explain the function and availability of community agencies

II. NURSING PLAN

A. Objectives

1. To allay the fear and anxiety in leaving the security of the hospital
2. To ensure continuity of care in the home by instructing the patient and his family so that they will fully understand the treatments that the physician desires
3. To understand the psychosocial aspects related to the patient's readjustments following hospitalization, to increase the nurse's effectiveness in working with the patient and his family

B. Patient Preparation

1. Planning for dismissal should begin on admission, when the nurse should assist the patient in setting goals, both short-term and long-term, in regard to future health. Of primary importance may be the home situation to which the patient will be returning, the amount of responsibility he must assume after discharge, the amount and type of assistance he will have, and his expected physical limitations after hospitalization. If assistance or follow-up is needed, arrangements should be made prior to dismissal. If treatments (such as irrigations, soaks, injections) are to be carried out at home, the person responsible should be taught early in hospitalization, so that he or she will have time to develop some degree of skill in technique. Also, this will give the nurses time to evaluate his competence and the patient's tolerance, so adjustments may be made as needed.
2. In preparation for dismissal, nursing personnel should strive to keep the patient's personal belongings in close proximity, especially if the patient is transferred from one room or unit to another.

C. Equipment

1. Wheelchair or cart, if condition warrants
2. Patient's personal belongings

III. IMPLEMENTING NURSING INTERVENTION

A. Therapeutic Aspects

1. Actual discharge of the patient must be preceded by a written order

from the physician. At this time, he may give the patient instructions. The nurse should be present so that she can reinforce and clarify the physician's instructions and answer questions as necessary.

2. The actual dismissal procedure varies among hospitals. Nursing personnel must assume responsibility for seeing that the patient receives diet instructions, prescriptions, follow-up, return information, and so forth. They must also be sure that the patient and family understand any restrictions imposed by the physician and the reason for them. Hospital personnel should assist the patient in packing and should double-check all drawers and shelves, bathroom, closets, and so on for any of the patient's belongings. The patient should be escorted from the unit in a cordial, pleasant manner. It is usually desirable for the patient to leave by wheelchair, because in the excitement of going home, he may overestimate his capabilities.

B. Communicative Aspects

1. *Observations*

   a. Sometimes a patient may wish to be dismissed against the physician's orders. If so, he should sign a "Dismissal Against Medical Advice" form and fully understand the meaning of it. If he refuses to sign, he cannot legally be kept in the hospital. The physician is to be notified in either case.

   b. When the physician desires a medication to accompany the patient home, he will write a prescription. The nurse should reinforce any instructions given by the physician.

2. *Charting*

   a. Indicate time of dismissal, condition, and mode of departure.

   b. The nurse will check to see that the physician's order is noted, and the chart is signed out with a signature before it leaves the unit.

DATE	TREATMENT	TIME	OBSERVATIONS	SIGNATURE
5/20		1000	Dismissed via wheelchair, accompanied by M. Doe, N.A., and wife. Condition apparently improved and appears to be happy about going home. Digitoxin 0.1 mg sent home with patient. Instructed to take 0.1 mg once a day. Appointment made to return to district clinic in one week to see physician. Dietitian instructed patient and wife concerning bland diet.	F. White, R.N.

3. *Referrals*

  a. If the patient will need assistance at home, he may be referred to a visiting nurse agency.

  b. Some areas have a meal delivery service which could help provide hot meals for patients who live alone, until they are able to cook for themselves.

C. Teaching Aspects—Patient and Family

1. Instruct the patient or family regarding care and treatment.

2. Reinforce teaching of special procedures.

3. Instruct the patient on any expected side effects of procedures, treatments, or medication.

IV. EVALUATION PROCESS

A. Did patient or family understand the treatments the physician desires?

B. Did the patient leave with a warm feeling toward the hospital?

C. Does the patient understand when he is to return to the physician's office?

D. Did the patient follow the normal recovery sequence and timetable for the problem causing his hospitalization?

43

Douche (Internal Vaginal Irrigation)

I. ASSESSMENT OF SITUATION

A. Definition

Irrigation or flushing of the vaginal canal

B. Terminology

None

C. Rationale for Actions

1. To cleanse and disinfect the vagina and adjacent parts in preparation for surgery

2. To relieve pain, soothe inflamed, congested tissue and stimulate relaxed tissue

3. To reduce offensive odors by deodorizing the vagina

4. To contribute to the mental and physical comfort of the patient

5. To apply medication to mucous surfaces

II. NURSING PLAN

A. Objectives

1. To reduce the patient's anxiety during an embarrassing treatment

2. To provide for the patient's comfort and privacy

3. To observe the condition of the genitoperineal area

4. To report the physical and emotional effects of the treatment

5. To teach patient self-care

B. Patient Preparation

1. A distended bladder can cause discomfort during a vaginal treatment and predispose to trauma. The patient should void immediately prior to the procedure.

2. The patient should understand why the douche is being done and should participate in the procedure to the extent she is able.

C. Equipment

1. Vaginal irrigation tray, including douche bucket, tubing, douche nozzle, towels, and gloves

2. Bottle of antibacterial cleanser

3. Water-soluble lubrication

III. IMPLEMENTING NURSING INTERVENTION

A. Therapeutic Aspects

1. The temperature of the douching solution should be 105° F.

2. The patient should be in a dorsal recumbent position on a bedpan (Fig. 43-1,A). Draping is accomplished with a bath blanket in triangular fashion.

3. Proper body alignment facilitates relaxation. Remove all but one pillow from beneath the patient's head.

4. Microorganisms on the external genitalia may be decreased by giving perineal care.

5. Sterile equipment reduces the number of pathogenic organisms in the field of work. The douche tray is placed at the foot of the bed and opened onto a sterile towel. The douche can is set upright, with the tubing clamped. A sterile towel is placed over the pubic area. Antibacterial cleanser is then poured over the cotton balls. The douche

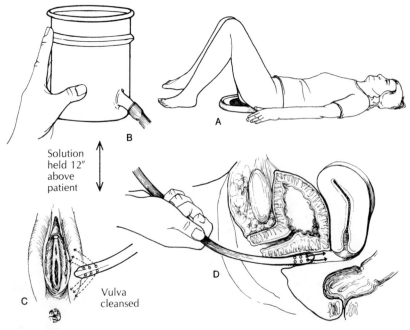

FIGURE 43.1

can is filled with 500 to 1,000 ml of solution (Fig. 43-1,B). The nurse dons sterile gloves.

6. Friction may cause trauma to delicate tissues. Lubrication of the douche tip reduces friction and may be accomplished by the application of a water-soluble jelly, such as K-Y jelly.

7. Transfer of organisms from external genitalia to vagina and cervix occurs during treatment. When normal vaginal flora are reduced by disease or trauma, the tissue is susceptible to pathogens. The labia are separated and cleansed with a new sterile cotton ball for each downward stroke. The tube should be unclamped and the air expelled from the tubing. The douche tip should be examined for nicks and cracks (Fig. 43-1,C).

8. The vaginal canal is curved, so the douche nozzle should be inserted into the vagina, downward, then upward toward the coccyx (Fig. 43-1,D).

9. Excess pressure may force infectious material into the uterus. The irrigation can should be held 12 inches above the level of the vagina. The folds of the vagina may be cleansed by gently moving the douche tip forward and backward along the vaginal tract.

10. Gravity will facilitate outflow of the solution. The head of the bed may be elevated for a few minutes, unless contraindicated.

11. Dry skin promotes comfort and reduces bacterial growth; the genitalia should be dried thoroughly.

B. Communicative Aspects

1. *Observations*

   a. Include signs, symptoms, behavior, and complications.

2. *Charting*

   a. Record appearance, behavior, and conversation.

DATE	TREATMENT	TIME	OBSERVATIONS	SIGNATURE
4/28	Douche given	0900	Patient placed in dorsal recumbent position. Draped, and external genitalia cleansed with Zephiran. Nozzle inserted into vagina gently. Water retained for 2 to 3 minutes. Solution drainage clear; expelled by patient. Perineal area dried with sterile towel.	B. Smith, L.V.N.

3. *Referrals*

   Not applicable

C. Teaching Aspects—Patient and Family

1. Patient should be cautioned against taking douches, unless they are ordered. The solution may wash away protective secretions.

2. If douching is ordered for home use, instructions should be given to patient and family on preparation of solution, height of container, position to assume during douche, and so forth. Also explain sterilization and storage of equipment.

IV. EVALUATION PROCESS

A. Was the patient's anxiety reduced?

B. Did the patient understand and cooperate in the treatment?

C. Was a therapeutic nurse-patient relationship maintained, contributing to improved opportunities for communication?

D. Was the purpose for which the douche was administered achieved?

E. Was sterility maintained?

F. Was the patient adequately screened and draped?

44
Dressings, Surgical

I. ASSESSMENT OF SITUATION

A. Definition
The process by which a soiled dressing is removed, the wound cleansed, and a sterile dressing applied

B. Terminology
None

C. Rationale for Actions
1. To absorb drainage
2. To splint or immobilize wound and surrounding tissue
3. To protect the wound from mechanical injury
4. To promote hemostasis, as by a pressure dressing
5. To prevent contamination by body excreta
6. To provide physical and mental comfort

II. NURSING PLAN

A. Objectives
1. To allay fear and anxiety regarding the wound
2. To observe and evaluate the healing process
3. To prevent or reduce infection
4. To note and record wound size, appearance and characteristics of drainage, as well as complications, such as pain, fever, and anorexia

B. Patient Preparation
1. Fear of the suture line breaking open creates tension and anxiety and may predispose to immobility on the part of the patient. The nurse should explain that sufficient tension has been applied to the wound by the sutures to prevent breaking when the patient turns, coughs, or hyperventilates

C. Equipment
1. Dressing cart or dressing tray
2. Dressings, as indicated
3. Suture set

4. Antiseptic solution

5. Waxed bag, for disposal of contaminated dressings

III. IMPLEMENTING NURSING INTERVENTION

A. Therapeutic Aspects

1. To prevent contamination, handwashing should be carried out before and after dressing change. To remove dressing, loosen tape and remove outer dressing by touching outer surface only. The inner dressing should be removed with forceps.

2. An intact covering is a defense against invasion by pathogens. The dressings should be secured with adequate tape. If the dressing adheres to the wound, it may be moistened with saline to facilitate removal.

3. Dressings should be discarded in a waxed bag. Wax prevents fluid leaking through the sides of the bag, which could contaminate other surfaces.

4. The use of a disinfectant on and around the wound decreases the number of microorganisms and thus lessens the danger of infection. If permitted, the wound should be cleaned with a cotton ball or gauze pad and antiseptic working from the wound outward for an area of 2 inches. A sterile pad is used after each stroke. Sterile forceps should be used for this cleansing process (Fig. 44-1). Remember, the forceps used for removing dressings and cleansing the wound are contaminated; be sure the forceps do not come in contact with the wound.

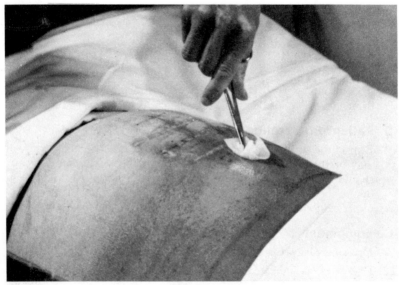

FIGURE 44.1

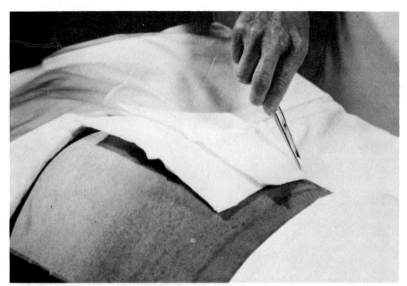

FIGURE 44.2

5. A dry, sterile dressing inhibits the spread of microorganisms by inhibiting capillary action. The wound should be covered with a dry,
sterile dressing, using sterile forceps (Fig. 44-2). A nonpenetrable
substance, such as a Telfa pad, may be used next to the skin, to prevent its sticking to the wound and the subsequent trauma when it is
removed. The next layers will serve mainly to absorb drainage, and
their thickness will depend on the amount of drainage anticipated.
Large, bulky dressings should be avoided. An alternative would be
more frequent changing of the moderately sized dressing. Added padding may be needed over drains (Fig. 44-3).

6. The dressing should be taped securely in place. Paper tape and silk
tape cause less skin reaction and are more easily removed than adhesive tape. If frequent dressing changes are necessary, Montgomery
strips may be applied (Fig. 44-4). They are placed on both sides of
the wound and have holes in the inner tips. The dressing is secured
by gauze strips tied between strips on opposite sides of the dressing.
To remove the dressing, the gauze is simply untied. These may be
made from 1- or 2-inch tape.

7. The patient should be left in a clean, comfortable environment. The
waxed bag containing the soiled dressing should be disposed of in a
covered container outside the patient's room.

B. Communicative Aspects

1. *Observations*
   a. Observe the wound to see that the edges are in close approximation.

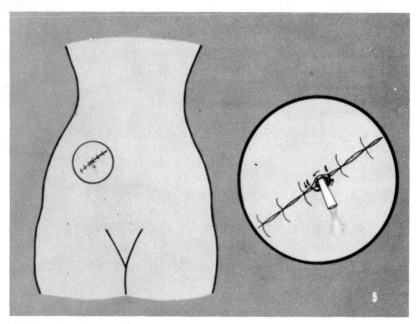

FIGURE 44.3

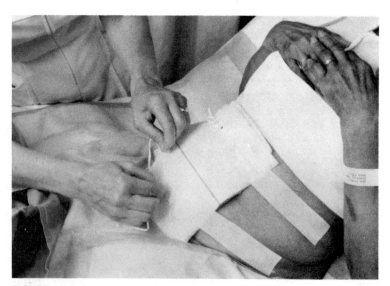

FIGURE 44.4

b. Observe the wound for signs of inflammation and infection, such as redness, swelling, pain, heat, foul odor, or loss of function of the body part.

c. Note the character (color, type, odor) and amount (estimate in ml if practical) of the drainage.

2. *Charting*

DATE	TREATMENT	TIME	OBSERVATIONS	SIGNATURE
5/19	Dressing change	0800	Abd dressing changed. Incision cleansed with Zephiran chloride. Moderate amount (approximately 30 ml) serosanguineous drainage. Wound edges in close approximation without signs of inflammation. Sterile dressing applied, secured with nonallergenic tape. Patient anxious, states, "Won't my stitches split when I cough?" Explanation given to patient and family about suture tension.	F. White, R.N.

3. *Referrals*

a. If the patient will need dressings after dismissal from the hospital, he should be told what kind of dressings to buy and where to get them.

b. If the patient has cancer, he may have his dressings furnished by the local chapter of the American Cancer Society.

C. Teaching Aspects—Patient and Family

1. Instruct patient and family to keep their fingers away from the wound and from the part of the dressing next to the wound.

2. If the patient is to go home with dressings:

a. Explain the procedure for changing dressings to both patient and family, emphasizing sterile technique.

b. Instruct patient and family to report to the physician any change in drainage or wound appearance.

c. Instruct patient and family about proper technique for discarding dressings.

IV. EVALUATION PROCESS

A. Do the patient and family understand the procedure?

B. Is the patient mentally and physically comfortable?

C. Has the healing process been noted?

D. Was aseptic technique maintained in order to prevent or reduce infection?

E. Has the appearance of the wound and drainage been noted?

45

Enema (Lower Bowel Irrigation) and Rectal Tube

I. ASSESSMENT OF SITUATION

A. Definition

The process of introducing a stream of solution into the rectum or lower colon and draining it off by natural or artificial means; the rectal tube facilitates expelling gas

B. Terminology

1. *Retention enema:* solution introduced into lower bowel but not expelled. It may serve as a local medication or soothing agent. It may also be retained so the body can absorb it to bring about sedation, hydration, or nourishment. The type of solution may cause fluid to be withdrawn from the body, as in the case of cerebral edema. Retained fluids may also help cool the body or stop local hemorrhage.

2. *Nonretention enema:* solution given with the intention of its being expelled within a few minutes, along with feces, gas, and other substances

3. *Harris flush* (up and down flush): lower bowel irrigation which promotes the expulsion of flatus from the intestines. This is especially helpful with postoperative patients, whose intestinal tracts have been at rest and now need assistance in reestablishing normal peristalsis.

4. *Feces:* body wastes, including food residue, bacteria, epithelium, and mucus, discharged from the bowels by way of the anus

5. *Flatus:* gas in the digestive tract

6. *Anus:* outlet of the rectum

7. *Rectum:* lower portion of the large intestine, about 5 inches long in the adult. It is located between the sigmoid flexure and the anus.

8. *Colon:* the large intestine, from cecum to rectum; 4 to 6 feet long in the adult and divided into ascending, transverse, and descending sections

9. *Peristalsis:* a progressive contraction movement which occurs involuntarily in hollow tubes of the body, especially the alimentary canal. Distention of the tube increases peristalsis. The contraction and relaxation of the musculature forces contents through the tube.

C. Rationale for Actions

1. To cleanse or remove accumulated solids or gases from the lower bowel

2. To stimulate peristalsis in the bowel

3. To soothe and treat irritated mucosa

4. To supply fluids and nourishment to the patient

5. To decrease body temperature through coolant contact with the proximal vascular system

6. To stop local hemorrhage

7. To decrease cerebral edema

8. To introduce medication into the system

II. NURSING PLAN

A. Objectives

1. To carry out the treatment as quickly and efficiently as possible, to prevent trauma and undue discomfort and embarrassment

2. To educate the patient and family, when appropriate, in principles of establishing and maintaining normal bowel function

3. To observe and record carefully the patient's reactions and the results of treatment

4. To ensure a safe atmosphere and optimal cooperation by proper positioning and use of side rails and organizing and checking equipment beforehand

B. Patient Preparation

1. The descending colon is on the left side; gravity aids the flow of solution into it. Position the patient on the left side, flat in bed, if not contraindicated. Explain procedure to the patient. If he is unable to retain the solution, enema may be given on bedpan. Have the patient flex his knees, the top one higher than the bottom one.

2. Poor muscle tone of the anal sphincter may cause seepage or nonretention of solution, so a bedpan should be placed next to the patient.

3. If the patient will retain and expel the enema on a bedpan, a pad placed under the hips and buttocks prior to beginning the procedure may prevent soiling the bed linens.

C. Equipment

1. Disposable enema bag
2. Bath thermometer
3. Linen: hip pad, towel, bath blanket
4. Bedpan, bedside commode, and tissue (if patient cannot go to bathroom for expulsion)
5. Solutions as ordered
   a. The adult colon can hold 750 to 1,000 ml of solution.
   b. Temperatures of enemas vary:
      (1) Cooling enema to reduce fever: 95° F
      (2) Adult enema: 105° to 110° F
   c. Types of solutions:
      (1) *Liquid soap:* 1 packet to 1,000 ml water
      (2) *Saline:* 2 drams salt to 1,000 ml water
      (3) *Sodium bicarbonate:* 2 to 4 drams to 1,000 ml water
      (4) *G.S. or 1-2-3 (from pharmacy):* magnesium sulfate 50%, 30 ml; glycerine, 60 ml; and hot water, 90 ml
      (5) *Olive oil:* 2 to 5 ounces olive oil, warmed to 100° F. Retain 3 minutes.
      (6) *Paraldehyde:* dosage ordered in 2 ounces of water
      (7) *Chloral hydrate:* dosage ordered in 2 ounces of mineral oil
      (8) *Glycerine and water:* 3 ounces glycerine in 4 ounces of water
      (9) *Commercial solutions:* give as directed on package
6. Rectal tube
7. Water-soluble lubricant

III. IMPLEMENTING NURSING INTERVENTION

A. Therapeutic Aspects

1. Each agent or type of enema produces a specific action on the patient. The nurse must be sure the correct type is being used, according to the physician's orders, and is given in the appropriate manner.
2. Agents used to stimulate peristalsis act as mucosal irritants. They must be mixed thoroughly and correctly to avoid harmful local irritation.
3. Heat is effective in stimulating nerve plexuses in intestinal mucosa. The temperature of the environment, the length of the tubing, and the rate of fluid flow will influence the temperature of the solution. Solutions entering the rectum at body temperature or very slightly above will not injure normal tissue. Proper temperature is 105° to 110° F. This temperature must be checked with a bath thermometer.

4. Friction is reduced when a surface is lubricated. Coat last 2 to 3 inches of the enema tube with a water-soluble lubricant, such as K-Y jelly.

5. Air introduced into the colon before the solution may overly distend the walls, causing additional discomfort and peristalsis. Air must be expelled from the tubing before its insertion into the rectum. If the enema is to induce elimination, a small amount of air may make it more effective.

6. The anal canal is approximately 1 to 1½ inches long in the adult. Slow insertion of a lubricated tube minimizes spasm of the intestinal wall. In the adult, gently separate buttocks with one hand, instruct patient to take a deep breath and slowly insert tube 4 to 5 inches (Fig. 45-1). If any resistance is met, do not force tubing. Allow a little solution to flow, then insert tube further. If resistance is still met, report it to the physician.

7. Gravity causes the solution to flow from the reservoir into the rectum. The higher the elevation of the fluid, the faster the rate of flow and the greater the pressure in the rectum. The maximum elevation for an adult is 18 to 24 inches. Release the clamp and elevate the enema bucket slowly to start flow. The tube should be rotated gently to avoid contact with the colon wall.

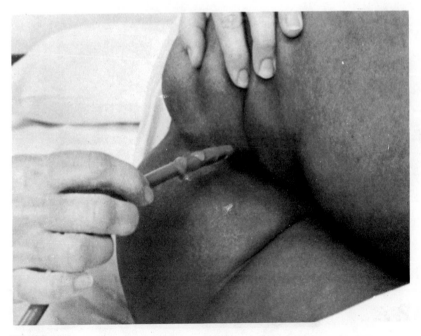

FIGURE 45.1

8. Distention and irritation of the intestinal wall produce strong peristaltic action, which is sufficient to empty the lower intestinal tract. If the patient complains of cramping or desire to expel enema prematurely, clamp the tube or lower the enema bag until the feeling subsides, then resume. In a retention enema, the nurse must be especially careful not to stimulate strong peristaltic action.

9. If tubing is not clamped after all of the solution is in, air may enter the colon, which causes additional discomfort. Tubing should be clamped before all of the solution is given.

10. In a Harris flush, lower the enema bag below bed level, before all solution has left tubing, to allow gravity to siphon solution from colon. Continue alternate raising and lowering of the enema bag until gas bubbles cease or the patient feels more comfortable and abdominal distention appears relieved (Fig. 45-2).

11. Solution that remains in the colon for the specified length of time should bring about the desired effects.

    a. *Nonretention enema:* the effect of an evacuative enema is enhanced if it can be retained 5 to 10 minutes. Encouragement from the nurse may be helpful. Have the bedpan ready or be prepared to assist the patient to the bathroom when he can no longer retain the enema.

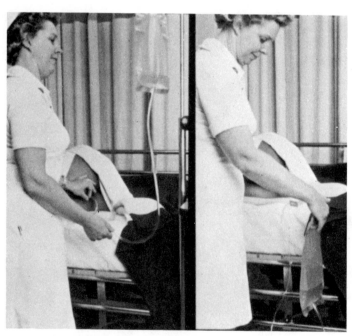

FIGURE 45.2

b. *Retention:* encourage the patient not to expel the enema for the time span ordered by the physician or until the solution is absorbed.

12. An enema may not be expelled if there is reduced neuromuscular response. The nurse must make a nursing diagnosis in this case. If after an hour there is no return, place the patient on his right side near the edge of the bed with the bedpan on a chair next to the bed. Remove the tubing from the enema bucket, place one end in the bedpan and reinsert the rectal end into the patient as before. Measure to be sure all of the solution is siphoned out. If the solution does not return, attach funnel to the end of tubing and fill tubing with warm water (105° F., adult). Reinsert tube as before. Allow a little fluid to run in, then quickly invert funnel into bedpan. Measure as noted earlier.

13. The patient's sense of well-being will be enhanced if he is left in a clean and fresh condition. If the patient is in bed, make sure he has tissue and signal light nearby. If he is able to go to the bathroom, make sure the call light is nearby and that he knows how to signal. The nurse should be sure that the patient and his linens are left clean. Allow a rest period afterward, as an enema can exhaust a patient. Reusable enema equipment should be labeled with the patient's name and stored in an appropriate place. The bedside area should be left neat and clean.

14. Rectal tube: A tube may be inserted into the rectum and left in place for the purpose of expelling gas and relieving distention. The tip is lubricated, and the same principles apply as were discussed earlier in enema administration; however, no fluid is instilled. The tube may be taped in place for approximately 20 minutes. The end of the tube may be placed under water, and the presence of bubbling will denote the fact that the gas is being expelled. A plastic bag or container should be secured over the end of the tube in case liquid feces are returned (Figs. 45-3, 45-4, 45-5).

B. Communicative Aspects

1. *Observations*

When the enema is expelled, the nurse should observe the color and consistency of the feces (hard, soft, loose). She should also observe the amount of fluid returned, general amount of flatus expelled (large, small) and the general reaction of patient (*e.g.,* tolerated well, appears exhausted). She should also note any abnormal findings, such as blood, mucus, pus, or worms. If the enema was the retention type, she should note if desired results were obtained (*e.g.,* did the patient appear sedated if sedation was given, or did local bleeding stop). The results should be described according to what was given and what the desired results were. If the patient was unable to expel a nonretention enema, whether or not the solution was siphoned off successfully should be noted.

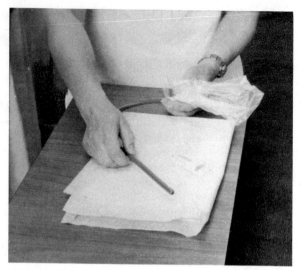

FIGURE 45.3

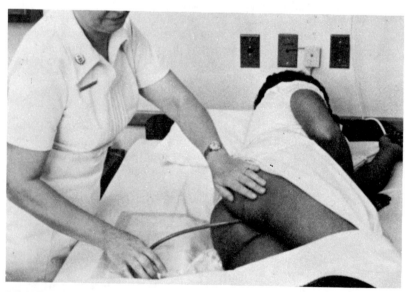

FIGURE 45.4

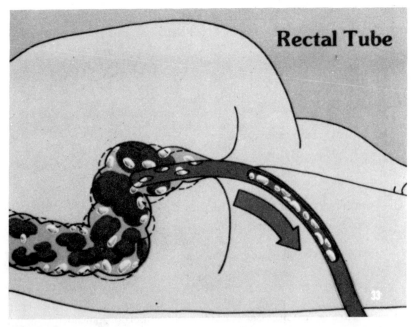

Rectal Tube

FIGURE 45.5

2. *Charting*

DATE	TREATMENT	TIME	OBSERVATIONS	SIGNATURE
5/5	Soap suds enema	0900	Patient took all of solution, without difficulty. Solution expelled in bathroom. States he feels all solution returned. Moderate amount hard, dark-brown stool noted in returned solution. Patient appears to have tolerated procedure well.	C. Allen, L.V.N.

DATE	TREATMENT	TIME	OBSERVATIONS	SIGNATURE
5/15	Harris flush	1000	Patient able to expel large amounts of flatus during procedure. Abdomen appears much less distended. Patient states he feels much better. All of solution returned.	D. Young, N.T.

DATE	TREATMENT	TIME	OBSERVATIONS	SIGNATURE
5/30	Olive oil retention enema	2100	3 oz olive oil at 100° F instilled in rectum and retained for 3 min. Moderate amt of hard, dark-brown stool returned, with no signs of bleeding. Patient's temp 99.8° F. Abdomen soft and patient says he feels better.	G. Ivers, R.N.

3. *Referrals*

Not applicable

C. Teaching Aspects—Patient and Family

1. If the patient will need enemas after discharge from the hospital, teach the patient or parents and family the correct technique. They should understand basic anatomy and know how often to give enemas and why.

2. Administration of an enema provides excellent opportunity for health teaching. Teach patient what constitutes normal elimination and why enemas are necessary. Explain the importance of adequate diet and fluids, exercise, and responding to the natural urge in the promotion of normal elimination.

3. A patient in the laxative or enema habit needs much reeducation, and success will be hard to come by. The nurse should explain the possibility of permanent damage to tissues if enemas or laxatives are used over a long period of time. The patient should understand that "normal" does not necessarily mean a daily bowel movement. Every individual has a different pattern of normality.

IV. EVALUATION PROCESS

A. Does the patient understand the importance of establishing regular bowel habits without dependence on enemas and laxatives?

B. Were modesty and privacy protected?

C. Were teaching opportunities utilized to demonstrate proper techniques?

D. Was the desired result of the treatment achieved?

E. Was the safety of the patient recognized and guarded throughout the procedure?

46
Eye, Irrigation of

I. ASSESSMENT OF SITUATION

A. Definition

The washing out of the conjunctival sac with a stream of liquid

B. Terminology

1. *Accommodation:* adjustment of the eye for seeing at different distances; the adjustment of the eye, whereby it is able to focus the image of the object on the retina. The contraction and relaxation of the ciliary muscles, reflex in nature, are necessary for accommodation.

2. *Asepsis:* a condition free from germs, free from infection, sterile

3. *Bactericidal:* being able to destroy bacteria

4. *Canthus:* the angle at either end of the slit between the eyelids; the external and internal canthus.

5. *Conjunctiva:* mucous membrane that lines the eyelids and is reflected onto the eyeball

6. *Conjunctival reflex (blinking):* an involuntary response; closure of the eyelids when conjunctiva is touched or threatened

7. *Cornea:* the clear, transparent anterior portion of the fibrous coat of the eye, constituting about one-sixth of its surface

8. *Contamination:* the introduction of disease germs or infectious material into or on normally sterile objects

9. *Dissemination:* as applied to disease organisms, scattered throughout an organ or the body

10. *Eyeball:* the body of the eye; a spherical organ situated in a bony cavity called the orbit.

11. *Eyelids:* two movable protective skin folds, which when closed, cover the anterior surface of the eyeball. The upper is the larger and more movable; it is raised by the superioris muscle. Cilia (eyelashes) are attached to both eyelids.

12. *Lacrimal duct:* the lacrimal apparatus consists of the lacrimal glands, lacrimal sac and the lacrimal duct. Tears constantly formed by the gland wash over the eyeball and keep the surface of the eye moist. Some of the tears are evaporated. Others find their way down the lacrimal sac and duct, which empties into the nasal cavity.

13. *Microorganisms:* minute living bodies not perceptible to the naked eye; usually refers to bacteria or protozoans

14. *Pathogen:* a microorganism or substance capable of producing disease

15. *pH:* the hydrogen ion (H+) concentration; a symbol used to express the degree of acidity or alkalinity. The normal pH of the blood is 7.35 to 7.45. The pH of a neutral solution is 7.0, at 25° C.

16. *Plexus:* a network of nerves or vessels

17. *Pupil:* the contractile opening at the center of the iris for the transmission of light. It contracts when exposed to strong light and when the focus is on a near object. It dilates in the dark and when the focus is on a distant object. Both pupils should be equal in appearance.

18. *Retina:* the structure which receives the image formed by the lens and is the immediate instrument of vision. It is a light-sensitive structure, on which light rays are focused. It extends from the point of-entrance of the optic nerve anteriorly to the margin of the pupil, completely lining the interior of the eye.

19. *Optic nerve:* the second cranial nerve, with a special sense of sight. It enters the eye through the dense, white fibrous outer coat of the eyeball. The nerve spreads out over the posterior two thirds of the inner surface of the globe on the thin layer of the retina. In it are situated the tiny nerve endings which, when properly stimulated, transmit visual impulses to the brain that are interpreted as sight.

C. Rationale for Actions

1. To remove a foreign body
2. To flush out an irritating chemical
3. To treat an inflammation of the conjunctiva; remove inflammatory secretions
4. To obtain antiseptic effects
5. To produce temperature effects
6. To prepare the eye for surgery

II. NURSING PLAN

A. Objectives

1. To allay fear and anxiety
2. To use measures to prevent infection and avoid further injury to the eye
3. To provide an environment restful to the eyes
4. To carry out the procedure as ordered by the physician
5. To teach the patient or his family the proper care of the patient's eyes and eye health

B. Patient Preparation

1. For maximum safety of the patient, all equipment used and the solution introduced into the conjunctival sac should be sterile. Aseptic technique must be followed. Precautions must be taken to prevent dissemination of the infection to the other eye, as well as to other persons. Thorough hand-washing is essential before and after the procedure. The nurse may desire to wear a mask and goggles. The unaffected eye should be covered during the procedure.

2. Gravity will aid the flow of solution away from the affected eye. The patient should sit comfortably or lie on his back, with his head tilted toward the side of the affected eye, so that the solution will flow from the inner canthus toward the outer canthus.

3. A sheet of plastic and a towel over the patient's shoulders will prevent wetting the clothing and bedding. If the patient is able, he may hold the basin to the side of his face to receive the return flow when he is in sitting position. In the lying position, place the curved basin at the cheek on the affected side to receive solution (Fig. 46–1).

C. Equipment

1. The prescribed solution

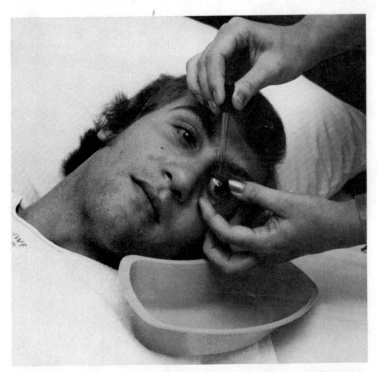

FIGURE 46.1

2. An irrigator

    a. An eye dropper is satisfactory when small amounts of solution are used.

    b. A soft rubber bulb syringe, flask, or irrigating can will do for larger amounts.

    c. Commercially prepared plastic irrigating bottles containing sterile ophthalmic solutions are available.

    d. Eyecups are not used as they can spread infection or cause injury.

III. IMPLEMENTING NURSING INTERVENTION

A. Therapeutic Aspects

1. Antiseptic solutions are chosen for their effect on the causative organism. The physician's order should be checked for specified solution, amount, and temperature. For cleansing purposes, physiologic saline is usually used.

2. Light causes pain in many eye conditions. The light should be arranged in a position to provide optimal illumination of the working area, without shining directly in the patient's eyes. An eye pad may be ordered to be worn between irrigations.

3. If the cornea or conjunctiva is touched, reflex blinking will occur. For this reason, it is difficult to hold the eyelids apart when eye treatments are carried out. The lids should be gently separated with the thumb and fingers of the left hand, to expose the conjunctival sac (Fig. 46-2). Pressure is exerted on the bony prominences of the cheek and brow, never on the eyeball.

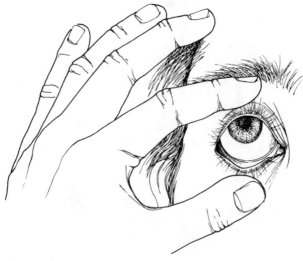

FIGURE 46.2

4. Irrigate the eye, using low pressure with sufficient force to gently remove secretions from the conjunctiva. The solution should flow steadily and should be repeated until the eye is free of secretions.

5. Any type of corneal stimulation gives rise to pain. The eyelid, lashes, and eye itself should not be touched with the irrigator.

6. Movement of the eye, when the lid is closed, helps move secretions from the upper to the lower conjunctival sac. The patient should close his eyes periodically throughout the procedure.

7. The patient may have the urge to rub or wipe his eyes with his fingers. To minimize this problem, the nurse should dry the eye and surrounding area with a sterile cotton ball on completion of the irrigation.

B. Communicative Aspects

1. *Observations*

   a. Appearance of the eye or eyes should be noted, especially redness, swelling, lacrimation, nature of discharge, and unequal, pinpoint, or dilated pupils. Appearance of returned irrigation solution is also important.

   b. Verbal complaints (headache, burning, smarting, photophobia, visual disturbances like blurring, pain) should be recorded.

   c. Overt behavior (blinking, frowning, squinting, rubbing the eyes) should be observed.

2. *Charting*

DATE	TREATMENT	TIME	OBSERVATIONS	SIGNATURE
3/21	Right eye irrigated with 30 ml sterile physiologic saline, 98° F, q.i.d.	0900	Right eye irrigated with 30 ml of sterile physiologic saline at 98° F. Returns cloudy. Large amount of yellow purulent discharge from eye before irrigation. Patient stated, "My eye smarts most of the time but feels better following irrigation." Wife present during irrigation; shown how to irrigate eye according to physician's directions.	F. White, R.N.

3. *Referrals*

   Not applicable

C. Teaching Aspects—Patient and Family

1. Explain the physician's directions to the patient or his family. Impress on them the necessity of following the directions.

2. Teach the patient or his family how to irrigate the eye and the importance of using the correct method.

3. Teach the patient eye health and how to protect the eyes from infection.

4. Instruct the patient's family and visitors how they can aid in the patient's recovery: engage in pleasant conversation near patient, identify self when entering the room if patient's eyes are bandaged.

5. Teach the patient the importance of returning for treatments if necessary and following the physician's directions exactly.

IV. EVALUATION PROCESS

A. Was the patient's anxiety alleviated?

B. Did the patient understand the purpose of the treatment and how it was going to be done before it was begun?

C. Were safety precautions used in carrying out the procedure?

D. Was the treatment given on time and in the manner ordered?

E. Was the procedure carried out with skill and gentleness?

F. Was the patient's head supported for maximum comfort throughout the procedure?

G. Is the environment subdued to provide maximum rest for the patient and minimal exertion of the eye muscles?

H. Has the purpose for which the eye irrigation was undertaken been achieved?

47

Fecal Impaction, Removal of

I. ASSESSMENT OF SITUATION

A. Definition

An abnormal accumulation of fecal material that forms a hardened mass in the lower portion of the bowel

B. Terminology

1. *Anus:* outlet of the rectum

2. *Feces:* body wastes, including food residue, bacteria, epithelium, and mucus, which are discharged from the bowel by way of the anus

3. *Peristalsis:* a progressive contractive movement that occurs involuntarily in hollow tubes of the body, especially the alimentary canal. The contraction and relaxation of the musculature forces material through the tube.

4. *Rectum:* the lower portion of the large intestine, about 5 inches long in the adult. It is located between the sigmoid flexure and the anus.

C. Rationale for Actions

1. To remove the fecal impaction
2. To assure the return of normal peristalsis
3. To restore normal fluid and electrolyte balance
4. To prevent rectal trauma and bleeding

II. NURSING PLAN

A. Objectives

1. To relieve the discomfort of impaction with minimal discomfort for the patient
2. To allow the patient adequate time to rest and recover from the procedure
3. To reassess the patient's bowel habits and dietary regimen to prevent future impaction
4. To teach the patient and family measures which will prevent recurrence

B. Patient Preparation

1. A clear explanation of what impaction is and why it must be removed should precede the initiation of treatment. The patient should be told that manual removal will cause discomfort, but once the impaction is removed, the rectal fullness and pain will subside.
2. A mild sedative may be given 30 minutes before the removal of the impaction to lessen the severity of discomfort. The bed should be well padded and the patient's personal clothing protected from soiling.

C. Equipment

1. Disposable pad or plastic sheet
2. Bedpan
3. Clean gloves
4. Lubricating jelly
5. Enema equipment (see Technique 45, Enema [lower bowel irrigation] and Rectal Tube)

III. IMPLEMENTING NURSING INTERVENTION

A. Therapeutic Aspects

1. Fecal impaction is easier to prevent than to treat. Unless the patient has been taking medication to decrease peristalsis, the presence of a fecal impaction usually indicates less than optimal nursing care. Preventive measures include adequate fluid intake, proper exercise, nutritious diet, judicious use of the proper laxatives, and cleansing enemas.

2. Elderly patients are especially prone to constipation and the formation of impactions; therefore, preventive measures should be undertaken early. Patients on prolonged bed rest may be predisposed to impaction formation. Barium sulfate used in various radiological examinations may enter the bowel and harden. Mentally confused patients may disregard the natural impulse to defecate, and hence impaction may occur. All of these patients must be carefully monitored to ensure regular bowel movements. Regularity refers to amount as well as frequency of bowel movements. Often liquid stool will be discharged around the impaction and may be misleading. These stools are usually foul-smelling and incontinent. This is an obvious indication of fecal impaction.

3. Fecal impaction is usually a dry, hard mass in the lower rectum. This hard mass results from a decrease in motility and advancement of the feces in the large bowel. During the delay caused by slow movement, more water than usual is reabsorbed into the intestine. Softening and lubrication may be accomplished by suppositories or oil retention enemas. This is usually followed by cleansing enemas until the impaction is removed.

4. If enemas fail to remove the impaction, digital removal may be necessary. The patient is usually placed in Sims's position. The bedpan should be nearby to receive the fecal material. Clean gloves should be used. The forefingers should be well lubricated to minimize friction and are then carefully inserted into the anal sphincter (Fig. 47-1). This will increase the patient's discomfort; however, concurrent explanation and encouragement may help him to endure the procedure. By digital manipulation, the mass can be broken up and removed manually, a piece at a time, to the bedpan (Figs. 47-2, 47-3). If the mass is very hard and large, it may be necessary to remove only a part of the total mass at a time.

5. After the impaction is removed, the rectal area should be cleaned and the patient should rest (Fig. 47-4).

B. Communicative Aspects

1. *Observations*

   a. The patient should be observed during digital removal of the impaction to assess his tolerance of the procedure. It may be neces-

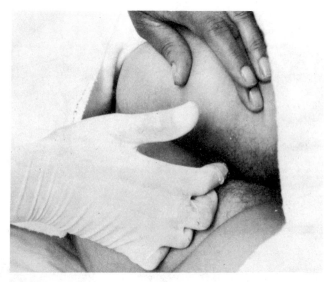

FIGURE 47.1

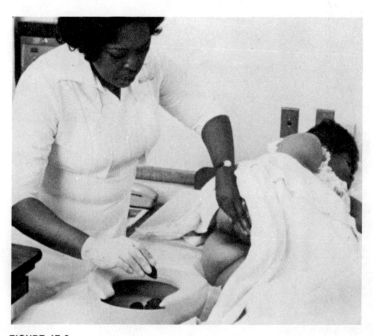

FIGURE 47.2

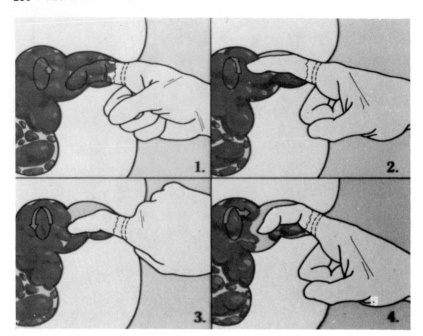

FIGURE 47.3

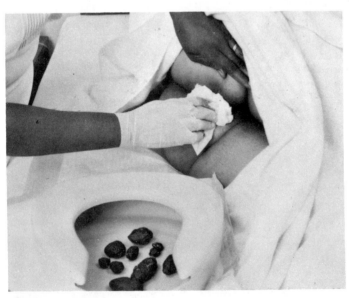

FIGURE 47.4

sary to remove part of the impaction and wait several hours before resuming, to allow the patient to rest.

b. The rectal area should be observed after removal of the impaction to make sure that the manual manipulation did not irritate the mucosa or an internal hemorrhoid, resulting in rectal bleeding.

c. The patient must be observed for regular bowel movements to ensure that the impaction will not recur.

2. *Charting*

DATE	TREATMENT	TIME	OBSERVATIONS	SIGNATURE
10/13	Oil retention enema	0700	4 oz. oil instilled. Pt. instructed to retain as long as possible. States she still feels fullness in rectal area but will hold enema solution	
	Fecal impaction removed	0800	Enema expelled with small amount liquid feces. Hard mass felt on digital rectal exam. Large fecal impaction removed manually. Pt. c/o great amount of discomfort during removal but seems relieved now and much less distended. No rectal bleeding. Is sleeping at this time.	J. Dillon, R.N.

3. *Referrals*

Not applicable

C. Teaching Aspects—Patient and Family

1. The patient should be taught to observe his own stools for amount, consistency, and frequency. A deviation resulting in less frequent stools or incontinent loose stools may indicate impaction.

2. Constipation with impaction occurs most frequently in immobilized or inactive patients who have inadequate water intake, seldom change position, and do not use their abdominal muscles. Knowledge of these causes may enable the patient to actively participate in impaction prevention by altering his behavior and modifying his diet to include suffiicient fluids, bulk, and appropriate foods such as fresh fruits and vegetables to promote motility and propulsion.

3. The patient and family should be instructed on the dangers of becoming laxative-dependent. Because of their availability and predictability, laxatives are often abused, especially by elderly people. The importance of balanced diet and adequate exercise should be stressed.

IV. EVALUATION PROCESS

A. Was the patient able to retain the oil retention enema?

B. Was the patient able to tolerate the manual removal of feces?

C. Did the patient seem receptive to preventive teaching instructions?

D. Was the entire impaction removed?

E. Is the abdomen less distended?

F. Was any rectal bleeding noted?

G. Has prevention of impaction recurrence been included in the plan of nursing care?

48

Foot Care

I. ASSESSMENT OF SITUATION

A. Definition

Preventive measures taken to avoid deformities of the feet

B. Terminology

1. *Plantar flexion (footdrop):* a deformity in which the foot bends at the ankle in the direction of the sole of the foot

2. *Claudication:* limping or lameness

3. *Metabolic process:* metabolic rate decreases as energy requirements decrease. Anabolism declines, catabolism accelerates. Thus nitrogen content increases in the body.

4. *Ischemia:* deficiency of blood in a part, due to functional constriction or actual obstruction of a blood vessel

5. *Inversion:* movement that turns the sole of the foot inward

6. *Anabolism:* any constructive process by which simple substances are converted by living cells into more complex compounds, especially in living matter

7. *Catabolism:* destructive process in which complex substances are converted by living cells into simpler compounds

C. Rationale for Actions

1. To prevent deformities of the feet

2. To prevent infection
3. To maintain comfort and cleanliness
4. To promote optimal peripheral circulation
5. To promote optimal metabolic functioning

II. NURSING PLAN

A. Objectives
1. To keep the patient as comfortable as possible
2. To prevent complications associated with prolonged bed rest
3. To remove potentially dangerous situations
4. To teach proper foot care to patient and family

B. Patient Preparation
1. Careful examination of the feet is an important part of routine care.
   a. Examine the skin closely—look for signs of nail disruption.
   b. Palpate carefully for any joint or phalangeal sensitivity.
   c. Note any stress or sensitive areas in joints and phalanges.
   d. Explain the need for daily foot care to the patient.
      (1) Bathe and massage feet daily.
      (2) Lubricate feet daily with lanolin-based cream.
      (3) Wear flat, ventilated shoes.
      (4) Wear socks free of lumps.
      (5) Avoid externally warming the feet. This may increase the metabolic demand beyond the level that the circulatory system can support, resulting in ischemic injury.
      (6) Never elevate feet above heart level.
   e. Perform knee, ankle, and foot exercises daily.
   f. Keep toenails trimmed square and smooth.
   g. In caring for bed patients, the nurse must fully understand the normal movements of the feet and ankles.

C. Equipment
1. Footboard
2. Basin and toenail clippers
3. Lanolin- or petrolatum-based cream

III. IMPLEMENTING NURSING INTERVENTION

A. Therapeutic Measures
1. The feet are particularly vulnerable to infection. Because of their distance from the main blood supply, they are often subject to problems,

especially in certain circulatory diseases (*e.g.*, peripheral vascular disease) and diabetes. However, proper foot care is important for everyone.

2. Prolonged bed rest places a severe strain on all parts of the body, especially the feet. To avoid the deformity known as plantar flexion, a footboard should be placed at the foot of the bed. The patient's feet should be flat against it, in the natural position (Fig 48-1). The footboard not only facilitates keeping the feet in the natural position, but also keeps the bed linens from pushing the tops of the feet downward. Padding may also be needed to keep pressure points from developing on the heel and the bony prominence of the ankle. Active and passive exercises involving the toes, feet, and ankles are also necessary, at least twice daily.

3. Muscular involvement is limited by the capacity of the circulatory system to provide glucose and oxygen and to eliminate lactic acid and carbon dioxide. Claudication is the result of poor circulation.

4. The feet should be kept clean. They should be immersed in water, even if a bed bath is being given (see Technique 27, Baths, Cleansing, for the method). A lubricant should be rubbed gently on the feet daily to prevent drying and cracking.

5. Toenails can be a source of foot problems. They should first be soaked in a basin of warm water to soften them. Toenails then should

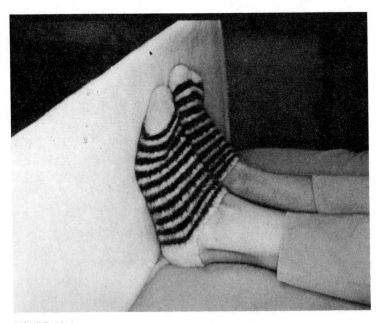

FIGURE 48.1

be trimmed carefully, straight across and not too short. This will help prevent trauma and ingrown toenails.

6. Properly fitting shoes are essential to good foot care. A powder may be used if the feet tend to perspire. Tight shoes are not only uncomfortable but predispose to ingrown toenails, corns, and poor circulation.

B. Communicative Aspects

1. *Observations*

   a. Watch for any cracking, breaks in the skin, and ingrown toenails. These should be attended to at once.

   b. Be sure that the patient's feet are flat against the footboard at all times.

   c. Avoid large concentrations of linens at the foot of the bed, since they weight heavily on the feet.

   d. Be sure the heels and ankle prominences are propped so that they do not lie directly against the mattress, predisposing to pressure sores (decubitus ulcers).

2. *Charting*

DATE	TREATMENT	TIME	OBSERVATIONS	SIGNATURE
5/1	Toenails trimmed	0930	Trimmed straight across after immersion in warm water for 5 minutes. No trauma noted. Feet propped against footboard.	L. Davis, N.T.

3. *Referrals*

   Not applicable

C. Teaching Aspects—Patient and Family

1. Teach the patient and family the importance of proper foot care. Encourage them to seek attention for foot problems.

2. Stress the importance of properly fitting shoes.

3. Show the proper method of cutting toenails and encourage the patient or family to follow this method at home.

IV. EVALUATION PROCESS

A. Did plantar flexion, pressure sores, or infection develop?

B. Were patient and family taught proper foot care prior to discharge?

49

Gastric Intubation (Decompression, Irrigation, Lavage, and Gavage)

I. ASSESSMENT OF SITUATION

A. Definition

The introduction of a tube into the stomach for therapeutic or diagnostic purposes. Tube types are:

1. *Levin:* a rubber or plastic, disposable, single-lumen tube
2. *Salem-Sump:* a plastic, disposable, double-lumen tube

B. Terminology

1. *Gastric lavage:* the administration and siphoning back of a solution through a catheter passed into the stomach
2. *Gastric gavage:* a method of artificial feeding by means of gastric intubation
3. *Gastric decompression (aspiration):* the removal of gastric contents, foods, fluids, or gas by means of a syringe or electric suction machine
4. *Intermittent:* ceasing at intervals

C. Rationale for Actions

1. To prevent or relieve abdominal distention
2. To aid in diagnostic procedures
3. To lavage the gastric system
4. To gavage the gastric system
5. To aspirate or decompress the gastric system

II. NURSING PLAN

A. Objectives

1. To allay the fears and anxieties of the patient, thereby gaining his confidence and cooperation
2. To maintain medical asepsis
3. To teach the patient and family the purpose of the treatment

4. To observe the signs and symptoms which might indicate displacement of the tube

5. To observe and accurately record the effects and results of the procedure

6. To maintain optimal patient comfort and security throughout the procedure

7. To observe for early signs and symptoms of complications and take appropriate action

B. Patient Preparation

1. Before insertion begins, the patient may be shown the tube as well as pictures and diagrams that will help him understand its functions.

2. A careful explanation to the patient will lessen anxiety and enhance cooperation.

3. The rubber tube should be placed in ice for 15 minutes before insertion. Cold causes rubber to be more rigid, making the tube easier to direct during insertion.

4. When the formula is to be administered by way of a nasogastric tube, it should be warmed to room temperature prior to administration, to decrease excessive peristalsis and prevent regurgitation.

C. Equipment

1. *Gastric intubation*

   a. Gastric tube, as ordered (adults, #12 to 16F, depending on size)

   b. Basin with ice, if rubber tube is ordered

   c. Disposable irrigation set

   d. Water-soluble lubricant

   e. Clamp

   f. Adhesive tape, ½ inch

   g. Safety pin

   h. Rubber band

   i. Glass of water with straw, if permitted

   j. Stethoscope

   k. Emesis basin

   l. Wipes

   m. Bath towel

2. Equipment as outlined above for gastric intubation applies also to decompression, irrigation, lavage, and gavage, with the following additions:

   a. *Gastric decompression*

   (1) Gomco Theromotic suction machine

(2) Air Shields suction machine

  b. *Gastric irrigation*

    (1) Solution, as ordered by physician

    (2) Disposable irrigation set

  c. *Gastric lavage*

    (1) Solution or antidote, as ordered by physician

    (2) Disposable irrigation set

  d. *Gastric gavage*

    (1) Asepto syringe

    (2) Formula, as ordered

    (3) Barium cup

    (4) Water

III. IMPLEMENTING NURSING INTERVENTION

A. Therapeutic Aspects

1. *Gastric intubation*

  a. Aseptic technique should be employed, owing to the sensitivity of the tissue involved. All measures to prevent injury and infection should be utilized.

  b. Swallowing is easier and the gag reflex is decreased as the tube passes through the nasopharynx when the patient is in a sitting position. High Fowler's position is best, unless there are medical contraindications. A towel may be placed over the patient's chest and an emesis basin kept nearby, in case passage of the tube stimulates vomiting. Passage of the tube is facilitated by lubricating the end of the tube.

  c. The tube will fall readily into the nasopharynx if the floor of the nasal passage is depressed. This can be accomplished by hyperextension of the head and neck (Fig. 49-1).

  d. The actual passage of the tube should be accomplished in firm, steady progression. To lessen stimulation of the gag reflex, pass the tube gently and firmly as the patient swallows. Depth to which the tube should be passed is measured from the bridge of the nose to the lower tip of the sternum. The patient should be told what is happening and how he can best aid tube insertion as the procedure progresses. If allowed, ice chips or a cup of water should be given to the patient. A pillow behind the shoulders will facilitate hyperextension of the head. The lubricated end of the tube is grasped in one hand, and the other hand may be used to gently elevate the tip of the nose to expose the nostril. The tube is inserted in a gentle, firm motion. Once the tube is in the nostril, the hand not holding the tube may be used to secure it, while the other hand is moved lower on the tube to get more length to in-

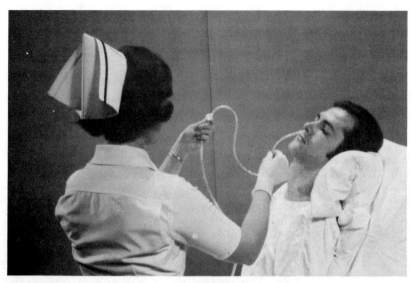

FIGURE 49.1

sert. When the tube reaches the throat, a sip of ice or water will facilitate movement into the esophagus. Once past the gag center, the tube should be passed quickly into the stomach to the predetermined depth.

e. The mucous membrane of the gastrointestinal tract is easily damaged and thus a likely site for infection. The tube should *never* be forced if an obstruction is encountered. It may be removed and reinserted in the other nostril. Persistent obstruction or complaints of severe pain necessitate cessation of intubation efforts and notification of the physician.

f. Assurance of proper positioning of the tube in the stomach is essential. The stomach is never empty; it always contains at least a small amount of gastric juice. Presence of tube in the stomach can be verified by: obtaining gastric content on aspiration; auscultation by stethoscope over the epigastric area as air is inserted through the tube; or submersion of the open end of the tubing under water—continuous bubbling indicates the tube is in the lungs.

g. The patient should be left with a feeling of comfort and security. Fasten the tube to the patient's nose with a small piece of adhesive tape. He should be told that although he needs to be careful not to jerk or pull the tube, normal activity, such as turning and talking, will not dislodge the tube. He will need frequent oral hygiene and lubrication of his lips to help eliminate the parched, dry feeling due to mouth breathing. Linen should be clean and fresh and all equipment returned to the proper places. A disposable irrigation tray should be labeled and left at the bedside for irrigation.

2. *Gastric decompression (aspiration)*

   a. Gastric suction is produced by an electric suction machine. It should be plugged in and turned on to assure proper functioning before being attached to the patient.

   b. Suction of ½ to 4 pounds per square inch may be used for gastric suction without causing injury to gastric mucosa. On a Gomco suction machine, the intermittent flow of current is indicated by the flashing on and off of a red light. The switch should be on "low" position, unless otherwise ordered.

   c. The suction bottle should be emptied every 8 hours or as often as necessary. The fluid intake must be evaluated in relation to the amount of fluid removed by gastric aspiration.

3. *Gastric irrigation*

   a. The gastric tube must remain patent (open). Any particles or secretions may be removed from the tube by disconnecting it from the suction machine, filling an irrigating syringe with the amount and type of solution ordered (usually 30 ml normal saline) and injecting the solution slowly into the tubing. The gastric tube acts like a siphon. The syringe is disconnected and the solution drains back into a basin, which is slightly below bed level.

   b. To prevent injury to the gastric mucosa, gentle pressure by way of the syringe may be applied if the solution does not return freely. When all the instilled solution has returned, the tubing is again fastened to suction. Any amount over or under the amount of fluid instilled should be recorded in the appropriate place on the intake and output record.

4. *Gastric gavage*

   a. A healthy nutritional state is maintained by the regular intake of a proper, balanced diet, which supplies all of the proper nutrients in adequate amounts. In some patients, this requires special formulas in specified amounts instilled by way of the gastric tube at intervals.

   b. The patient should be placed in as near normal position for eating as is possible for him and his condition. The head of the bed should be raised, if not contraindicated.

   c. Before instillation of any fluid into the tube, the nurse must be certain it is in the proper position. This is best checked by aspiration of gastric contents (Fig. 49-2).

   d. Excess air entering the stomach by way of the tubing adds to distention and discomfort. The formula should be poured slowly into the syringe barrel, keeping it half-full at all times. Distention, nausea, and excessive peristalsis may be prevented by the

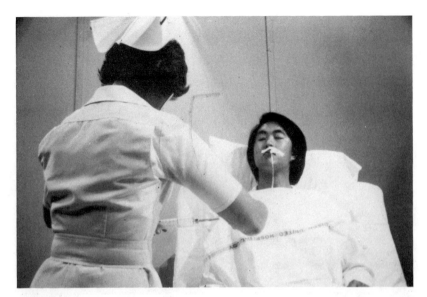

FIGURE 49.2

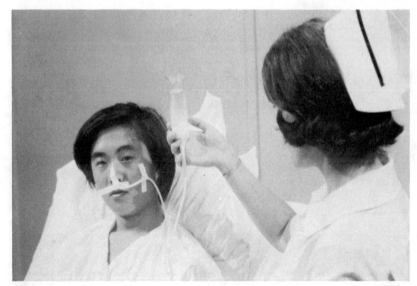

FIGURE 49.3

slow instillation of formula into the stomach. The speed of flow is determined by the height of the syringe. The formula should be allowed to flow by gravity; it should not be forced (Figs. 49-3, 49-4, 49-5).

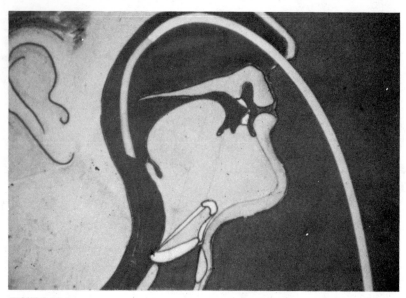

FIGURE 49.4

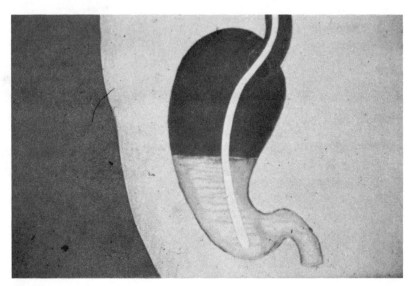

FIGURE 49.5

    e. To maintain patency, the tube should be flushed with 30 ml of water after the feeding, unless contraindicated. The syringe is then removed and the tube clamped to prevent air entering the stomach.

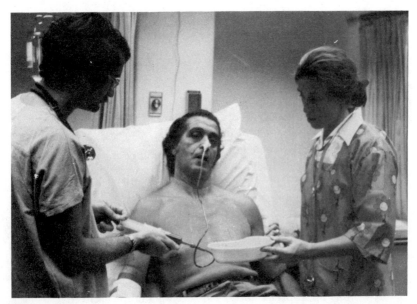

FIGURE 49.6

f. Good nutrition and comfort can be promoted by relaxation before, during, and after meals. Leave the patient in a comfortable position and a neat environment. Clean and replace equipment for the next feeding.

5. *Gastric lavage*

   a. A large amount of solution, approximately 500 ml in an adult, is necessary to flatten out the rugae of the stomach in order for the fluid to reach all parts of the mucous membrane. The solution or antidote should be injected by way of the tube in quantities sufficient to cleanse or neutralize the stomach contents. It should then be aspirated or allowed to flow back naturally (Fig. 49-6). A tube with a large lumen is necessary, owing to the size of particles and the thickness of gastric secretions. The nurse should continue washing the stomach until the return is consistently clear.

   b. Unpleasant aftertaste may be eliminated with fluid intake or a sweet-tasting substance, if this is allowed. The nurse should administer some type of oral hygiene after this procedure.

6. *Removal of the nasogastric tube*

   a. Clamping the tube cuts off air pressure and prevents any fluid from remaining in the tubing and entering the trachea. With the tube pinched, it should be withdrawn quickly and gently in one continuous motion.

b. The patient should be left in a clean and comfortable environment. He should be given a cloth to wash his face, and tape marks should be removed.

B. Communicative Aspects

1. *Observations*

   a. Gastric intubation

      (1) Examine drainage from tube.

      (2) Observe the patient for cyanosis, dyspnea, or coughing, as these may indicate that the tube has entered the trachea or lung and should be removed immediately.

   b. Gastric decompression

      (1) Observe the patient for nausea, vomiting, and distention, which indicate suction is not functioning properly or efficiently.

      (2) Observe the patient for signs and symptoms of fluid and electrolyte imbalance. These should be evaluated, investigated, reported, or treated with appropriate nursing measures.

      (3) The appropriate suction must be maintained effectively.

         (a) Ascertain if equipment is in good working condition.

         (b) Check patency of the tube.

         (c) Irrigate tube properly, as ordered.

      (4) Drainage must be observed carefully and any abnormalities reported promptly.

      (5) Accurate measurement and recording of drainage is mandatory.

   c. Gastric gavage

      (1) Observe for signs and symptoms of distention or regurgitation.

      (2) Observe patient's reaction to the treatment.

   d. Gastric lavage

      (1) Examine drainage from tube as to color, type, and appearance.

      (2) Observe effect of the treatment on the patient.

2. *Charting*

   a. Gastric intubation

DATE	TREATMENT	TIME	OBSERVATIONS	SIGNATURE
5/3	#16 Levin tube inserted	0900	120 ml clear, yellow fluid obtained. Very cooperative. No difficulty in passing. Complaining of lump in throat. Rinsed mouth with water.	F. White, R.N.

b. Gastric lavage

DATE	TREATMENT	TIME	OBSERVATIONS	SIGNATURE
5/9	#16 Levin tube inserted	1630	Tube inserted without difficulty. Stomach lavaged with 1,000 ml normal saline. 1,500 ml greenish-brown fluid returned. Tube removed. Appears calm and relaxed. Given mouthwash.	F. White, R.N.

3. *Referrals*

a. If gavage feeding is to be done on a long-term basis, and will be done by the family after the patient goes home, follow-up visits by a visiting nurses' association may help to allay the family's apprehension, to evaluate the patient's nutritional status, and to assure patency and proper insertion of the tube.

b. If the lavage procedure was for the purpose of removal of a harmful substance, the family should be advised of the nearest poison control center, if appropriate, for future reference. The family's knowledge of how to utilize poison control services may save a life.

C. Teaching Aspects—Patient and Family

1. Gastric intubation and decompression

a. Explain the procedure to the patient and family.

b. Encourage the patient to change position frequently to prevent rubbing constantly over the orifices of the eustachian tubes, causing irritation.

2. Gastric gavage

a. Explain the procedure to the patient or family.

b. If the patient is going home on tube feeding, teach the current method of feeding to the family.

3. Gastric lavage

a. If lavage is to remove poison from stomach, explain to patient and family if time allows. Tell them about the poison control center, if appropriate, after the procedure.

b. If lavage is for diagnostic study, explain purpose and expected results to the patient and family.

c. If lavage is a preparation for surgery, be sure the patient understands why it is necessary. Also utilize this time for preoperative teaching about coughing, turning, deep breathing, and so on.

IV. EVALUATION PROCESS

A. Did the patient cooperate?

B. Was the patient reassured while the tube was being passed?

C. Did the nurse impart confidence?

D. Was the procedure explained to the patient and family?

E. Was the patient made comfortable at the completion of treatment?

F. Is the charting pertinent and accurate?

G. If solution was used, was the amount sufficient?

H. Was entrance of air prevented while pouring the solution?

I. If suction was used, was it checked frequently for working efficiency?

J. Was good oral care given while the tube was in place?

K. Was lubricant used each time the tube was inserted?

L. Was the tube clamped before removal?

M. Was medical asepsis maintained?

N. Was the tube tested for placement?

O. Was the desired effect obtained?

50

Gown and Glove Procedure, Sterile

I. ASSESSMENT OF SITUATION

A. Definition

To maintain a sterile environment by donning gown and gloves in such a manner as to cover nonsterile areas without contaminating the outside of gown or gloves

B. Terminology

None

C. Rationale for Actions

1. To maintain sterile environment

2. To protect the patient from contamination

3. To minimize risk of infection

II. NURSING PLAN

A. Objectives

1. To don gown or gloves in such a manner as to ensure sterility

2. To maintain sterility throughout the procedure

B. Patient Preparation

Not applicable

C. Equipment

1. Sterile gown, if needed

2. Sterile gloves

3. Powder, if desired

4. Equipment pertinent to procedure

III. IMPLEMENTING NURSING INTERVENTION

A. Therapeutic Aspects

1. Any sterile procedure depends on the absence or reduction of micro-organisms. To accomplish this, thorough handwashing must be done prior to donning the gown or gloves. Preoperatively, a surgical scrub is done according to the policy of the individual hospital.

2. In the sterile gown procedure, the hands are dried with a sterile towel, which is held away from the body and discarded after use (Fig. 50-1). Gowns are packed with the inside out, so the nurse grasps the inside of the gown at the neck and lets it tumble open while held away from the body (Fig. 50-2). She then slips her hands into the armholes, while touching only the inside of the gown (Fig. 50-3). Someone else will reach inside the sleeves and pull them on, until the sleeves extend just beyond the fingertips. This second person ties the gown at the neck and waist, being careful not to touch the sterile front of the gown. The nurse is then ready to don the gloves. The nurse may go ahead and pull the sleeves on over the hands if someone else in sterile uniform is available to hold her gloves stretched open so she may gently plunge her hands inside them without touching the outside of the gloves.

3. In the closed glove procedure, gloves are opened with sterile forceps and are left lying on the sterile towel. With her gown on, hands extended through the sleeves only as far as the cuff seam (Fig. 50-4), the nurse grasps one glove through the gown sleeve and places it thumbside down on the palm side of the other arm, with the opening toward her hand (Fig. 50-5). The edge of the glove cuff next to her wrist is grasped with the fingers of the hand to be gloved, and the up-

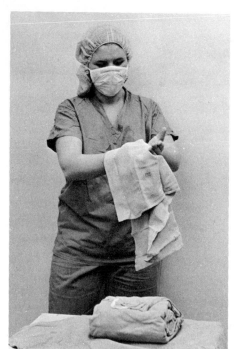

FIGURE 50.1

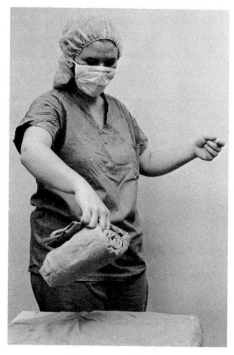

FIGURE 50.2

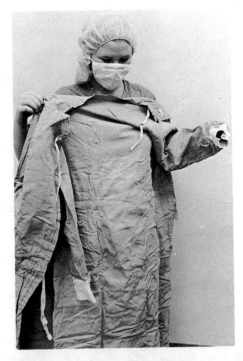

FIGURE 50.3

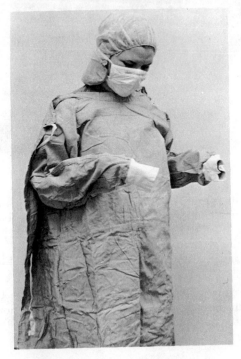

FIGURE 50.4

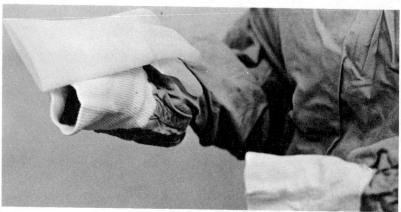

FIGURE 50.5

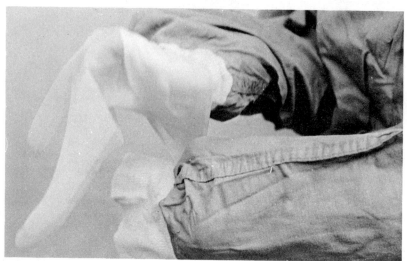

FIGURE 50.6

per edge of the glove cuff is grasped with the stillcovered free hand and pulled over the fingers and hand being gloved (Fig. 50-6). The sleeve is then pulled to draw the cuff into position over the wrist, automatically drawing the glove onto the hand. The second glove is applied in the same manner, using the gloved hand to assist (Fig. 50-7).

4. In the open-glove procedure, the gloves are opened and must be cuffed. With one hand the nurse grasps the cuff of the opposite glove and slips the fingers of the opposite hand inside. She pulls the glove

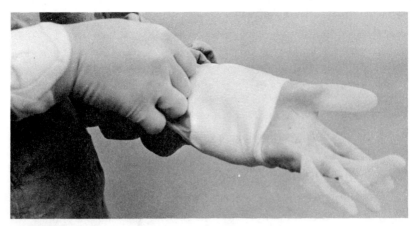

FIGURE 50.7

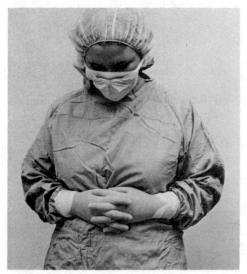

FIGURE 50.8

on by holding the cuff, being careful not to contaminate the outside of the glove and leaving the cuff turned. Then she slips the gloved fingers *under* the cuff of the other glove and inserts her ungloved fingers inside and pulls it on, leaving the cuff turned. The area inside the folded cuffs is considered sterile.

5. On completion of the procedure, the nurse must take care to keep her gloved hands in the sterile field (Fig. 50-8).

B. Communicative Aspects

1. *Observations*

   a. Observe for breaks in sterile technique during gown and glove application.

   b. Observe for tears in gloves and any wetness on gown, which are considered breaks in the sterile field.

2. *Charting*

   a. Chart for the procedure to be carried out.

3. *Referrals*

   Not applicable

C. Teaching Aspects—Patient and Family

1. Adequate explanation of why this is being done may eliminate the patient's anxiety.

2. If sterile procedures are to be done at home (e.g., catheterization, sterile dressing changes), the family must be instructed in the importance and techniques of maintaining sterility.

IV. EVALUATION PROCESS

A. Was the sterile technique strictly adhered to?

B. Was the patient cooperative?

C. Did any infections develop which might indicate poor technique?

51

Hair, Daily Care and Shampoo

I. ASSESSMENT OF SITUATION

A. Definition

Daily care or cleansing of the patient's hair and scalp

B. Terminology

None

C. Rationale for Actions

1. To promote mental and physical comfort

2. To maintain cleanliness of hair

3. To prevent tangling and matting of hair due to prolonged bedrest

II. NURSING PLAN

A. Objectives

1. To maintain a healthy atmosphere through cleanliness

2. To promote a feeling of well-being through the cosmetic effects of hair care

B. Patient Preparation

1. Many people cannot imagine how a shampoo can be done while a person is flat in bed. Adequate explanation prior to initiating this procedure will help the patient to understand and be more cooperative.

2. To avoid causing the patient to chill, the windows should be closed and the chance of drafts minimized. A bath blanket should replace the top covers, and a towel is placed across the chest and tucked around the neck and shoulders.

C. Equipment

1. Daily care
   a. Comb and brush
   b. Towel

2. Shampoo
   a. Shampoo basin
   b. Dryer, if available
   c. Three bath towels and a pad
   d. Two washcloths
   e. Plastic sheet or apron
   f. Shampoo
   g. Washbasin
   h. Cup

III. IMPLEMENTING NURSING INTERVENTION

A. Therapeutic Aspects

1. *Daily care*
   a. Cleanliness enhances attractiveness and self-esteem. Daily brushing of the hair aids in cleanliness, distribution of oil, and stimulation of circulation in the scalp.
   b. In giving hair care, consideration must be given to the patient's physical capabilities. If possible, the pillow is removed and a towel placed under the hair. The hair should be brushed as vigorously

as the patient's condition and desire warrant. It should then be attractively arranged as the patient wishes and the towel discarded. The brush and comb should be cleaned after each use.

2. *Shampoo*

a. The patient should be placed in a comfortable position to cause the least possible physical exertion. A pillow is placed under the patient's shoulders to elevate his head. Two towels with plastic in between go under his head. A pad is placed on the edge of the shampoo basin to reduce discomfort as it is placed under the patient's neck. A shampoo basin has an open spout on one side, which is placed over the edge of the bed (Fig. 51-1). The end is placed over a washbasin, which rests on a chair or table and catches the overflow from the shampoo basin. A long plastic bag, with both ends open, can substitute for the spout on the shampoo basin. The hair is brushed to remove tangles and then thoroughly wet with warm water. Shampoo is then applied and the hair lathered well. After a short rinse, the hair should be shampooed again. It is then rinsed thoroughly until all the shampoo is removed. The nurse must keep an eye on the rinse basin and empty it as necessary to avoid overflow.

b. Unbroken, healthy skin serves as the first line of defense against harmful agents. Avoid scratching the patient's scalp with sharp fingernails or rings.

c. The shampoo is applied and rinsed thoroughly twice. Water temperature should not exceed 105° F. so as not to injure the scalp. Matted or tangled hair may not be cut without written consent,

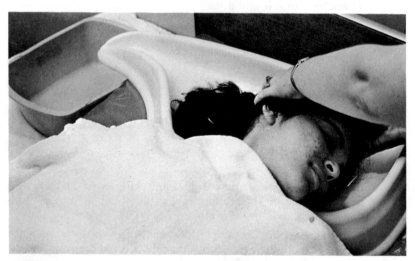

FIGURE 51.1

except in emergencies. Oils may be used to help comb out tangled hair before shampooing.

    d. Good grooming gives a person a sense of well-being. The hair should be dried, combed, and attractively arranged.

B. Communicative Aspects

1. *Observations*

    a. Observe the patient's reaction to and tolerance of the procedure.

    b. Abraded or broken areas on the scalp should be detected and reported.

2. *Charting*

DATE	TREATMENT	TIME	OBSERVATIONS	SIGNATURE
5/1	Shampoo	0945	Small scalp abrasion on left temporal area noted during hair care. Area appears reddened. Dr. D. notified. Tolerated procedure well.	G. Ivers, R.N.

3. *Referrals*

Not applicable

C. Teaching Aspects—Patient and Family

1. Teach importance of establishing and maintaining good daily hygiene habits.

2. Emphasize the importance of avoiding chills while shampooing the hair.

IV. EVALUATION PROCESS

A. Was the patient's comfort maintained throughout the procedure?

B. Does the patient seem more at ease and in better spirits?

C. Was the integrity of the skin maintained?

D. Was chilling avoided?

52

Handwashing

I. ASSESSMENT OF SITUATION

A. Definition

A measure carried out to remove pathogenic organisms from the skin

B. Terminology

1. *Asepsis:* absence of pathogenic bacteria
   a. Surgical asepsis: an attempt is made to render absolutely free from all microorganisms (sterile) every object that comes in direct or indirect contact with a wound.
   b. Medical asepsis: an attempt is made to prevent the transfer of pathogenic organisms from one person to another, but not all equipment is sterile.
2. *Clean:* free from all discernible soil or dirt; sanitary
3. *Contamination:* in medical asepsis, contact with an object that has living pathogenic organisms on it from someone other than the person handling the object. The physician, for example, contaminates his stethoscope when he places it on the chest of a child with scarlet fever.
4. *Detergent:* cleansing agent
5. *Infection:* growth of pathogenic microorganisms in any area of the body, giving rise to signs and symptoms of disease
6. *Microorganisms:* minute, living bodies, not perceptible to the naked eye; most are harmless, but a few are pathogenic.
7. *Pathogenic microorganisms:* microbes capable of producing disease
8. *Sterile:* free from microorganisms; aseptic

C. Rationale for Actions

1. To provide a defense against the direct or indirect spread of microorganisms from one person to another
2. To provide an aseptic hospital environment

II. NURSING PLAN

A. Objectives

1. To decontaminate or prevent contamination of the hands

2. To remove the maximum number possible of pathogenic organisms present on the skin

3. To prevent or reduce incidence of cross-infections

4. To teach personnel, patient, and family good personal hygiene

5. To minimize skin infections of the hands

B. Patient Preparation

1. The patient should understand when and how to properly accomplish thorough handwashing.

2. Frequent and effective handwashing should be encouraged and provided as part of the patient's hygiene at the following times:

   a. Prior to eating

   b. Following any activity in which the hands must come in contact with external genitalia, anal region, body discharges, and known dirty areas (*e.g.,* floor).

C. Equipment

1. Soap

2. Water

3. Paper towels

4. Lotion

5. Orange stick or nail file

III. IMPLEMENTING NURSING INTERVENTION

A. Therapeutic Aspects

1. Thorough handwashing should be encouraged by nursing personnel:

   a. Before and after giving personal care to a patient

   b. After contact with infective materials

2. Rinse so that water falls back into the sink, preventing further contamination of both the sink rim and floor (Fig. 52-1). For good body mechanics, the person should stand in front of the sink, with knees slightly bent. The soap and water controls should be within easy reach. Clothing should not touch the sink rim.

3. The water should be cool or lukewarm. Hot water removes more oil from the skin and thus is more drying.

4. Since normal skin acidity is a factor in controlling bacterial growth and preventing irritation, detergents that do not change the pH of the skin are desirable. The hands are wet with water. The application of soap to a wet skin surface, followed by friction, produces an optimal amount of suds (Fig. 52-2). These suds break up the accumulated surface mixture, which harbors bacteria.

5. Friction by rotary motion and rinsing under running water aid in the mechanical removal of bacteria. When the fingers and thumbs of

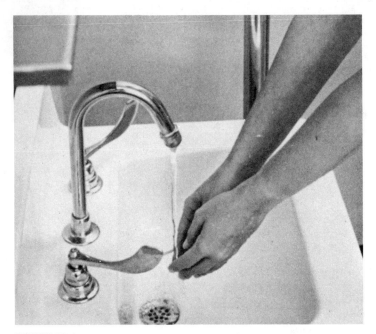

FIGURE 52.1

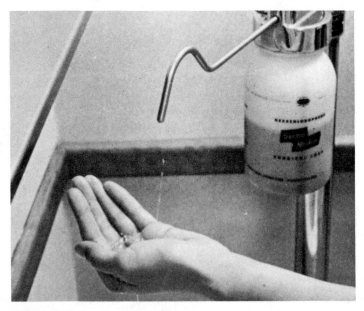

FIGURE 52.2

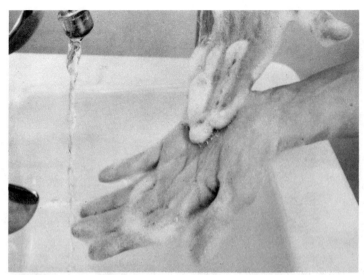

FIGURE 52.3

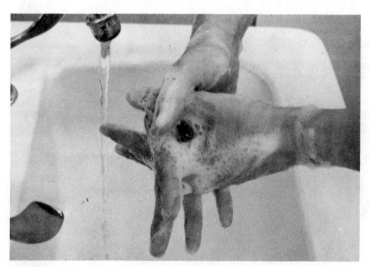

FIGURE 52.4

both hands are interlaced and moved back and forth, the interdigital areas are cleaned. Microorganism count is lower on smooth surfaces and higher in folds and under fingernails. The hands should be washed well for 20 to 25 seconds, using a rotary motion and friction. Ten friction motions to the palmar and dorsal aspects of the hands and fingers, to the fingers interlaced to cleanse the interdigital spaces, and on the palmar and dorsal aspects of the hands and fingers can be done in 25 seconds (Figs. 52-3, 52-4, 52-5).

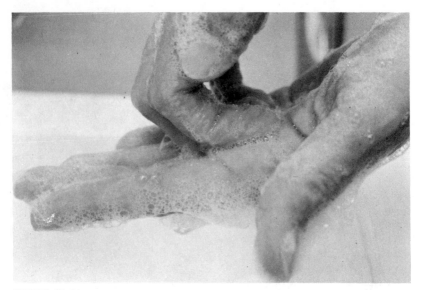

FIGURE 52.5

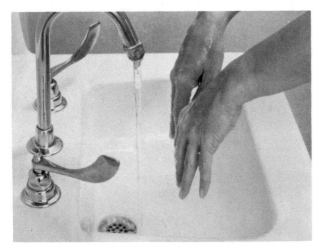

FIGURE 52.6

6. Hands and wrists should be rinsed under running water, allowing water to flow from the elbows to the finger tips (Fig. 52-6). Surface bacteria should run into the sink rather than up the forearm. Water aids in the removal of organisms.

7. Clean, well-trimmed fingernails are essential to minimizing the opportunity for bacteria to accumulate and grow under the nails. Clean fingernails with nail file or orange stick, as indicated (Fig. 52-7).

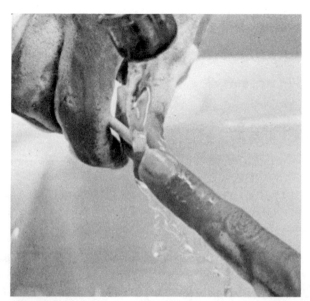

FIGURE 52.7

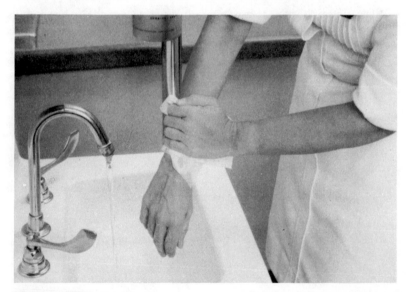

FIGURE 52.8

8. All microorganisms need moisture for growth. Hands should be dried from fingers to forearms (clean to dirty), with a clean paper towel (Fig. 52-8). The faucet handles are considered contaminated and should be turned off with a dry paper towel.

9. Frequent handwashing destroys the natural oils and causes drying and cracking of the skin. If the skin surface is kept intact, bacterial invasion and possible secondary infection are prevented. Hand lotion should be applied.

B. Communicative Aspects

Not applicable

C. Teaching Aspects—Patient, Family, and Hospital Personnel

1. Handwashing is a must for all hospital personnel on arrival to the unit and prior to leaving.
2. Handwashing is most essential before and after caring for any patient and at indicated intervals during care.
3. No jewelry other than the wedding band should be worn because bacteria can become lodged in the crevices. Watches should have a stretch band, which will allow it to be pushed up on the arm during handwashing and other procedures.
4. Manicuring and cleaning the fingernails should be done prior to working hours as a part of daily hygiene.
5. Manicuring also prevents hangnails and skin abrasions.
6. Keep skin irritations to a minimum. When frequent handwashing is necessary, a change of assignment may be indicated if irritation is severe.
7. Skin irritation predisposes to secondary infections. Rubber gloves help to protect open skin areas from becoming infected.
8. Instruct patients and their families on the principles of good hand-washing techniques.

IV. EVALUATION PROCESS

A. Has a proper handwashing routine been established and is it being followed?
B. Has teaching of patients, family, and personnel been thorough and effective?
C. Are the hands clean?
D. Has the hospital-acquired infection rate been reduced?

53

Hot and Cold Applications

I. ASSESSMENT OF SITUATION

A. Definition

Physical agents applied to an area of the patient's body which bring about a change in tissue temperature, locally or systemically, for a therapeutic purpose. Reactions to heat and cold are modified by mode and duration of application, degree of heat and cold applied, condition of the tissue, and surface of the body covered by the application. Types of applications are:

1. *Dry applications*

   a. *Aquamatic (K-Matic) pad:* a rubber pad with tubular construction that can be filled with distilled water. An electric control unit heats the water and keeps it at an even temperature. The temperature is set by using a plastic key. This pad permits the maintenance of a constant temperature at the level prescribed by the physician; therefore, it is both safer and more effective than a hot water bottle or electric heating pad.

   b. *Freezabag:* a rubberized or plasticized flat bag containing a chemical substance that is frozen and used as a cold dry application to a body surface. It must be covered with a protective covering before application.

   c. *Heat cradle:* a metal cradle in which several electrical sockets are installed for luminous bulbs; a means of providing radiant heat.

   d. *Heat lamp:* a goose-neck lamp containing a 60-watt light bulb, applied 18 to 24 inches from body site (Fig. 53-1). The heat lamp provides dry heat radiation.

   e. *Heating pad:* the heating element of an electric pad consists of a web of wires that convert electrical current into heat (Fig. 53-2).

   f. *Hot water bag:* a rubber or plastic device filled with water (temperature ordered by the physician) and applied to a body site for heat conduction (Fig. 53-3). (See Terminology for ranges of temperature.)

   g. *Ice bag or collar:* a rubber or plastic device filled with ice chips and covered with a protective fabric before application to the patient's body site. Vasoconstriction of peripheral vessels is caused by cold application. (See ranges of temperature in Terminology for further information.)

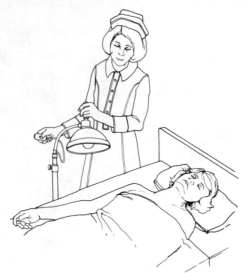

FIGURE 53.1

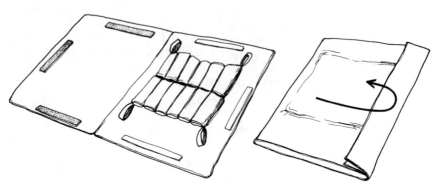

FIGURE 53.2

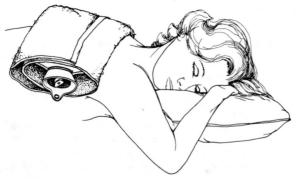

FIGURE 53.3

h. *Ice glove:* a rubber glove filled with ice chips, covered with light covering and applied to a body surface. It is usually used in a postoperative oral surgery patient.

2. *Moist applications*

a. *Alcohol or cold sponge baths:* a means by which reduction of body temperature occurs from evaporation. Cool water or a combination of cool water and alcohol is applied to the skin.

b. *Compresses:* may be either moist (gauze) dressings or washcloths. A compress is usually applied to smaller body areas and has to be changed frequently. Compresses may be either hot or cold, sterile or unsterile, as designated by the physician.

(1) *Hot compresses* utilize the principle of heat conduction and can be sterile or unsterile moist applications. Generally, gauze is soaked in the solution designated by the physician. The excess fluid is wrung out of the gauze to be applied. Sterile precautions are indicated when the compress is to be applied to an open wound or to an organ, such as the eye, to prevent entrance of microorganisms. An insulating, waterproof cloth is placed over the compress, to aid heat retention. Hot compresses hasten the suppurative process and improve circulation.

(2) *Cold or ice compresses* are usually made of gauze or washcloths. The application of cold to open wounds or to lesions that may rupture requires sterile technique. Cold diminishes the formation and absorption of bacterial poisons. It also causes vasoconstriction, decreased tissue metabolism, and sensory anesthesia. It is thus used in contusions, sprains, strains, and for controlling hemorrhages. Cold compresses might also be used for an injured eye, headache, tooth extraction, or hemorrhoids. The material used for application is immersed in a basin (clean or sterile, as ordered) that contains pieces of ice and a small amount of water or ordered solution. If the sterile technique is used, the sterile solution bottle is set in the bowl of ice. Compresses should be changed frequently.

c. Packs are usually applied to an extensive area of body surface. They may be either cold or hot, sterile or unsterile, as designated by the physician. Examples are as follows:

(1) *Hot pack* (foment) is a piece of heated, moist flannel or towel that is applied to a patient's skin in order to provide superficial heat. The effect of moderate heat is vasodilation, lessened viscosity of the blood, increased tissue metabolism, and relief of pain, congestion, inflammation, swelling, and muscle spasms. Application to open wounds or lesions that may rupture advocates the sterile technique. A heating device may be used to keep the pack warm. If the sterile procedure is ordered, the solution, towels, and dry covering must be sterile, as

well as the rubber gloves or forceps used for wringing them dry. Use a sterile bath thermometer for testing; if not available, pour sterile solution into clean container, and test the temperature with a regular bath thermometer. Discard the solution after testing; do not use it on the patient.

(2) *A cool wet pack* is composed of bath towels, moistened in water cooled with a small amount of ice chips. After wringing, the towels are applied full length to cover the anterior and posterior trunk of the body and each extremity. The temperature of the water is maintained at 75° F. Ice bags may be placed at the axillae, groin, and head (Fig. 53-4). The cool wet pack is used to reduce body temperature by evaporation. If the sterile procedure is ordered or necessitated because of an open wound, the solution, towels, and dry covering must be sterile; also, sterile rubber gloves or sterile forceps are used for wringing the pack. Use a sterile bath thermometer for testing; if not available, pour sterile solution into a clean container, and test the temperature with a regular bath thermometer. Discard the solution after testing; do not use it on the patient.

(3) *Ice packs* are used occasionally to lower body temperature or the temperature of a patient's limb prior to surgery. It is a method of hypothermia and should be used with caution. Large plastic bags of ice are placed around the patient, with one between the legs. Rectal temperature readings are taken every 5 minutes. An ice cap may be applied to the head. Lower body temperatures are used for checking inflammation and suppuration by decreasing blood supply, slowing cellular metabolism, and inhibiting microbial activity. Extreme cold can destroy tissue if the application is continued for a long time.

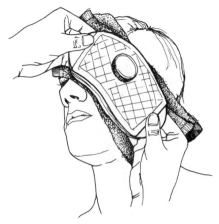

FIGURE 53.4

d. *A soak* usually refers to the immersion of a part of the body, such as a foot or a hand, or it may refer to wrapping the part with gauze and saturating it with fluid. If the sterile technique is used, all articles and solutions must be sterile.

B. Terminology

1. *Anesthesia:* no feeling or sensation
2. *Conduction:* the passage of heat from molecule to molecule, as through a metal
3. *Congestion:* an abnormal accumulation of fluid in a part
4. *Erythema:* redness of the skin, due to congestion of capillaries
5. *Evaporation:* a means by which water leaves the body surface, reducing body heat
6. *Exudate:* a substance produced on or in a tissue by a disease or vital process
7. *Hypothermia:* artificially lowering the body temperature
8. *Inflammation:* a condition of the tissues in reaction to injury
9. *Insulator:* a material or substance that prevents or inhibits conduction, as of heat
10. *Medical asepsis:* microorganisms are kept within a well-defined area, and any articles or materials removed from this area are immediately rendered free of bacteria, so they cannot transfer the infection.
11. *Metabolism:* activity which takes place within the cells. It has two phases: *catabolism,* in which the glucose derived from carbohydrates and ketones and glycerol derived from fat are broken down into carbon dioxide, water, and energy; and *anabolism,* in which the energy from catabolism is used in the synthesis of enzymes and proteins needed by the body cells.
12. *Microorganism:* minute living bodies, not perceptible to the naked eye
13. *Pathogen:* an organism or material capable of producing disease
14. *Radiation:* the transfer of heat from warm objects to cool objects in the form of electromagnetic waves
15. *Ranges of temperature:* cool, 65° to 80° F.; cold, 59° to 65° F.; very cold, below 55° F.; hot, 105° to 115° F.; warm, 100 ° to 105° F.; tepid, 80° to 98° F.
16. *Sterile technique:* absence of any microorganism. Sterile technique demands the utilization of sterile equipment and supplies.
17. *Surgical asepsis:* refers to practices carried out in order to keep an area free of unnecessary organisms
18. *Suppuration:* the formation of pus

C. Rationale for Actions

1. Heat applications are ordered by the physician to:
   a. Effect vasodilation
   b. Soften exudate
   c. Increase suppuration
   d. Relax tissue
   e. Reduce pain
   f. Increase temperature
   g. Increase metabolism
   h. Increase circulation away from a congested area

2. Cool or cold applications are ordered by the physician to withdraw heat from tissue in order to:
   a. Effect vasoconstriction
   b. Reduce inflammation
   c. Reduce temperature
   d. Produce local anesthesia
   e. Decrease metabolism

II. NURSING PLAN

A. Objectives

1. To understand and relate the principles of hot or cold applications to the individual's prescribed treatment
2. To carry out the application with expediency and detailed care
3. To reassure and inform the patient regarding application
4. To follow safety measures prior to, during, and following application

B. Patient Preparation

1. The patient should be prepared in advance for the difference in temperature. The nurse should bring all equipment to the bedside and offer explanations as she applies the prescribed application. The patient should know the purpose and expected outcome of the procedure.

C. Equipment

1. *Aquamatic pad*
   a. Aquamatic pad
   b. Distilled water
   c. Aquamatic key
   d. Fabric covering
   e. Patient thermometer (to take temperature, pulse, and respiration before, during, and after treatment)

2. *Freezabag*
   a. Freezabag
   b. Fabric for covering Freezabag
   c. Patient thermometer

3. *Heat cradle*
   a. Heat cradle, with bulbs
   b. Screen, for privacy
   c. Patient thermometer

4. *Heat lamp*
   a. Gooseneck lamp
   b. 60-watt bulb
   c. Screen, for privacy
   d. Patient thermometer

5. *Heating pad*
   a. Electric heating pad
   b. Protective covering for heating pad
   c. Patient thermometer

6. *Hot water bag*
   a. Hot water bag
   b. Protective covering for hot water bag
   c. Graduated flask, for water
   d. Bath thermometer
   e. Patient thermometer

7. *Ice bag or collar*
   a. Ice bag or collar
   b. Protective cover for ice bag
   c. Ice chips
   d. Patient thermometer

8. *Ice glove*
   a. Ice bag, collar, or glove
   b. Ice chips
   c. Basin
   d. Protective covering
   e. Patient thermometer

9. *Alcohol or cold sponge bath*
   a. Bath thermometer

b. Bath blanket for patient

c. Basin

d. Solution (water, with or without alcohol, as ordered)

e. Washcloths and towel

f. Patient thermometer

10. *Compresses*

a. *Sterile compresses*

(1) Sterile solution, as ordered

(2) Bath thermometer (to test solution temperature, pour sufficient amount in unsterile container and test with regular bath thermometer; discard; do not use on patient)

(3) Sterile gauze squares or sterile washcloths

(4) Sterile basin

(5) Sterile forceps or sterile rubber gloves for application

(6) Sterile towels for covering gauze

(7) Patient thermometer

b. *Clean compresses*

(1) Solution, as ordered

(2) Bath thermometer

(3) Gauze squares or washcloths

(4) Clean towel for insulation over gauze

(5) Plastic material for insulation over gauze

(6) Clean rubber gloves for applying compresses

(7) Patient thermometer

11. *Hot pack or foment*

a. Towels

b. Solution, as ordered

c. Basin

d. Bath blanket for patient

e. Bath thermometer

f. Waterproof cover (plastic)

g. Dry pack or covering (towels)

h. Patient thermometer

12. *Cool wet pack*

a. Bath towels, for moistening

b. Ice chips

c. Basin

d. Towels for dry pack or covering

    e. Bath thermometer

    f. Rectal thermometer for patient

    g. Waterproof cover (plastic)

13. *Ice packs*

    a. Rectal thermometer for patient

    b. Plastic bags

    c. Protective coverings for bags

    d. Ice cap

    e. Ice chips

    f. Bath blankets

    g. Screen, for privacy

14. *Soaks*

    a. Solution, as ordered

    b. Basin, for immersion

    c. Towels

    d. Screen, for privacy

    e. Gauze, if ordered

    f. Patient thermometer

III. IMPLEMENTING NURSING INTERVENTION

A. Therapeutic Aspects

1. *Hot/warm/cold/cool moist packs or compresses*

    a. The application of heat or cold to open wounds or lesions which may rupture demands a sterile technique to alleviate further contamination from the transfer of microorganisms. The nurse should wash her hands carefully before application. Sterile gloves or sterile instruments must be used to apply sterile applications.

    b. Absorbent and loosely woven fibers will hold moisture. Woolens, flannels, or towels may be used for hot/cold applications to large surface areas. Gauze squares and washcloths may be used for small surface areas. The patient's temperature, pulse, and respiratory rate serve as guides to his reaction to heat. Vital signs should be taken prior to, during, and after application.

    c. Woolens and flannels absorb water slowly. The solution should be tested prior to immersion as a safety measure in assuring correct temperature.

    d. Air will reduce the temperature of a hot pack or compress by evaporation. The patient should be fully prepared so that a minimum of time will be expended in the application of the pack or compress. The skin area under a heated application may be lubricated with petroleum jelly.

e. The degree of vasodilation indicates the intensity of the heat or cold. If the application is very hot, it may contract cutaneous vessels and decrease blood supply. Warm applications lead to increased blood supply and muscle relaxation. The application should be placed lightly on the skin and lifted after a few seconds to inspect for erythema or paleness. The first reaction to cold is vasoconstriction of the cutaneous vessels, causing coolness and paleness. The skin should be observed closely throughout the procedure for signs indicating the need for modification of temperature.

f. Air spaces between the skin and the pack will reduce the effect of the application, since air is a poor conductor of heat. The pack or compress should be wrapped around the site, molding it to the skin surface. Insulation and covering will prevent heat and moisture loss. The moist pack should be covered with a dry pack and a waterproof covering. The weight of a massive pack often restricts movement and causes fatigue. Positioning the patient in proper alignment promotes comfort.

2. *External application of dry heat*

a. Because of the possibility of burns and the physiological changes that occur throughout the body when heat is applied locally, (*i.e.*, vasodilation of peripheral blood vessels, increased respiratory rate, fall in blood pressure, decrease in body heat production, and increase in leukocytes), it is imperative to obtain a specific order from the physician. The order should contain the method of application, the temperature, and the duration. Vital signs, including temperature, should be taken prior to the application of heat.

b. *K-Matic pad*: distilled water is used in mechanical devices requiring water to prevent mineral formation. The reservoir should be filled ⅔ full and turned end-to-end to release air bubbles, which could interfere with even heat conduction. The heating pad should be covered to prevent burns. After applying to the skin, the nurse should watch for erythema or undesirable side effects.

c. *Electric heating pad*: crushing or creasing the wires in the pad may impair function, causing portions of the pad to overheat, resulting in burns or fire. Pins should be avoided in securing the pad to reduce danger of electrical shock. No type of electrical equipment should be used in the presence of oxygen. A protective covering over the pad acts as an insulator, as dampness from a wet dressing or perspiration from the patient's wet skin could create a short circuit. The patient may become accustomed to the temperature, due to depression of peripheral nerve endings. He should be instructed not to elevate the setting on the pad, however, as burns may result.

d. *Hot water bag*: heat is applied by conduction. Air should be expelled from the bag, as it is a poor conductor of heat. The bag is filled ⅔ full. It should be covered with a heavy fabric cover to slow heat transmission, absorb perspiration, and lessen the danger of burning.

e. *Heat lamp:* heat lamps employ the principle of radiation. They are used to increase hyperemia (blood circulation), thereby increasing the supply of oxygen and nourishment to tissues. The skin should be dry and clean, to lessen the danger of burning. A 60-watt bulb is usually used 18 to 24 inches from the area of skin to be treated. The light should be placed to the side of the patient rather than over him, because of the danger of its falling. It should never be placed under bed linen, because of the fire hazard involved. The area should be checked every 5 minutes during treatment. The recommended duration of treatment is 15 to 20 minutes. Signs of untoward reaction are redness and pain. The skin should be moist, warm, and pink at the conclusion of the treatment.

f. *Heat cradle:* A heat cradle provides radiant heat, which is less localized than a heat lamp. The top sheet may be used to cover the cradle to hold in heat and prevent cooling by circulating air. The treatment duration is usually 10 to 15 minutes, with the heating element 18 to 24 inches from the skin.

3. *External application of cold:* cold produces vasoconstriction and reduces tissue metabolism. Cold has an anesthetic effect on the skin, and the patient may become unaware of impulses from the skin which normally serve to warn that tissue damage is occurring. A protective covering is essential to prevent tissue trauma, provide comfort, and provide for absorption of moisture, which condenses on the outside of the bag.

4. *Body soaks:* the soak provides warmth, cleanses the area, hastens suppuration, and applies medication to a designated area. Equipment is usually sterile, because soaks are most often applied to an open wound. The physician should specify site, duration, temperature, technique, type, and purpose of soak. Soaking dressings prior to removal lessens trauma to healing tissues. The affected area should be immersed slowly, in order to acclimatize the patient to the temperature of the solution. The patient should be placed in a position of comfort, to avoid fatigue and muscle strain. Duration of treatment is usually 20 minutes. The temperature of the solution and condition of the patient should be checked every 5 minutes. The heat of the solution will cause some vasodilation and erythema.

B. Communicative Aspects

1. *Observations*

   a. Prior to, during, and after any type of moist or dry application, the patient should be observed for signs and symptoms involving the skin and mucous membranes; these should be investigated, evaluated, reported, or treated with appropriate nursing measures. This is of particular importance when the patient:

(1) Is at the extremes of age

(2) Is known to have delicate or sensitive skin

(3) Has impaired circulation

(4) Is subject to having irritating substances on the skin or mucous membranes (*e.g.,* perspiration, urine, feces, gastrointestinal secretions, various exudates)

(5) Depends on others for physical care or protection (*e.g.,* infants and young children, the weak or debilitated, mentally incompetent, unconscious, immobilized, or bedridden)

(6) Has an appliance or equipment in contact with the skin or mucous membranes (*e.g.,* traction, casts, braces, various tubes).

(7) Has an injury or disease condition that affects the skin or mucous membranes

b. In addition, during hot/cold applications, observe the abnormal circulatory changes, such as excessive or prolonged redness, whiteness, or cyanosis.

c. Verbal complaints of discomfort by the patient warrant careful observation. If indicated, the treatment should be discontinued and reported appropriately.

2. *Charting*

a. Duration

b. Frequency

c. Times, as ordered

d. Temperature of solution

e. Time and duration

f. TPR before, during, and after treatment

g. Appearance of site

h. Behavior and comments of patient

DATE	TREATMENT	TIME	OBSERVATIONS	SIGNATURE
4/8	Warm compresses	0800	Compresses applied with K-Matic pad, 95° F. to rt anterior forearm. TPR before treatment, 98.6, 80, 24. States he is familiar with treatment to be done.	
		0810	States he is comfortable. T 99, P 80, R 24. Skin on rt anterior forearm appears slightly pink.	

DATE	TREATMENT	TIME	OBSERVATIONS	SIGNATURE
		0820	Compresses removed. Skin appears pink at compress site. No other overt observation of rt anterior forearm. T 99, P 80, R 24. Stated, "That sure made my arm feel better." Fluids offered and taken.	B. Smith, L.V.N.

3. *Referrals*

   Not applicable

C. Teaching Aspects—Patient and Family

1. If the treatment is to be continued at home, the nurse should tell the patient how the application is prepared and what to substitute for the hospital's equipment.

2. The patient or family should be taught the adverse signs and symptoms of prolonged or improper administration of hot and cold applications.

IV. EVALUATION PROCESS

A. Was the patient in a comfortable position during and after the treatment?

B. Was the equipment sterile, if need be?

C. Was the application renewed as often as necessary?

D. Was adequate observation made during the treatment?

E. Did the nurse understand the method and show skill in the application?

F. Was adequate explanation given to the patient and family?

G. Was the charting pertinent and accurate?

H. Was adequate observation made during the treatment to avoid complications?

I. Was the objective of the application accomplished?

54

Incontinent Patients, Care of

I. ASSESSMENT OF SITUATION

A. Definition
Those unable to control the discharge of urine or feces

B. Terminology
1. *Anal sphincter:* the constricting circular muscle that closes the anus
2. *Overflow or paradoxical incontinence:* urine builds up in the bladder until the pressure causes dribbling, which stops when the excess pressure has been relieved
3. *Total incontinence:* the bladder is unable to store any urine, and dribbling is almost constant

C. Rationale for Actions
1. To prevent secondary problems due to incontinence
2. To instigate a bladder or bowel training program as early as possible

II. NURSING PLAN

A. Objectives
1. To keep the patient as clean and dry as possible
2. To avoid embarrassing the patient
3. To assist the family and patient to accept the condition and involve them in the retraining program

B. Patient Preparation
1. Any retraining program involving the systems of the body is slow, tedious, and time-consuming. The patient should understand at the outset what is expected of him and should participate in the formation of goals. This will allow him to cooperate more fully and to feel self-satisfaction when a goal is reached.

C. Equipment
1. Incontinence pads
2. Urinal

III. IMPLEMENTING NURSING INTERVENTION

A. Therapeutic Aspects

1. *Bladder incontinence*

    a. The usual pH of urine is between 5.5 and 7.0, which is acidic. For this reason, urine can be a cause of tissue breakdown if the skin is not kept clean and dry. This is a difficult task with the incontinent patient. It is usually desirable to absorb the urine with diapers or incontinence pads, but this can be very embarrassing to the patient. The word "diaper" should never be used; "pad" is a better choice. These pads should absorb as much urine as possible and should be changed frequently, at which time the perineal area should be cleaned and dried.

    b. Urinary incontinence is associated with the dependence of early childhood. Thus, many patients feel embarrassed and insecure. The nurse should *never* speak in a condescending or criticizing manner to incontinent patients. A pleasant, positive approach is the best way to get a bladder training program underway.

    c. An indwelling catheter is an easy, simple way to solve the nurse's problems with incontinence, but it does little to return the patient to a state of equilibrium. Catheters are also known to be a major cause of bladder infection. Therefore, they should be used only as a last resort, and then only for the patient's well-being, not the nurse's convenience.

    d. A positive approach to a bladder training program can be invaluable in acquiring patient cooperation. Some examples of bladder training include offering the bedpan at regular or pre-set intervals, limiting fluids to certain times followed by an attempt to void, and clamping the catheter for progressively longer intervals prior to its removal. The objective is to rebuild bladder musculature slowly by gradually reestablishing normal voiding patterns.

    e. Every effort should be made to keep the patient's environment pleasant and odor-free. Frequent changes of incontinence pads and cleaning the area help. Also, internal consumption of some juices, such as cranberry juice, reduces the odor.

2. *Bowel incontinence*

    a. Fecal incontinence is usually related to an impairment of the anal sphincter itself or to the nerves that control it. The goals of the nurse should be to prevent tissue breakdown and to assist the patient in regaining whatever control he can. The patient should be kept clean. A pad may need to be applied and should be changed as soon as evacuation occurs. It should not be called a "diaper."

    b. Fecal incontinence is an embarrassing situation. The nurse should show acceptance of the patient as a human being and never make him feel insecure or childish.

c. Fecal incontinence is not a condition to which all must resign themselves immediately. However, it is unkind to set unrealistic, unattainable goals for the patient. He will get discouraged but must be reassured and encouraged to keep trying. The training program may include the use of suppositories or enemas. Sitting on the commode in the normal position facilitates evacuation. Regularity and consistency are important parts of a bowel-training program.

B. Communicative Aspects

1. *Observations*

   a. The incontinent patient must be watched closely for soiling, so he can be kept clean and dry, to minimize adverse reactions.

   b. The nurse should be alert to early signs of tissue breakdown.

   c. Watch for early signs of willingness and readiness to begin a training program.

2. *Charting*

   a. Chart any abnormal findings.

   b. Record bowel and bladder training progress.

3. *Referrals*

   Regularly scheduled visits from a professional nurse to assess the patient's physical condition and progress of the bowel or bladder training program may be indicated after the patient is discharged.

C. Teaching Aspects—Patient and Family

1. Bowel and bladder training programs require patience and cooperation. The family should be involved, if feasible. Stress must be placed on positive occurrences, and continual encouragement of the patient is necessary.

2. If the incontinent patient is to go home, the family should be instructed on how to keep him dry and clean, to prevent complications.

IV. EVALUATION PROCESS

A. Has the patient accepted his condition?

B. Has a bladder or bowel training program been instituted and adhered to? How much success has been attained?

C. Did tissue breakdown occur?

55

Intake and Output, Recording

I. ASSESSMENT OF SITUATION

A. Description
The accurate measurement of fluids taken into and released from the body; abbreviated "I&O"

B. Terminology
None

C. Rationale for Actions
1. To determine the general condition of the patient
2. To aid in formulation of a diagnosis
3. To assess the need for fluid increase or restriction
4. To gain early clues to potentially dangerous physical situations

II. NURSING PLAN

A. Objectives
1. To record intake and output accurately
2. To report discrepancies to the physician
3. To elicit patient cooperation in keeping the I&O record

B. Patient Preparation
1. Patient cooperation is essential if the I&O is to be accurate. If the patient understands why it is being kept, he is much more likely to cooperate.
2. If the patient can get up to go to the bathroom, a bedside commode or a receptacle to fit inside the commode to catch the urine should be made available as soon as the patient is placed on I&O.

C. Equipment
1. I&O record slip
2. Pencil

III. IMPLEMENTING NURSING INTERVENTION

A. Therapeutic Aspects

1. Many changes in clinical conditions are manifested in discrepancies in the intake and output record (*e.g.*, edema, diaphoresis). An accurate I&O is essential in the diagnosis and treatment of many diseases. Administration of a diuretic is an excellent example of the importance of keeping an accurate I&O record. Followup doses are often based on the I&O record. I&O plus daily weight can give a good indication of the progress of therapy.

2. Accurate measurements are essential. A conversion record is located in Technique 59 Medications, administration of. The nurse should also know the number of ml of liquid in such consumables as a bowl of Jell-O, ice cream, and cereal. Urine should be measured in a graduated cylinder. It is important that the patient not void with a bowel movement, as this renders the output record unreliable. Basins which partially cover the commode and catch the urine but not the feces are available. A receptacle can also be held over the perineum to catch the urine.

3. Urinary incontinence makes accurate output measurement impossible. However, the number of voidings and approximate amount (*i.e.*, large, moderate, small) should be recorded.

B. Communicative Aspects

1. *Observations*

   a. Intake includes:

   (1) Anything liquid by mouth

   (2) IV fluids and clysis

   (3) Gastric feedings and irrigation fluids above the amount removed

   (4) Foley catheter irrigation above the amount removed

   (5) Peritoneal dialysis fluid

   b. Output includes:

   (1) Emesis

   (2) Urine

   (3) Blood loss (approximate)

   (4) Drainage from incisions, wounds, and so forth (approximate)

   (5) Gastric aspiration

   (6) Fluids withdrawn from the body, such as paracentesis, thoracentesis, surgical drainage bags, and so on

   c. Gross discrepancies between intake and output should be called to the physician's attention.

2. *Charting*

a. I&O should be recorded for each shift, as well as each 24 hours.

INTAKE

DATE / TIME	ORAL	LEVIN	IRRIGATION	PARENTERAL	TOTAL
7-3	30 ml ice chips	400 ml	0	1,000	1,430
3-11	50 ml ice chips	400 ml	0	1,000	1,450
11-7	0	450 ml	0	1,100	1,550
Total, 24 hrs	80 ml	1,250 ml	0	3,100	4,430

OUTPUT

URINE VOIDED	CATHETER #1	#2	LEVIN	OTHER	TOTAL
0	800	0	800	0	1,600
0	950	0	600	0	1,550
0	700	0	1,000	0	1,700
0	2,450	0	2,400	0	4,850

3. *Referrals*

Not applicable

C. Teaching Aspects

1. Many patients can assist in keeping their own I&O if they are properly instructed.
2. Patients should understand the reason for I&O.

IV. EVALUATION PROCESS

A. Did the intake correlate with the output? If not, was it called to the physician's attention?

B. Did the patient actively participate in keeping the record?

C. Was the patient well hydrated?

D. Was regular elimination encouraged?

56

Intestinal Decompression, Assisting With

I. ASSESSMENT OF SITUATION

A. Definition

The insertion of a long tube into the intestinal tract to aspirate intestinal contents. Types of tubes are (Fig. 56-1):

1. *Miller-Abbott tube*

    a. 10-foot biluminal tube: 1 lumen for introducing air, water, or mercury to inflate the balloon; the other for drainage

    b. Metal tip and balloon on the end of the tube

    c. Balloon inflated after insertion

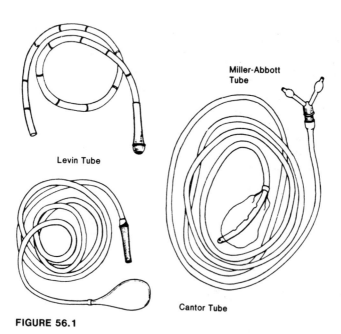

Levin Tube

Miller-Abbott Tube

Cantor Tube

FIGURE 56.1

2. *Cantor tube*
   a. 10-foot, single-lumen tube
   b. Balloon at the tip of the tube
   c. Mercury injected into the balloon before insertion
3. *Levin tube*
   a. A rubber or plastic, disposable single-lumen tube
   b. A rubber or plastic, disposable double-lumen tube (Salem-Sump)

B. Terminology

Decompression: the removal of pressure, gas, and fluids from the intestinal tract

C. Rationale for Actions

1. To remove gas and fluids in the prevention and treatment of distention of the intestines
2. To stimulate peristalsis
3. To locate and relieve obstruction

II. NURSING PLAN

A. Objectives

1. To allay fears and anxieties of the patient
2. To assist the physician in inserting the tube
3. To maintain patency of the tube to insure proper function
4. To provide comfort for the patient
5. To maintain fluid and electrolyte balances
6. To observe for signs and symptoms that indicate incorrect placement of the tube
7. To keep an accurate record of:
   a. Drainage: amount, color, and type
   b. Intake and output
   c. Effects produced by the treatment
8. To teach patient and family the purpose of the treatment

B. Patient Preparation

1. The suction machine should be tested prior to the procedure.
2. Gastrointestinal intubation is unpleasant and tedious for the patient. He is likely to be much more cooperative if he has a thorough explanation prior to beginning the procedure. The patient should be sitting up, if he is able. The physician may use a topical local anesthetic to minimize discomfort. The patient should be told to relax and breath through his mouth during the procedure.

C. Equipment

1. Gastrointestinal tube, as ordered by physician
2. Basin with ice
3. Disposable irrigation set
4. 5 to 10 ml of mercury
5. Local anesthetic, as ordered
6. 10-ml syringe
7. Glass of water, with straw
8. Emesis basin
9. Wipes
10. Suction machine
11. Adhesive tape, ½ inch
12. Rubber band
13. Water-soluble lubricant
14. Irrigating solution, as ordered

III. IMPLEMENTING NURSING INTERVENTION

A. Therapeutic Aspects

1. Gastrointestinal tubes are longer than the common nasogastric (Levin) tubes, because they must be passed into the actual intestinal tract. To encourage their passage from the stomach, they may have a balloon filled with air (Miller-Abbott) or mercury (Cantor) at the tip. The balloons serve the same purpose as a portion of food does, *i.e.*, stimulating peristalsis and encouraging tube passage. Prior to insertion, the tube should be lubricated sparingly, to reduce friction, and chilled well, to make it easier to handle. The mercury is inserted into the Cantor tube prior to insertion, by way of a needle injection into the balloon. The balloon on the Miller-Abbott tube is inflated through the air lumen after it reaches the stomach. Actual insertion is the same as for a Levin tube (see Technique 49, Gastric intubation).

2. Once the tube is in place, it must be secured with tape. This should be done in such a way as to promote optimum comfort yet assure it will not come loose. It is essential to avoid pressure on the nostril. The tube should not be taped, however, until it has been fully advanced to the desired level. The tube is then connected to suction. The patient should be able to move about in bed without risk of dislodging the tube.

3. To maintain fluid and electrolyte balances, the patient's fluid intake should be evaluated in relation to any fluid from the gastrointestinal tract. When a patient has a tube draining fluid from the body into a container, the drainage must be measured and recorded accurately. Accurate I&O is essential.

4. The weight of the mercury carries the balloon through the gastrointestinal tract by gravity. Position and activity aid in the passage of the tube. The patient may lie on his right side with his back in Fowler's position, then on his left side and progress to ambulation in an effort to facilitate tube advancement.

5. Breathing through the mouth causes the lips and tongue to become dry and cracked. Frequent oral hygiene should be provided. Lubrication of the lips may aid comfort.

6. To remove the tube, the balloon is deflated in the Miller-Abbott tube. The tube is withdrawn slowly, at 10 minute intervals, about 6 inches each time. Once it reaches the stomach, it may be withdrawn in a rapid steady motion, as a nasogastric tube would be. It should be clamped during removal to prevent aspiration. If any resistance is met, the physician should be notified. The Cantor tube is removed in 6 inch increments, as well, until the bag of mercury is visible in the throat. It is removed through the mouth, and the tube is then pulled out of the nose. Thorough oral hygiene will be needed after removal.

B. Communicative Aspects

1. *Observations*
   a. Assess the patient for signs and symptoms of fluid and electrolyte imbalances.
   b. Observe amount, color, consistency, and odor of the drainage.
   c. Observe effects of treatment on the patient.

2. *Charting*

DATE	TREATMENT	TIME	OBSERVATIONS	SIGNATURE
5/27	#16 Miller-Abbott tube connected to suction. Vaseline to lips.	0900	Inserted by Dr. D. to the "S" mark. 5 ml Hg instilled into balloon. 200 ml thick, brown fluid obtained. Placed on rt side. Following doctor's departure, appeared very apprehensive. Sat and talked briefly with him. Appears more relaxed.	G. Ivers, R.N.
		1000	Tube advance 1 inch, as ordered.	G. Ivers, R.N.

3. *Referrals*
   Not applicable

C. Teaching Aspects—Patient and Family

1. Explain procedure, equipment, and purpose prior to beginning the procedure, at the level of the patient's understanding.

2. Explain why the patient will lie on right side, then back, then left side, to facilitate tube progression.

IV. EVALUATION PROCESS

A. Were safety measures applied to prevent injury or infection?

B. Was patient reassured while the tube was being passed?

C. Is the patient clean and comfortable?

D. Is the charting pertinent and adequate?

E. Is the suction apparatus functioning properly?

F. Is the suction machine on "low" position?

57

Intravenous (IV) Infusion Administration

I. ASSESSMENT OF SITUATION

A. Definition

The introduction of a solution, blood or blood derivatives directly into a vein, by way of an angiocath, intra-cath, butterfly, or scalp vein needle (Fig. 57-1).

B. Terminology

1. *Angiocath:* a needle within a plastic tubing. The needle is removed after insertion in the vein; the plastic tube remains in the vein for infusion.

2. *Butterfly needle:* a small needle used for unstable veins; so named because of the butterfly wing appearance of the upper portion of the appliance, used for guidance during insertion and anchorage during infusion.

3. *Intra-Cath:* a large bore needle with a plastic catheter which is threaded through it after venipuncture. The needle is removed from the injection site, and the plastic catheter remains in the vein.

4. *Dripmeter:* a chamber between bottle and tubing with which to observe rate of infusion

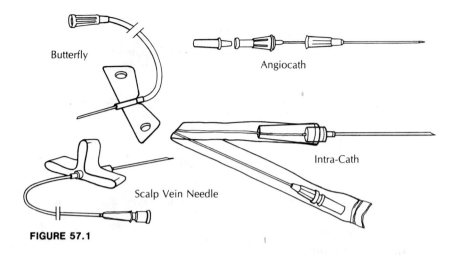

Butterfly

Angiocath

Intra-Cath

Scalp Vein Needle

FIGURE 57.1

5. *Microdripmeter:* a chamber between bottle and tubing which allows for accurate counting of drops
6. *Unit of blood:* 500 ml of blood in a container
7. *Derivatives (blood):* constituent parts (of whole blood)

C. Rationale for Actions

1. To restore or maintain fluid and electrolyte balance
2. To provide for basic nutrition
3. To provide a vehicle to administer medication

II. NURSING PLAN

A. Objectives

1. To make patient as comfortable as possible
2. To prevent infection or complications
3. To allay patient's fears and apprehensions
4. To observe closely for adverse reactions
5. To teach patient and family safety precautions
6. To report desired or undesired effects
7. To recognize the signs and symptoms of a blood reaction

B. Patient Preparation

1. Proper identification of the patient prevents error. A medicine card should be made for each bottle of fluid that the patient receives. The card should be checked with the patient's room number, bed card, and identity bracelet. To minimize fear, an adequate explanation should be given as to reason and method of administration. Having

equipment completely assembled before entering the patient's room will enhance his feeling of well-being.

2. Since the application of external tubing will impair mobility, the patient should go to the bathroom, if his condition permits, before the intravenous puncture is made.

3. Placement of a towel under the arm to be used will decrease the possibility of soiling the bed linens or patient gown.

C. Equipment

1. Intravenous solution, as ordered by physician
2. IV tubing, with attached drip chamber
3. Intravenous tray, with alcohol sponges, tourniquet, and adhesive or paper tape
4. Covered armboard
5. Intravenous standard
6. Needles: 20-gauge, 1-inch long or 19-gauge, 1-inch long
7. Butterfly needles (sizes #16 and #19)
8. Scalp vein needles
9. Sterile disposable angiocath (size as ordered, #14, #16, #18, and so forth)
10. Additional equipment needed for Intra-Cath:
    a. Sterile disposable Intra-Cath (size as ordered)
    b. Sterile 4x4 dressings

III. IMPLEMENTING NURSING INTERVENTION

A. Therapeutic Aspects

1. Air bubbles should not be introduced into the bloodstream during intravenous therapy. The bottle of fluid should be hung with tubing intact and flushed of all air bubbles. The drip chamber should be at least half full.

2. A tourniquet is applied above the intended site of injection (Fig. 57-2). This causes constriction of the vessels, resulting in engorgement and distention of the veins, making them more accessible. Only venous return should be impaired; a pulse below the tourniquet should still be palpable.

3. Circulation to a part may be increased by positioning, active and passive exercise, or the application of heat. If the vein is not distended and easily palpable, the nurse may lightly pat the area, have the patient open and close his fist, lower the extremity below the level of the heart, or apply a warm towel.

4. The skin should be thoroughly cleansed with an alcohol sponge at

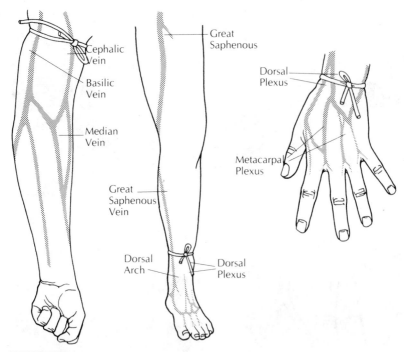

FIGURE 57.2

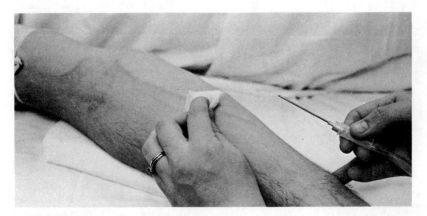

FIGURE 57.3

and around the injection site to prevent the entrance of pathogens (Fig. 57-3).

5. The pressure needed to pierce the skin is sufficient to force the needle through the vein. The needle should be held at a 45° angle,

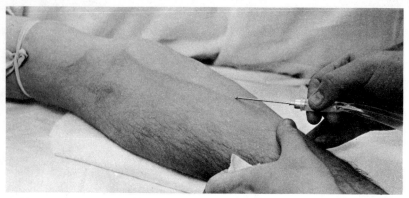

FIGURE 57.4A

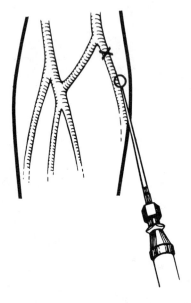

FIGURE 57.4B

bevel up, in line with and alongside the vein (Fig. 57-4). The needle should be inserted through the skin, about ½ inch below the intended site of vein puncture.

6. Following the course of the vein prevents the needle from puncturing it. When the needle is through the skin, lower the angle until it is almost parallel with the skin. The needle may then be inserted into the vein. The free hand may be used to palpate or control the vein while the needle is being introduced into it.

7. Increased venous pressure, due to the tourniquet, will cause blood to back into the needle when the vein is punctured. If a butterfly or regular needle is used, it should then be inserted another ½ or ¾ inch into the vein. Angiocaths and Intra-Caths are threaded while the vein is distended.

8. The increased venous pressure is relieved by release of the tourniquet.

    a. *Angiocath:* Remove inner metal needle, leaving the plastic tube in place in the vein.

    b. *Intra-Cath:* Withdraw metal needle from the skin and cover with plastic protector. Withdraw stylet from Intra-Cath.

9. Blood will clot in the needle or catheter if not in motion with other blood and fluid. Intravenous tubing should be connected immediately and the fluid allowed to flow.

10. Pressure of the wall of the vein against the needle opening will decrease or stop the flow of fluid. The needle may be supported with a cotton ball to keep it in the desired position.

11. Normally, venous pressure is greater than atmospheric pressure. IV fluids flow from an area of greater to lesser pressure and by gravity. The fluid should thus be hung 18 to 24 inches above the infusion site.

12. Since the smooth structure of the vein does not offer resistance to needle movement, the needle must be anchored with tape.

    a. *Angiocath:* anchor directly with tape.

    b. *Intra-Cath:* cover insertion site with sterile gauze, 4×4, and tape securely. Tubing should also be anchored, to prevent tension on the needle.

13. Three major factors influence the rate of flow: pressure gradient, size of tubing, and viscosity of fluid. The desired rate may be regulated by a screw clamp on the tubing.

14. Careless movements of the extremity may cause tension on the vein and possible dislodgment of the needle or catheter. The arm may be restrained on an armboard. The restraint should be loose enough, however, to avoid interference with fluid flow or normal blood flow in the lower part of the extremity.

15. To discontinue the infusion, the clamp is tightened to stop the flow of fluid. Holding the needle to prevent tissue trauma, the tape is removed and the needle or catheter is gently pulled straight out. Pressure is applied to the infusion site with an alcohol sponge to prevent bleeding or contamination. Unless oozing of blood continues, a bandage or dressing is unnecessary. The nurse should not immediately flex the patient's arm, since it has been immobilized for some time.

16. Special considerations for the transfusion of blood:

    a. Since agglutination and hemolysis of red cells may occur as a result of mixing incompatible blood groups, a type and cross-match should precede any blood administration.

b. Improper storage of blood and blood derivatives may cause cell destruction or pathogenic growth. The blood should be obtained from the lab immediately prior to its administration. Blood should not be kept out of storage for more than 1 hour.

c. Proper checking of blood prevents error, thereby decreasing chance of adverse effects. Blood units should be checked by two persons, an R.N. and another person of legal age. Both should sign the blood card which remains with the blood and, after transfusion, becomes a part of the medical record. The blood should be checked for the patient's name, room number, hospital number, physician's name, blood type, bag number, and Rh factor. The expiration date and VDRL are also checked.

d. Special tubing is used to administer blood. It has a filter to remove any small clots and prevent their entering the vein.

B. Communicative Aspects

1. *Observations*

a. Check infusion frequently for proper flow rate. Very rapid infusion is usually contraindicated because of the danger of causing too great a load on the circulatory system.

b. Observe to see that the solution continues to flow into the vein. If the needle or catheter slips out of the vein, the solution will flow into subcutaneous tissue, causing swelling as the fluid collects. This is referred to as "infiltration" and necessitates discontinuing the IV and restarting at a different site. If there is a question about whether the needle or catheter is still in the vein, a tourniquet can be applied above the needle and the IV infusion momentarily turned off. If blood runs into the tubing, the needle or catheter is still placed properly.

c. Any sign of redness, tenderness, or pain at the site of injection or path of the vein should be promptly reported. This indicates inflammation of the vein.

d. If more than one bottle of solution is ordered, the nurse attaches the additional bottles. The addition should be connected as soon as a bottle becomes empty; otherwise, there is danger of the line becoming filled with air or occluded, due to clotting in the needle or catheter.

e. If any medications are added to the bottle, a label is applied to the bottle, indicating drug, dosage, and time that the medication was added. The date and signature of the person adding medication should also be included.

f. Patients receiving blood should be observed closely for transfusion complications. These include:

(1) Hemolytic reactions

(2) Allergic reactions

(3) Febrile contamination

(4) Bacterial contamination

(5) Circulatory overloading

(6) Abdominal pain or cramping

g. If a reaction occurs:

(1) Discontinue the blood.

(2) Take patient's vital signs stat and as often as indicated.

(3) Notify physician immediatly.

(4) Send urine specimen and remaining blood or empty blood bag to lab, along with completed blood reaction form.

2. *Charting*

a. An entry should be made on the nurses' notes regarding the starting and maintaining of infusions. Vital signs should be taken and charted at the beginning of the infusion to serve as a baseline, should complications occur.

b. The accurate amount of fluid infused should be included on the IV record.

c. Infusion record

DATE	INFUSION	TIME START	FINISH	MEDICATIONS	RATE	SITE OF INJECTION
5/5	500 ml whole blood #4259	0930	1230		60 gtt per min.	L. forearm

d. Nurses' notes

DATE	TREATMENT	TIME	OBSERVATIONS	SIGNATURE
5/5		1300	Complaining of itching over body. Small reddened areas noted on chest; Dr. B. notified.	
		1305	T 100; P 84; R 20	
		1310	U.A. spec and empty blood bag sent to lab.	F. White, R.N.

3. *Referrals*

Not applicable

C. Teaching Aspects—Patient and Family

1. Instruct the patient and family to report any generalized discomfort or pain and swelling at the site of injection to nurse.

2. Explain to the patient and family the approximate length of time that infusion will last and to use a call light when assistance is needed to meet their needs.

3. Ask the family to notify the nurse if the solution ceases to drip in the chamber.

IV. EVALUATION PROCESS

A. Is the patient in a comfortable position and free of pain and fear?

B. Do the patient and family understand the procedure and what to expect?

C. Is an accurate intake and output record being kept and functioning of apparatus being recorded during each shift?

D. Does the intake and output record indicate the fluid balance?

E. Was the transfusion completed successfully?

F. Does the patient indicate any signs or symptoms of complications?

G. Was a sterile technique used in starting the infusion?

H. Were baseline vital signs recorded and compared with later vital signs to assure physiological well-being?

58

Isolation

I. ASSESSMENT OF SITUATION

A. Definition

Measures instituted to prevent the spread of microorganisms among hospital patients, staff, and visitors

Types are:

1. *Strict isolation:* used to prevent the transmission of highly communicable diseases which may be spread by either direct or airborne means

2. *Respiratory isolation:* used to prevent transmission of organisms by

direct contact or from droplets that are coughed, sneezed, or breathed into the environment

3. *Protective isolation:* used to prevent contact between potentially pathogenic microorganisms and uninfected persons who have impaired resistance

4. *Enteric precautions:* used to prevent the transmission of diseases which may be contracted through contact with feces

5. *Wound and skin precautions:* used to prevent personnel and patients from contracting infections via direct contact with wounds or heavily contaminated articles

B. Terminology

1. *Barrier technique:* medical aseptic practices observed to control the spread of and destroy pathogenic organisms. Mechanical barriers are set up to keep the organism confined to a certain area (*e.g.,* unit, room). "Barrier technique" is used interchangeably with the word "isolation."

2. *Communicable:* transmissable from person to person, either directly or indirectly

3. *Concurrent disinfection:* the destruction of pathogenic organisms as soon as possible after they leave the body

4. *Contaminated:* having come in contact with infectious agents or materials; applies to persons and objects

5. *Cross-infection:* a second communicable disease superimposed on a person already in the hospital for a first condition

6. *Immunity:* possessing specific antibodies to resist infection; may be active, passive, natural, or acquired

7. *Incubation period:* the development of an infection, from the time it gains entry into the body until the time of appearance of the first signs and symptoms

8. *Isolation:* the separation of persons with communicable diseases from others for a specified time

9. *Susceptibility:* the opposite of immunity; possessing no specific antibodies to resist infection

10. *Terminal cleaning:* the cleaning of a room and its contents following recovery, transfer, or death of persons who inhabited it and had a communicable disease

C. Rationale for Actions

1. *Strict isolation:* To prevent the spread of an infectious microorganism

2. *Respiratory isolation:* To prevent the spread of infection transmitted by the airborne route

3. *Protective isolation:* To protect susceptible persons from environmental contamination

4. *Enteric precautions:* To prevent the spread of microorganisms found in fecal material

5. *Wound and skin precautions:* To prevent the spread of microorganisms found in certain wounds and skin conditions

II. NURSING PLAN

A. Objectives

1. *Strict Isolation, Respiratory Isolation, Enteric Precautions, and Wound and Skin Precautions:*

   a. To assist in identifying the etiologic agent and establishing a diagnosis

   b. To control and prevent the spread of infection

   c. To provide physiological support and symptomatic relief

   d. To teach the patient, visitors, and ancillary hospital personnel the essentials of infection prevention and control

   e. To prevent fear, boredom, and loneliness for the patient while maintaining optimum isolation conditions

2. *Protective Isolation*

   a. To protect the patient from cross-infection by strict adherence to isolation precautions

   b. To provide physiological support and symptomatic relief

   c. To assist the patient, family, and visitors in acceptance of and adherence to isolation procedures by thorough explanation and positive reinforcement

   d. To prevent fear, bordom, and loneliness for the patient while promoting his comfort and safety

B. Patient Preparation

1. Since all isolation precautions require some type of restrictive interaction between the nursing staff and the patient, a thorough explanation in the earliest phase of treatment may reduce the patient's fears and misgivings. The explanation should be given in simple terms at a level befitting the patient's age, education level, and physical readiness to understand.

2. In every culture, there are some physical conditions, states of health, or disease processes which have negative connotations. The nurse must help dispel the stigma associated with communicable disease by showing ready acceptance of the patient as a person. She should help to clarify any misconceptions that the patient or his family may have regarding his illness.

C. Equipment

1. *Strict Isolation and Respiratory Isolation*

   a. In the room

(1) Three lined wastebaskets (one at the door, one in the bathroom, and one at the bedside) to receive contaminated tissues

(2) Paper towels in the bathroom dispenser

(3) Germicidal soap in the bathroom

b. Outside the room

(1) Strict or Respiratory Isolation card on door

(2) Box of disposable masks

2. *Protective Isolation*

a. In the room

(1) Lined wastebasket at the door

(2) Sphygmomanometer and stethoscope should be clean and should be left in the patient's room until isolation is terminated.

(3) Thermometer should remain in the room in disinfectant which is changed every 3 days.

(4) Mattresses and pillows should have plastic covers and should be cleaned with disinfectant immediately prior to admission of the patient.

b. Outside the room

(1) Protective Isolation card on door

(2) Isolation cart containing masks, clean or sterile gowns, caps, and shoe covers

3. *Enteric Precautions*

a. In the room

(1) Soap for handwashing

(2) Lined wastebasket in bathroom and at door

(3) Thermometer in disinfectant

b. Outside the room

(1) Enteric Precautions card on door

(2) Isolation cart containing gowns, gloves, impervious paper or plastic bags for dressings, and linen bags marked "Isolation"

4. *Wound and Skin Precautions*

a. In the room

(1) Lined wastebasket at bedside and in bathroom

(2) Antiseptic soap for handwashing

(3) Thermometer in antiseptic solution

b. Outside the room

(1) Wound and Skin Precautions card on door

(2) Isolation cart containing clean gowns, masks, and gloves, and linen bags marked "Isolation"

III. IMPLEMENTING NURSING INTERVENTION

A. Therapeutic Aspects

1. Loneliness is an unpleasant and usually avoided emotional experience, accompanying real or imagined isolation from others. The awareness that one is not alone is basic to psychological homeostasis. The staff should make frequent visits to the isolated patient's room to let him know someone is nearby. It is not necessary to gown and glove each time, simply open the door and speak to the isolated person frequently.

2. Emotions may be controlled or manipulated by diverting attention from events causing the emotional reaction. Periods of diversion are especially important for isolated patients, who cannot participate in the normal social interaction of the nursing unit. Watching television and reading are other helpful diversions.

3. Pathogenic organisms escape from the body by way of the respiratory, gastrointestinal, and urinary systems. They may also be released from draining wounds, skin lesions, and body cavities. Dressings from boils, abscesses, and so forth should be wrapped securely in paper and burned immediately. Discharges from the nose and throat are collected in tissue and deposited in a paper bag attached to the patient's bed. All disposable items, such as drinking cups, straws, and solid food wastes, should be placed in large, waxed bags, closed tightly, and burned. Nondisposable items, such as dishes and instruments, should be washed in warm soapy water, rinsed, dried, and packed in paper sacks, to be autoclaved. Contaminated bed materials such as linens and gowns should be placed in a marked linen bag, securely fastened, and labeled "contaminated." All of these are removed from the room by the double-bagging method. (See #11, below.)

4. Cleanliness discourages the growth of pathogenic microorganisms. The patient should be bathed daily, not only to provide soothing comfort and relaxation and to retard the pathogenic processes, but also to give the nurse an opportunity to observe for skin rash, pressure areas, and so forth. Body discharges should be cleaned away quickly and completely.

5. Clean items, surfaces, and areas become contaminated when brought into contact with contaminated objects. The nurse must identify the clean and contaminated areas. In strict isolation, areas outside the isolation room are clean, and inside the patient's room, the bathroom, and any article therein are contaminated. A gown is worn over the clothes of persons entering an isolation room (Fig. 58-1). It must overlap itself in the back and fasten, to ensure adequate protection. To remove the gown, untie it at the waist and neck (Figs. 58-2, 58-3). Wash hands thoroughly (Fig. 58-4), and pull off one sleeve by slipping fingers under the cuff (Fig. 58-5). Remove the second sleeve by grasping through the first sleeve (Fig. 58-6).

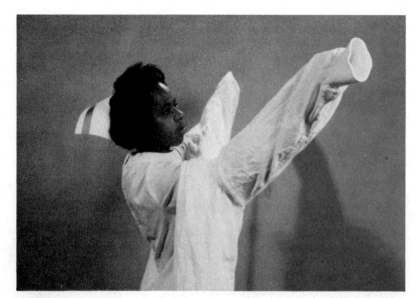

FIGURE 58.1

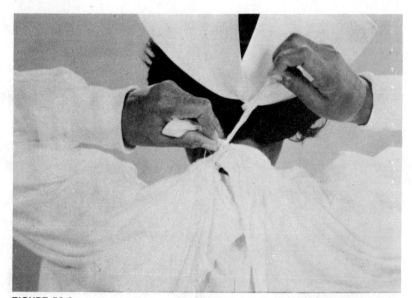

FIGURE 58.2

Fold outer contaminated surfaces together (Fig. 58-7) and discard in linen hamper (Fig. 58-8).

6. In Protective Isolation, the outside of the room is considered contaminated and the inside is clean. When entering, a clean or sterile

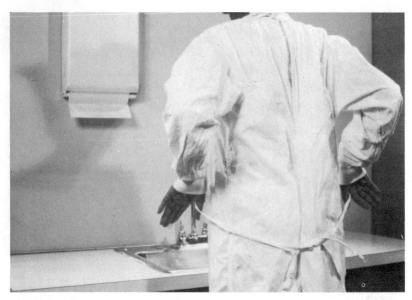

FIGURE 58.3

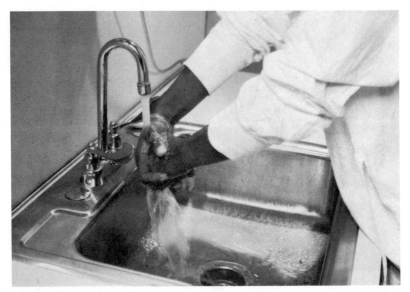

FIGURE 58.4

gown should be worn each time. The outside of the gown must not be exposed to contaminated surfaces prior to entry into the room in an effort to protect the susceptible patient. (See Technique 50,

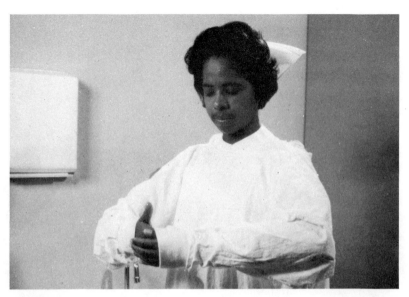

FIGURE 58.5

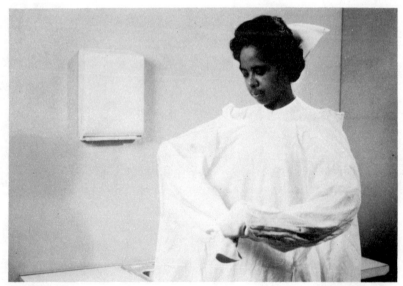

FIGURE 58.6

Gown and glove procedure, sterile.) Hair covering, shoe coverings, gloves, and masks may also be indicated (Figs. 25-9, 25-10).

7. In Enteric Precautions and Wound and Skin Precautions, items in the room that come in contact with potentially infectious pathways

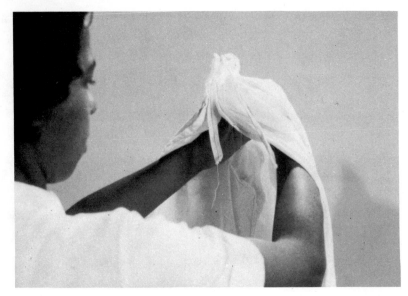

FIGURE 58.7

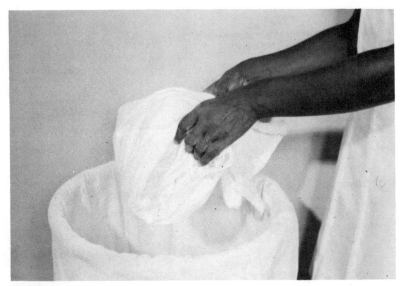

FIGURE 58.8

are considered contaminated. These pathways include oral-fecal secretions and the infected wound or skin area or secretions.

8. Organization of equipment and nursing actions minimizes the
chance of transfer of microorganisms and conserves time and en-

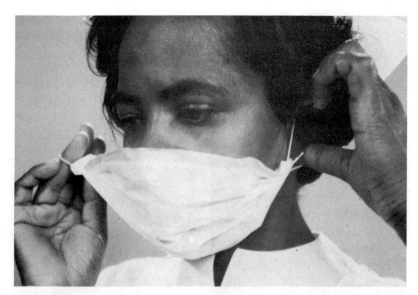

FIGURE 58.9

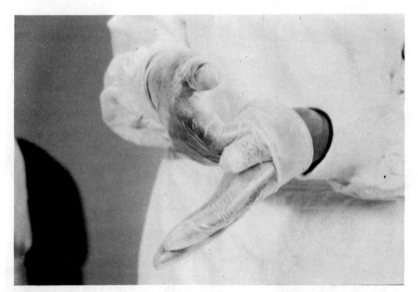

FIGURE 58.10

ergy. All equipment should be gathered prior to entering the isolation room. Unnecessary trips in and out of the room should be
avoided. A thermometer, sphygmomanometer, and stethoscope
should be left in the room until the patient is dismissed.

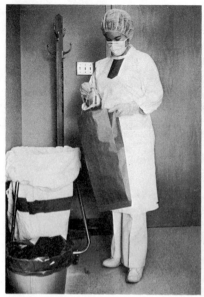

FIGURE 58.11

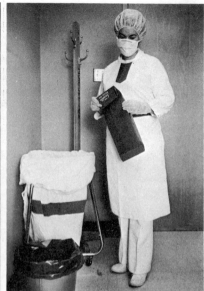

FIGURE 58.12

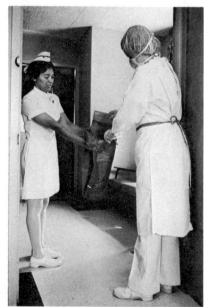

FIGURE 58.13

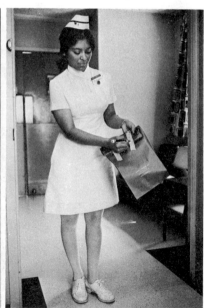

FIGURE 58.14

9. Moisture provides a better breeding environment for pathogens than does a dry surface. Each mask should be worn only 1 time and must be changed at least every hour to prevent contamination. Dishes which have been washed should be dried thoroughly before being placed in paper bags to leave the room.

10. Fresh air dilutes the concentration of airborne microorganisms. Proper ventilation can be achieved by open windows when feasible. The mobility of microorganisms from person to person is increased when suspended in air. The nurse should avoid shaking linens or dry dusting in an isolation room. The door of the room should remain closed.

11. All living organisms can be killed by exposure to moist heat at a temperature of 121°C. (250°F.) for 15 minutes. This is accomplished by autoclaving nondisposable contaminated articles. These articles must be removed from the room by the double-bagging method. Double-bagging means the "contaminated" nurse puts the article in a paper bag and closes it (Figs. 58-11, 58-12), and a "clean" nurse stands on the outside of the room and makes a cuff around the top of a clean bag. She holds this bag at the doorway protecting her hands by placing them under the cuff. The "contaminated" nurse inside the room places bagged items inside the cuffed bag (Fig. 58-13), which is then closed securely and taped shut with autoclave tape by the clean nurse. It is labeled with contents, date and "Isolation" (Fig. 58-14), and sent to the appropriate area.

12. Running water mechanically washes away organisms. Soap emulsifies foreign matter and lowers surface tension. Handwashing before and after contact with each patient is the single most important means of preventing the spread of infection (Fig. 58-15).

13. Disposable needles and syringes should be used on all patients in isolation. The used needles should be placed in prominently labeled, puncture-resistant containers.

14. Transporting patients in isolation

   a. Strict Isolation

     (1) The service to which the patient is being transported should be notified in advance of his contagious condition.

     (2) The patient should wear a clean isolation gown.

     (3) A clean cotton blanket should be placed around the patient, leaving his face exposed. He should wear a mask.

     (4) A Strict Isolation card should be attached to the stretcher or wheelchair.

   b. Respiratory Isolation is the same as Strict Isolation, except that a blanket need not be wrapped around the patient.

   c. Protective Isolation

     (1) Transporting should not be done because of the inherent possibility of infection.

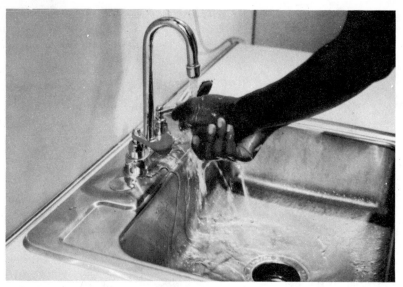

FIGURE 58.15

(2) If absolutely necessary, complete enclosure in sterile linen, front and back, with assurance of uninhibited breathing would be the optimal means of protection during transport.

d. Enteric and Wound and Skin Precautions

(1) Adequate covering and padding of the infectious pathways are usually adequate protection.

15. Specific disease entities as well as in-depth and detailed discussion of isolation may be found in the manual of the Public Health Services Center For Disease Control called *Isolation Techniques for Use in Hospitals*, 2nd edition, 1975, published by the U.S. Department of Health and Human Services.

B. Communicative Aspects

1. *Observations*

a. When diarrhea is present, the frequency, amount, and character of each stool should be noted.

b. Temperature, pulse, and respiration should be measured at least every 4 hours. Any sudden drop or rise in temperature should be reported at once. A change in the rate or volume of the pulse may be the first sign of serious complications.

c. The skin should be noted for any signs of rash, pressure areas, or other effects of prolonged convalescence.

d. The patient's emotional response to being isolated, his acceptance or rejection of it, is important.

e. Frequently, infectious processes are accompanied by fever, nausea, vomiting, and diarrhea. Accurate recording of intake and output is necessary to see that fluids and electrolytes remain in balance.

2. *Charting*

DATE	TREATMENT	TIME	OBSERVATIONS	SIGNATURE
4/9	Range of motion exercises	0800	Remains in strict isolation. Cheerful and visiting with nurse. Skin remains clear, without broken areas. No more diarrhea.	L. Davis, N.T.

3. *Referrals*

a. Information can be received by the patient or his family by writing to the following address:

(1) Governmental

Center for Disease Control, Public Inquiries, 1600 Clifton Rd., Atlanta, Ga. 30333

U.S. Department of Health and Human Services, U.S. Public Health Service, Washington, D.C. 20201

(2) International

World Health Organization (Regional Office for the Americas), 525 23rd St., N.W., Washington, D.C. 20037.

(3) Voluntary

The American Public Health Association, Inc., 1015 15th St., N.W., Washington, D.C. 20005.

C. Teaching Aspects—Patient and Family

1. The patient with a respiratory infection can be taught to fold several thicknesses of tissue and place them in a cupped hand to receive sputum. These should be disposed of in a paper bag, to be burned (Fig. 58-16).

2. The family must be taught the gowning technique. They should be instructed on the infectious processes, because the better their understanding, the more conscientious they will be.

D. Rehabilitation

1. Rehabilitation must begin in the acute phase of the disease. Proper positioning with support may prevent contractures and minimize orthopedic handicaps.

2. Be alert to significant signs of complications, as prompt therapy may prevent permanent disability.

3. Active and passive exercises, if not contraindicated, may help preserve muscle tone and relieve fatigue during prolonged convalescence.

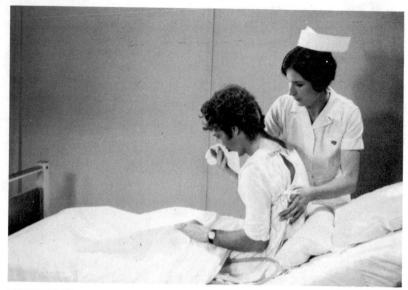

FIGURE 58.16

4. Occupational therapy can create diversion and teach the patient self-help activities.

IV. EVALUATION PROCESS

A. Has the infecting agent been isolated and identified?

B. Has aseptic technique been maintained?

C. Has the family understood and adhered to hospital policy regarding isolation technique?

D. Has the patient enjoyed a state of independence and a feeling of security and acceptance?

E. Has the patient been protected from hospital-acquired infections?

F. Has the patient maintained his previous weight? Has he received prompt and complete relief of associated symptoms?

G. Have persons exposed to the disease before the patient was isolated been referred to their physicians or the public health department for observation or treatment?

59

Medications, Administration of

I. ASSESSMENT OF SITUATION

A. Definition

The process by which drugs are given to a patient. Types are:

1. *Oral administration:* The process of administering drugs in the liquid or solid state (tablet, capsule), for absorption from the gastrointestinal tract

2. *Inhalation administration:* The process of administering drugs in the gaseous or vapor state, for absorption from the respiratory tract

3. *Topical administration:* The process of administering drugs in liquid (lotion, liniment), semi-solid (ointment, cream), or solid state (lozenges, suppositories), for absorption from the skin or mucous membranes

4. *Parenteral administration:* The process of administering drugs in solution or suspension by injection. Types include:

   a. Intradermal: a very small amount of solution (usually 0.1 ml) is injected just below the surface of the skin in the form of a wheal, for local rather than systemic effect (*e.g.,* Tb skin test, local anesthetic).

   b. Subcutaneous or hypodermic (H): a small amount (0.5 to 2.0 ml) of highly soluble medication is injected into the loose connective tissue under the skin for the purpose of administering a drug when (1) the oral route is not feasible (*e.g.,* the drug is destroyed by gastric juices, the patient cannot tolerate oral drugs, a more rapid effect than that of oral administration is desired) or (2) a slower, more sustained action is desired than with the IM route.

   c. Intramuscular (IM): a fairly large amount (up to 5 ml*) of solution or suspension is injected into the muscle body when (1) a more rapid absorption is desired than with the subcutaneous route or (2) the drug is irritating to the subcutaneous tissues or dangerous if injected intravenously. Intramuscular Z-track is a special IM injection in which the subcutaneous tissues are pulled

---

* Occasionally larger amounts (15 ml) of isotonic solutions, such as blood or gamma globulin, are injected into the gluteus maximus. The nurse may want to divide amounts of even less than 5 ml into 2 injections if the patient is emaciated.

aside during injection and allowed to return to normal position after injection, thus sealing off the needle track and preventing irritating or staining drugs (such as dextran iron complex [Imferon]) from leaking into the subcutaneous tissues.

d. Intravenously (IV): Varying volumes of completely soluble solutions are injected directly into the vein for immediate absorption.

B. Terminology

None

C. Rationale for Actions

1. To aid the body in overcoming an illness
2. To relieve symptoms of illness
3. To promote health and prevent disease
4. To aid in diagnosis
5. To hydrate the body cells and tissues

II. NURSING PLAN

A. Objectives

1. To allay fear and anxiety of the patient regarding the administration of the drug and its effect on his condition
2. To administer drugs according to the "Five Rights":
   a. The right drug
   b. The right dose
   c. The right route
   d. The right time
   e. The right patient
3. To observe, report, and record desired therapeutic effects, precautions taken, and untoward reactions of the drug administered

B. Patient Preparation

1. Before any medication is administered, a complete drug allergy history should be taken. The patient should know what drugs he is receiving and the expected effects. He should also be told about any side effects that he should anticipate.
2. Before giving oral medications, the nurse should be certain that the patient has fresh water. If the medication is highly unpalatable, as are many cancer chemotherapeutic drugs, the nurse should offer juice or nectar to the patient when taking this drug, if not contraindicated due to diet or incompatability.
3. If the drug being given is to have a relaxing, tranquilizing, or sedating effect, the patient should first void and the room be darkened and free of stimuli before the medication is given.

C. Equipment

1. *For all drugs:*

   a. Medication card

   b. Medication, as ordered

   c. Tray for carrying medication to patient

2. *Additional equipment:*

   a. For oral drugs, paper cup or medicine glass

   b. For inhalation drugs, atomizer or inhaler

   c. For topical drugs:

      (1) Glove* or applicator for lotions, liniments, and creams

      (2) Glove* and lubricant for suppositories or special applicator provided with drug

   d. For parenteral drugs:

      (1) Alcohol sponge

      (2) Syringe, according to volume of solution

      (3) Needle:

         (a) *Intradermal:* ½-inch, 25-gauge

         (b) *Subcutaneous:* ½-to 1-inch, 25-to-23-gauge

         (c) *Intramuscular:* 1½-inch, 20-gauge, depending on solution and muscle size

      (4) Tourniquet for intravenous injections

III. IMPLEMENTING NURSING INTERVENTION

A. Physician's Order

1. All medications, including placebos, are given only by a physician's order.

2. All orders should include the name of the drug, dose, route, and time. If the route is not specified, the medication is to be given orally.

B. Preparation of Medications

1. It is the nurse's responsibility to be familiar with the drugs that she administers. She should review drug literature carefully on any unfamiliar drug, with regard to usual dose, route, and precautions or untoward effects. If in doubt about any drug ordered, consult the team leader, head nurse, or physician.

2. Check medication label with care 3 times during preparation of each medication:

   a. When container is removed from shelf (Fig. 59-1).

---

* Sterile gloves are used when the area of application is an open wound and for administration of urethral suppositories.

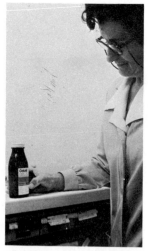

FIGURE 59.1

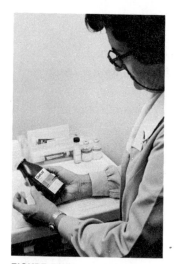

FIGURE 59.2

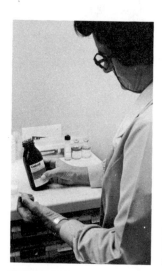

FIGURE 59.3

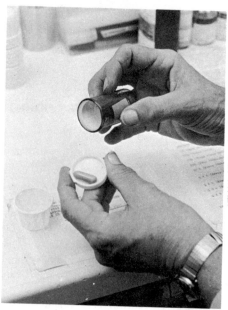

FIGURE 59.4

    b. While pouring or measuring dosage of medication (Fig. 59-2).

    c. Before container is replaced on shelf (Fig. 59-3).

3. Solid, stable dosage forms may be poured one hour before administration.

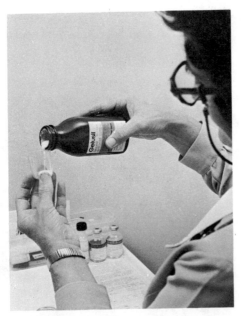

FIGURE 59.5

4. Preparation of dosage forms
   a. *Tablets, capsules:* Pour desired number into cap of bottle and from there into medicine cup (Fig. 59-4). *Do not* touch medications with fingers or return medications to container from cup.
   b. *Liquids:* Shake thoroughly, unless contraindicated on label. Pour medication with cup on level surface at eye level and with label in view (Fig. 59-5). Pour until the *bottom* of the meniscus is level with the desired amount marked on the cup. Use appropriately marked cup or syringe; *do not* estimate doses between marked lines. Wipe the edge of the bottle before replacing cap, so the cap does not stick.
   c. *Topical and inhalation drugs:* Prepare according to label.
   d. Injections
      (1) *From vial:* Cleanse rubber stopper thoroughly with alcohol sponge (Fig. 59-6). Inject air into vial in an amount equal to the solution to be withdrawn (Figs. 59-7, 59-8).
      (2) *From ampule:* File one side of the indented neck (Fig. 59-9) and, with the filed side toward you, break off the top of the ampule away from you, holding the top with a sponge (Fig. 59-10). If the ampule has a colored line around the neck, there is no need to file it (Fig. 59-11). The ampule may be inverted to facilitate withdrawal (Figs. 59-12, 59-13).

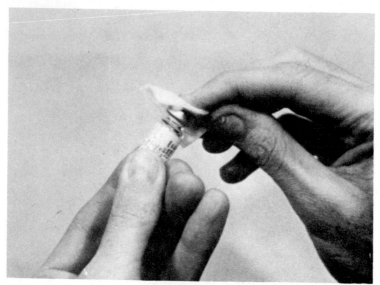

FIGURE 59.6

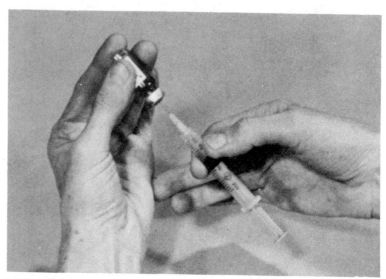

FIGURE 59.7

(3) *From tablet:* Pour tablet from container directly into disassembled glass syringe. Insert plunger and crush tablet. Draw diluent into syringe, being careful not to inject any of the tablet into diluent container. (If in doubt about contaminating solvent, discard.) Shake syringe until tablet dissolves in diluent.

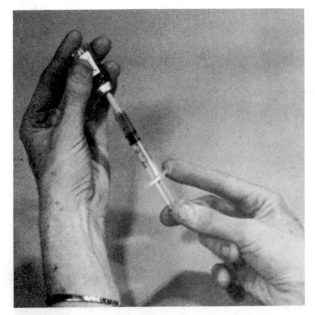

FIGURE 59.8

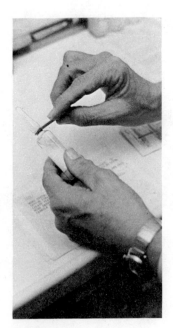

FIGURE 59.9

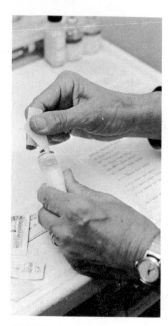

FIGURE 59.10

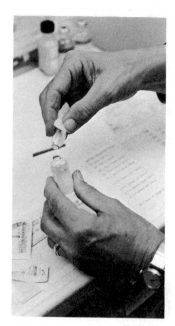

FIGURE 59.11

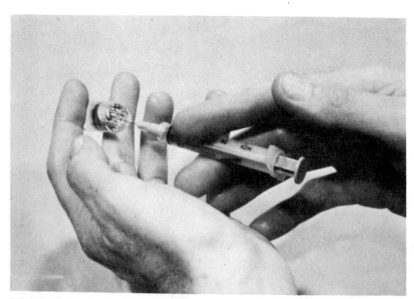

FIGURE 59.12

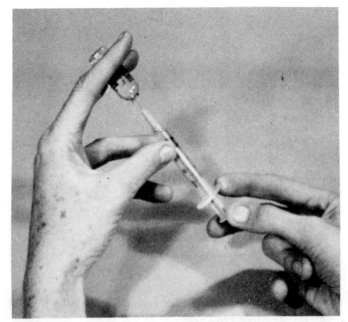

FIGURE 59.13

    e. Do not give drugs that have changed color, consistency, or odor.

    f. Do not give medications from containers unlabeled or with defaced labels. Only a pharmacist may fill bottles or change labels.

    g. Exercise caution in mixing medications. Do not give if they change or form a precipitate when mixed.

C. Nurses must use caution when converting from one system of measurement to another.

1. There are several methods of converting units, but all depend on knowing the basic equivalents:

$$
\begin{aligned}
64 \text{ to } 65 \text{ mg} &= 1 \text{ gr} \\
0.064 \text{ g} &= 1 \text{ gr} \\
1 \text{ g} &= 15 \text{ gr} \\
30 \text{ g} &= 1 \text{ oz} \\
1 \text{ ml} &= 15 \text{ m (minims)*} \\
30 \text{ ml} &= 1 \text{ fluid oz}
\end{aligned}
$$

*Both 15 m and 16 m are commonly used. There are exactly 15.43 m in 1 ml.

2. Any problem in conversion may be solved by making a proportion:

$$\frac{g}{gr} = \frac{g}{gr} \quad \text{Example: Convert 0.008 g to gr}$$

$$\frac{g}{gr} = \frac{g}{gr}$$

$$\frac{0.064 \text{ g}}{1 \text{ gr}} = \frac{0.008 \text{ g}}{x \text{ gr}}$$

$$0.0064 \text{ x} = 0.008$$

$$x = \frac{0.008}{0.064} = \frac{1}{8}$$

$$x = \frac{1}{8} \text{ gr}; \ 0.008 \text{ g} = \frac{1}{8} \text{ gr}$$

3. Summary, conversion:

    a. *Grams to grains:* $\dfrac{0.064 \text{ g}}{1 \text{ g}} = \dfrac{\text{known g}}{x \text{ g}}$

Or divide the number of grams by 0.064, or multiply the number of grams by 15.

    b. *Grains to grams:* $\dfrac{0.064 \text{ g}}{1 \text{ gr}} = \dfrac{x \text{ g}}{\text{known gr}}$

Or multiply the number of grains by 0.064, or divide the number of grains by 15.

    c. *Grams to ounces:* divide the number of grams by 30.

    d. *Ounces to grams:* multiply the number of ounces by 30.

    e. *Fluid ounces to milliliters:* multiply the number of fluid ounces by 30.

    f. *Milliliters to minims:* multiply the number of milliliters by 15.

    g. *Minims to milliliters:* divide the number of minims by 15.

4. Weight and liquid measures

    a. Approximate equivalents

    b. Always try to visualize the quantity with which you are concerned.

      (1) 1 m is about the size of a drop of water.

      (2) 1 g is approximately the weight of a drop of water.

      (3) 1 fluid dr is approximately a teaspoonful.

      (4) 1 teaspoonful of water weighs about 1 dr.

      (5) 1 oz almost fills a medicine or whiskey glass.

5. Table of approximate equivalents

    a. Weights

| APOTHECARY UNITS | | METRIC UNITS | | HOUSEHOLD |
Weight	Liquid	Weight	Liquid	UNITS
1 g	1 m	0.064 g	0.010 ml (or cc)	1 drop
15 g	15 m	1 g	1 ml	15 drops
1 dr (or 60 g)	1 fluid dr (or 60 m)	4 g	4 ml	1 t (or 60 drops)
1 oz	1 fluid oz	30 g	30 ml	2 T
1 lb	12 oz	360 g	360 ml	2 teacupsful
	1 pt	500 g	500 ml	2 glassesful
	1 qt	1 kg	1 liter or 1,000 ml	4 glassesful
	1 gal	4 kg	4 liter or 4,000 ml	16 glassesful

METRIC	APOTHECARY
30 g	1 oz (480 gr)
4 g	1 dr (60 gr)
1 g	15 gr
0.64 g (600 mg)	10 gr
0.32 g (300 mg)	5 gr
0.096 g (90 mg)	$1\frac{1}{2}$ gr
0.064 g (60 mg)	1 gr
0.048 g (50 mg)	$\frac{3}{4}$ gr
0.040 g (40 mg)	$\frac{2}{3}$ gr
0.032 g (30 mg)	$\frac{1}{2}$ gr
0.022 g (20 mg)	$\frac{1}{3}$ gr
0.016 g (15 mg)	$\frac{1}{4}$ gr
0.012 g (12 mg)	$\frac{1}{5}$ gr
0.010 g (10 mg)	$\frac{1}{6}$ gr
0.008 g (8 mg)	$\frac{1}{8}$ gr
0.0064 g (6 mg)	$\frac{1}{10}$ gr
0.005 g (5 mg)	$\frac{1}{12}$ gr
0.004 g (4 mg)	$\frac{1}{15}$ gr
0.0032 g (3 mg)	$\frac{1}{20}$ gr
0.0022 g (2 mg)	$\frac{1}{30}$ gr
0.0015 g (1.5 mg)	$\frac{1}{40}$ gr
0.0012 g (1.2 mg)	$\frac{1}{50}$ gr
0.001 g (1 mg)	$\frac{1}{60}$ gr
0.0008 g (0.8 mg)	$\frac{1}{72}$ gr
0.0006 g (0.6 mg)	$\frac{1}{100}$ gr
0.0005 g (0.5 mg)	$\frac{1}{120}$ gr
0.0004 g (0.4 mg)	$\frac{1}{150}$ gr
0.0003 g (0.3 mg)	$\frac{1}{200}$ gr
0.00025 g (0.25 mg)	$\frac{1}{250}$ gr
0.0002 g (0.2 mg)	$\frac{1}{300}$ gr

b.Volume

	METRIC	APOTHECARY
	30 ml (or cc)	1 fluid oz (490 m)
	10 ml	2½ fluid dr
	4 ml	1 fluid dr (60 m)
	1 ml	15 m (16m)*
	0.6 ml	10 m
	0.3 ml	5 m
	0.06 ml	1 m
	500 ml	1 pt
	1,000 ml (1 liter)	1 qt

D. Administration of Medications

1. Routine medications should be administered within 30 min of the designated time. Caution should be exercised in giving such medications as antibiotics and chemotherapeutic agents at the designated time in order to maintain blood levels.

2. Stat and pre-op orders must be given exactly on time.

3. The nurse who prepares the medication should also administer and chart it.

4. Identify the patient before administering any drug by checking the medication card with the bed card and the patient's ID band and by calling the patient by name (Figs. 59-14, 59-15, 59-16, 59-17).

5. If the patient refuses the drug, report to the team leader, discard the dose down the sink, and chart the reason for refusal.

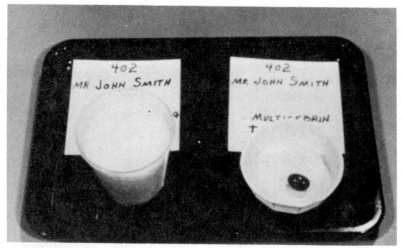

FIGURE 59.14

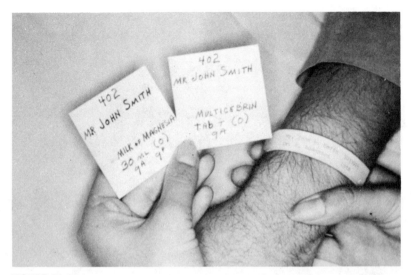

FIGURE 59.15

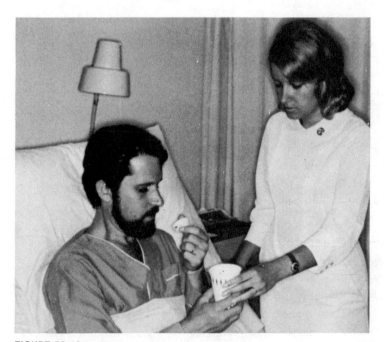

FIGURE 59.16

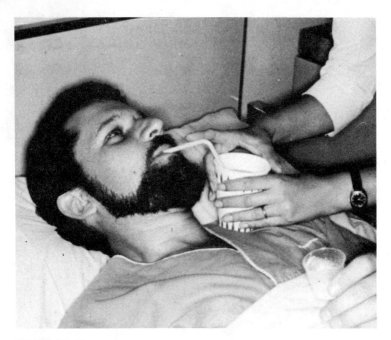

FIGURE 59.17

6. If the patient vomits soon after oral medications, attempt to identify the medications. Report to the physician, and do not repeat the medications unless ordered.

7. Medications should not be left at the bedside, with the following possible exceptions:

   a. Antacids

   b. Cough syrups (non-narcotic)

   c. Eye medications

   d. Inhalants

   e. Lotions, ointments

   f. Nitroglycerin

E. Special Precautions for Special Drugs

1. Two qualified persons should check dosage on insulin, anticoagulants, digitalis preparations, and IV medications.

2. Digitalis preparations

   a. Note pulse rate before giving drug (Fig. 59-18).

   b. Notify the physician before giving the drug if the apical pulse is below 60.

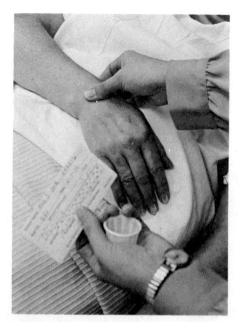

FIGURE 59.18

3. Heparin
   a. 0.1 ml of air is injected following the heparin to prevent leaking and hemorrhage into intradermal layers.
   b. Always inject into subcutaneous tissues of abdomen or iliac crest, as these sites are away from major muscle groups, reducing the possibility of hematoma.
   c. *Do not* draw back on plunger to check vein insertion, as this causes the needle to waver and produces a hematoma.
   d. Never massage the site, for fear of rupturing small vessels and causing a hematoma.
4. Insulin
   a. Rotate sites according to a definite plan (Fig. 59-19).
   b. When mixing regular and long-acting insulins, draw up the regular insulin first, to avoid contaminating it with the insoluble long-acting insulin. (Regular insulin should be kept clear, so it can be given IV in an emergency.)
5. Narcotics
   a. Record respirations before giving narcotics, as most narcotics have a selective depressant action on the respiratory center. A respiration rate of below 12 is considered too depressed for administering a narcotic.

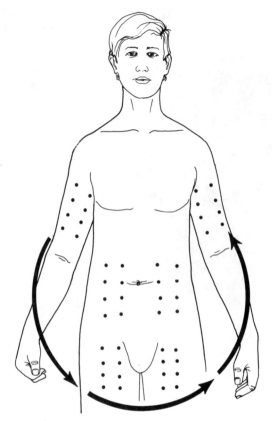

FIGURE 59.19

    b. The nurse shall also record pulse as an indicator of pain and to show its relationship with the respirations.

6. Paraldehyde is always given with a glass syringe, since it reacts chemically with plastic.

7. PRN: Check patient record to ensure that sufficient time has elapsed since last dose. Chart immediately after giving a dose and record reason for giving.

F. Therapeutic Aspects

1. Oral drugs—solids

    a. The nurse should avoid handling the oral medication and should introduce it into the patient's mouth with the cup, in order to avoid contamination.

    b. Stimulation of the back of the tongue produces the swallowing reflex. Therefore, if the patient has difficulty swallowing tablets, they should be placed far back in his throat.

    c. Fluids administered with a drug facilitate swallowing and hasten absorption from the gastrointestinal tract.

2. Oral drugs—liquids

    a. Dilution of a drug hastens its absorption. All liquid drugs should be diluted with ½ oz water or juice, except cough syrups, oils, and antacids.

    b. Some drugs harmful to tooth enamel, such as acid (corrosive) and iron (staining), hydrochloric acid, liquid iron preparations, and other potentially destructive drugs, should be given with a straw.

3. Inhalation drugs should be administered according to label directions.

4. Topical drugs—ophthalmic

    a. The patient should be positioned with his head back, since a dependent position aids gravitational flow. The eyelid should be cleansed of secretions prior to administration of medication.

    b. Pressure on the eye structure itself may cause damage. The patient should be instructed to open his eyes and look up. The eyelid is then held open by gentle pressure on the bony prominences.

    c. The cornea is very sensitive and may be easily damaged. Medication should be directed into the lower conjunctiva rather than directly on the corneal surface.

    d. Absorption of the excess drug by way of the nose and pharynx may lead to toxic symptoms. Using a sterile cotton ball, the nurse should gently press over the inner canthus to prevent the medication draining down the lacrimal duct.

    e. Once the medication bottle is opened, it is not sterile. To prevent spread of microorganisms, no part of the eye should be touched with the applicator.

5. Topical drugs—otic

    a. Straightening the ear canal allows the solution to reach all areas of the canal cavity. To accomplish this, the patient should be in a recumbent position on the unaffected side. Pull the ear up and back gently to allow the drops to fall to the side of the canal. The patient should remain lying on the unaffected side for several minutes, to allow the solution to reach all areas of the canal cavity.

6. Topical drugs—nasal

    a. Hyperextension of the head enables the medication to be better absorbed into the nares.

    Since microorganisms are spread by direct contact, care should be taken to see that the dropper does not come in contact with nostril mucosa. This is accomplished by gently raising the tip of the nostril to insert the drops (Fig. 59-20).

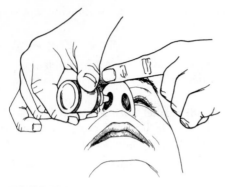

FIGURE 59.20

7. Topical drugs—liquids and semi-solids
   Apply according to label directions.

8. Topical drugs—solid, sublingual
   The rich blood supply under the tongue creates an avenue of rapid absorption. The tablet should be placed under the patient's tongue to dissolve.

9. Topical drugs—suppositories
   a. *Urethral suppository:* Microorganisms introduced into the urethra can ascend to the kidneys, causing renal infection. The perineal area should be cleansed and the suppository inserted using sterile technique (see Technique 35, Catheterization, Urethral).
   b. *Vaginal suppository:* The vagina has no sphincter to prevent the suppository from running out after it has melted. The patient should be placed in lithotomy position, with the hips slightly elevated. After lubricating the suppository, it should be inserted as far into the vagina as it will go. The medicine may be inserted by hand (covered by a sterile glove) or by an applicator. The patient should remain with hips elevated for 5 minutes.
   c. *Rectal suppository:* The anal canal is approximately 1 in long in the adult. Insertion of the suppository 2 in ensures passing the internal sphincter and facilitates retention. The buttocks should be spread and the lubricated suppository inserted with a clean gloved finger (Figs. 59-21, 59-22).

10. Parenteral drugs, intradermal injection
    a. The medial forearm gives a good visualization of the response to testing media.
    b. The skin should be cleansed with an alcohol sponge, using firm circular motions moving from the center outward. The needle is inserted with the bevel up at a 15° angle until just the tip is un-

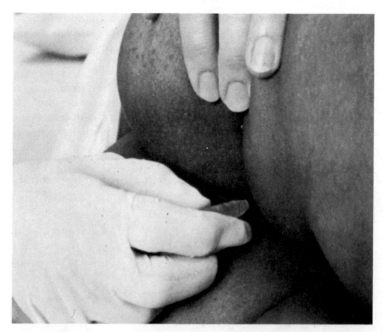

FIGURE 59.21

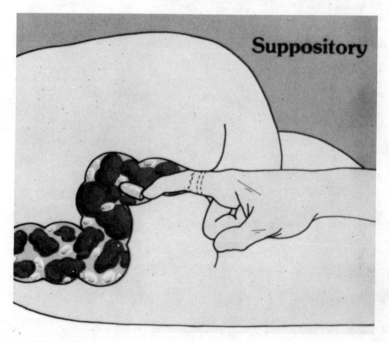

FIGURE 59.22

der the outer layer of skin (Fig. 59-23A, B). Injection of the solution should cause formation of a small blister or bleb.

11. Parenteral drugs, subcutaneous (hypodermic) injection

a. See previous cautions on insulin and heparin.

b. Any surface with loose connective tissues free from large blood vessels and nerves is acceptable. Usual sites are the outer aspects of the thighs. These sites are poorly supplied with sensory nerves and cause less pain than other sites. Rotation of sites lessens irritation and improves absorption (Fig. 59-24).

c. Microorganisms normally found on the skin may be removed by cleansing with an alcohol sponge in a circular motion from the center outward.

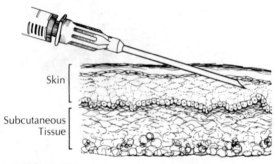

Skin

Subcutaneous
Tissue

FIGURE 59.23A

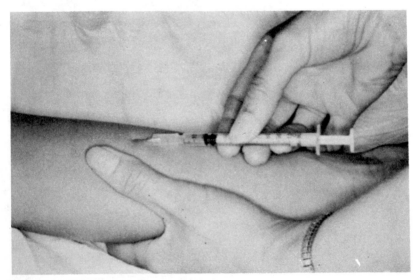

FIGURE 59.23B

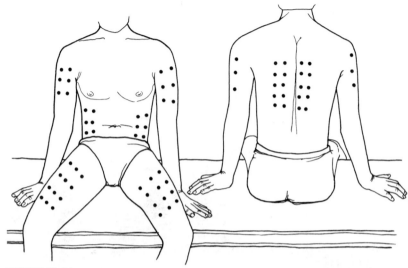

FIGURE 59.24

d. Elevating the subcutaneous tissue helps prevent the needle from entering the muscle. The tissue surrounding the injection site should be held in a cushion fashion. Subcutaneous tissue is abundant in well-nourished persons and sparse in emaciated or dehydrated persons.

e. The needle should be inserted at an angle between 30 to 90 degrees, depending on the amount and turgor of the tissue (Fig. 59-25A,B).

f. Injection of solutions into compressed tissue causes pressure against nerve endings and pain. Once the needle is inserted, the tissue should be released.

g. Substances injected into a blood vessel are absorbed immediately, possibly endangering the patient. The plunger of the syringe should be pulled back gently to determine if the needle is in a blood vessel. If blood appears, withdraw the needle partway and insert in a different direction, testing again to see if the needle is in a vessel. When no blood appears, inject the solution slowly.

h. The needle should be quickly withdrawn, to prevent tissue pulling and pain. Gentle rubbing of the area with an alcohol sponge aids in distribution and absorption of the solution.

12. Parenteral drugs, intramuscular injection

a. Approximately 0.2 or 0.3 ml of air should be drawn into the syringe after the medication has been drawn up. The lighter air bubble rises to the top of the heavier solution. This cleanses the needle and prevents leakage of irritating solution back into the subcutaneous tissues as the needle is withdrawn.

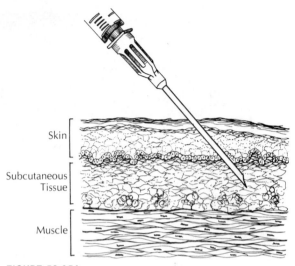

Skin

Subcutaneous Tissue

Muscle

FIGURE 59.25A

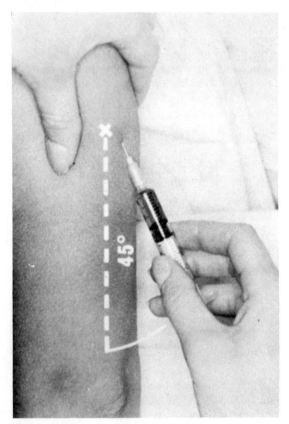

FIGURE 59.25B

b. The patient should assume a comfortable position; injection into a tense muscle causes pain (Fig. 59-26A,B). Drawing in a deep breath may help the patient relax. The injection site should be in a large muscle away from large blood vessels and nerves. Usual sights include the dorsogluteal, ventrogluteal and vastus lateralis

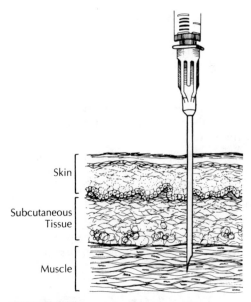

Skin

Subcutaneous Tissue

Muscle

FIGURE 59.26A

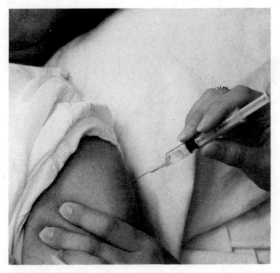

FIGURE 59.26B

(anterolateral thigh) in the adult. The deltoid and anterior thigh may also be used (Fig. 59-27).

c. Stimulation of peripheral nerves helps minimize the initial reaction when the needle is inserted. This can be accomplished by gently tapping the selected site with the fingers several times.

d. Microorganisms normally found on the skin may be removed by cleansing with an alcohol sponge in a circular motion, from the center outward.

e. Muscle tissue is vascular, and intramuscular solutions injected intravenously could endanger the patient. Pulling back on the plunger will help verify that the needle is not in a vein. If no blood appears, the medicine should be injected slowly to prevent pain. Quick removal of the needle minimizes pain and tissue trauma. Massaging the injection site aids in the distribution and adsorption of the medication.

13. Parenteral drugs, intramuscular Z-track. Same procedure as for IM injection, except:

a. The gluteus maximus is a large muscle, able to absorb irritating substances. It is the only site considered adequate for the Z-track method.

b. Compress the subcutaneous tissue. This helps ensure the needle enters muscle tissue. Then displace the subcutaneous tissue later-

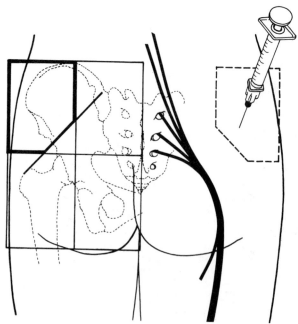

FIGURE 59.27

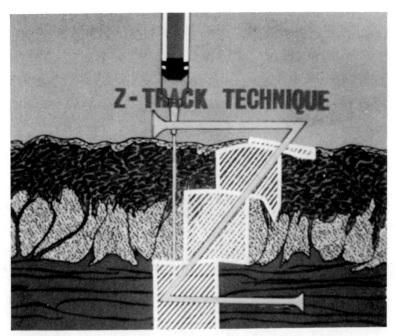

FIGURE 59.28

ally before injection, causing the needle tract to be sealed off when the tissues are relaxed after injection (Fig. 59-28).

c. Before releasing the tissue, wait 10 sec after injection of the medication. This delay and a 0.2 to 0.3 ml air bubble help seal off the injected fluid and prevent leakage back into subcutaneous tissue.

d. *Do not massage* the injection site. Tissue compression may force the solution back along the needle path and into the subcutaneous tissues.

14. Parenteral drugs, intravenous injection (see also Technique 57, Intravenous (IV) Infusion Administration)

a. Absorption by way of the vascular system is immediate. The literature should be reviewed carefully regarding suitability of drugs for IV use, dilution requirements, and safe rate of administration.

b. Diluent used for previous drugs may have been accidentally contaminated by these drugs. The medication should be diluted according to directions, using an unopened sterile vial of diluent.

c. Pathogens present on IV tubing may be forced directly into the bloodstream by the needle. For IV injection when patent IV infusion is present, the rubber portion of the IV tubing is cleansed with alcohol. The IV is clamped and the needle (25-gauge) inserted through the self-sealing double wall. For direct IV injection, the skin is cleansed with an alcohol sponge and venipuncture is made. Frequent aspiration of blood will ensure that the needle is in the vein.

    d. Too rapid absorption of drugs may cause toxic reactions or shock. The drugs should be injected slowly, at a rate specified by the drug literature. Following an IV medication, the IV tubing is unclamped, and patency is reestablished.

G. Communicative Aspects

1. *Observations*

    a. After the administration of any drug, the patient's reaction should be observed for: desired results, such as reduction of pain and fever; expected side effects, such as dryness of the mouth, and vertigo; untoward reactions, such as anaphylactic reactions.

2. *Charting*

    a. All medications given must be charted somewhere in the patient's legal record.

    b. Any reactions and pulse and respirations for narcotics are charted in the nurses' notes.

    c. If, for any reason, a scheduled dose is omitted, explanation is made in the nurses' notes.

DATE	TREATMENT	TIME	OBSERVATIONS	SIGNATURE
6/20	IM narcotic	1000	Demerol 75 mg given for pain in incision area. P 96, R 22.	
		1030	Sleeping quietly now. R 14. Pain apparently decreased.	B. Smith, L.V.N.

DATE	TREATMENT	TIME	OBSERVATIONS	SIGNATURE
8/14		0800	Digitoxin 0.1 mg p.o. withheld due to pulse of 52 and regular. Dr. D. notified. ECG done as ordered. Condition appears stable with no dyspnea or cyanosis.	C. Allen, L.V.N.

3. *Referrals*

Not applicable

H. Teaching Aspects—Patient and Family

1. If the patient is to be sent home with medication, he and his family need to know how to give the medication and what reactions to report to the physician.

2. If the patient has an untoward reaction to a drug, he needs to know the name of the drug (including trade and generic names) and that he should caution medical personnel about his allergy in the future.

3. Most patients should know what drugs they are receiving—it is their right. It is best that this be explained by the physician. The professional nurse, in certain situations, may need to explain the medications. The patient may need to know only the classification of the drug (blood pressure pill, antibiotic, pain shot), but sometimes it is vital for him to know the name (Digitalis, Regular or Lente Insulin, for instance).

IV. EVALUATION PROCESS

A. Is the patient mentally and physically comfortable?

B. Was the right drug given to the right patient at the right time in the right dose by the right route?

C. Does the patient or family understand what is necessary for them to understand?

D. Were precautions taken to guard against adverse reactions?

E. Was the desired effect achieved?

60

Oral Hygiene

I. ASSESSMENT OF SITUATION

A. Definition

The process of cleaning and freshening the teeth, gums, and mouth

B. Terminology

Dentures: artificially constructed teeth

C. Rationale for Actions

1. To keep the teeth, gums, and mouth in good condition
2. To freshen the mouth and relieve it of offensive odors
3. To prevent sores and infections
4. To provide a sense of well-being and comfort

II. NURSING PLAN

A. Objectives

1. To carry out oral hygiene measures as often as necessary to maintain a healthy, fresh mouth

2. To observe the teeth, gums, and mucous membranes carefully for early signs of soreness and infection

3. To teach the patient and family good oral hygiene and preventive care

B. Patient Preparation

A person must be motivated before he will accept and carry out daily oral hygiene. A great deal of patient teaching on the importance of good mouth care and preventive dentistry will enhance the patient's desire to care for his teeth properly.

C. Equipment

1. Toothbrush and toothpaste

2. Curved basin

3. Towel

4. Cool water and cup

5. Mouthwash

6. Medicated swabs, if needed (*e.g.,* lemon and glycerin)

7. Bulb syringe, if needed

III. IMPLEMENTING NURSING INTERVENTION

A. Therapeutic Aspects

1. Transmission of microorganisms may be avoided if proper hand-washing technique is utilized before and after oral hygiene is carried out. Oral care is usually given at the time of the daily bath to enhance overall comfort, and whenever deemed necessary or desirable by the patient or the nurse.

2. If the patient cannot sit up, he should be turned on his side with his face along the edge of the pillow. A towel and curved basin under his chin will serve as a receptacle for the rinsing water.

3. The toothbrush should have stiff bristles, to enable pressure to be placed on the gingivae (gums). Since warm water softens the bristles, the toothbrush should be rinsed with cool water before applying a strip of toothpaste to it.

4. The oral cavity contains a balanced biological system of microorganisms. Oral care should be designed to remove retained food debris, rather than to remove all organisms from the mouth. Brushing in the direction of tooth growth will facilitate removal of food particles, as well as stimulate the gums. One section of the mouth should be done

at a time. Bristles should be parallel to tooth surface, free edges up, and should extend beyond gum line. Turning bristles toward teeth, with one sweeping stroke, brings the tips firmly over gum tissue and tooth surface (Fig. 60-1, A-K). Repeat this stroke 5 times in each section of the mouth, both inside and out.

5. The gum tissue is sensitive, so care must be taken not to cause bleeding due to too much force.

6. The patient should rinse his mouth with cool water or mouthwash, to facilitate removal of loosened food particles and toothpaste, as well as to leave a fresh, clean taste in the mouth.

7. The unconscious patient

   a. Aspiration of fluids can occur if body alignment is not altered to facilitate drainage. The patient's head must be turned well to the side. The teeth are brushed gently in the above manner. A padded tongue blade may be used to gently separate the upper and lower teeth, for better exposure.

   b. Careful irrigation of the mouth with a bulb syringe and small amounts of water, followed by quick and complete retrieval of all rinsing solution, will help remove food particles. Extreme care to avoid aspiration of fluids into the trachea is mandatory.

   c. Mucous membranes tend to dry quickly when the patient is not receiving oral fluids, is mouth-breathing, or is receiving inhalation gases, such as oxygen. Mouth care may thus need to be done as often as every hour.

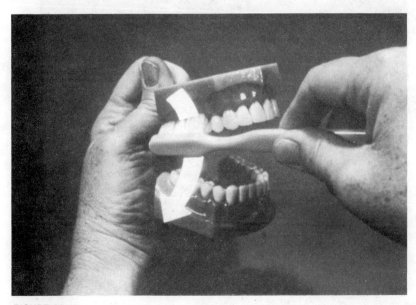

FIGURE 60.1A

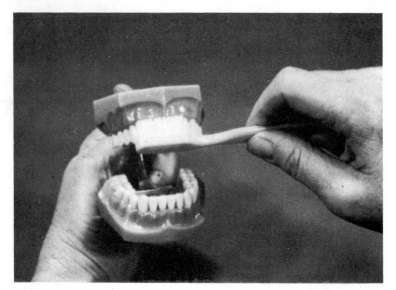

FIGURE 60.1B

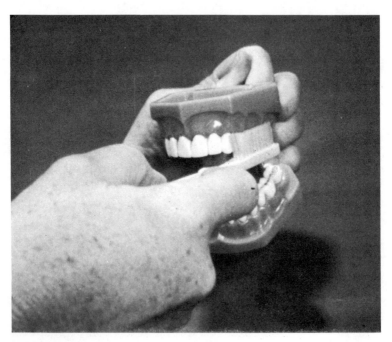

FIGURE 60.1C

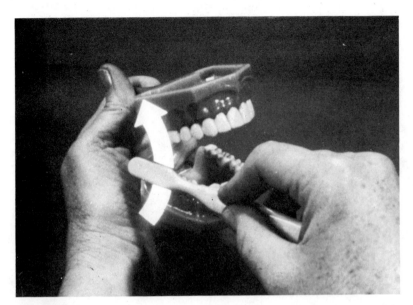

FIGURE 60.1D

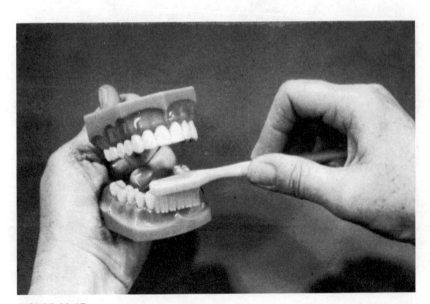

FIGURE 60.1E

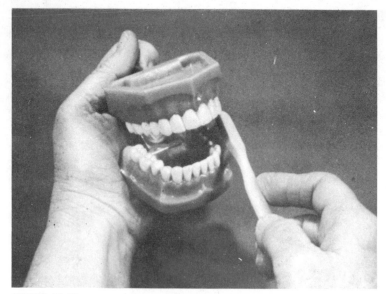

FIGURE 60.1F

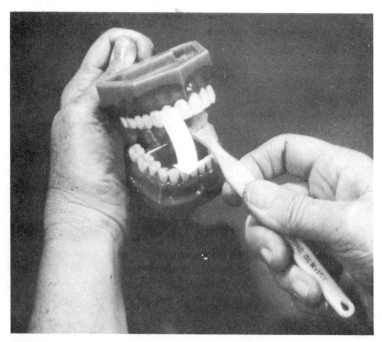

FIGURE 60.1G

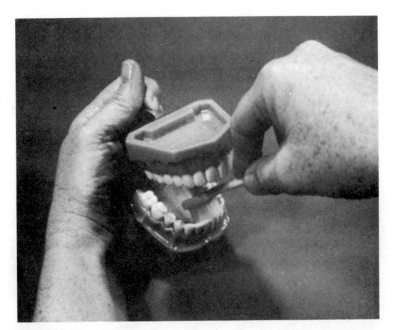

FIGURE 60.1H

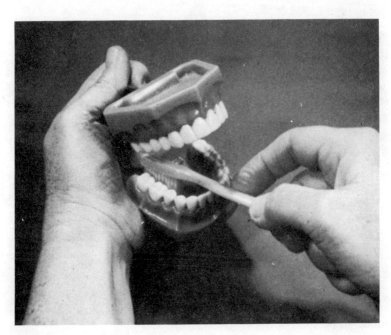

FIGURE 60.1I

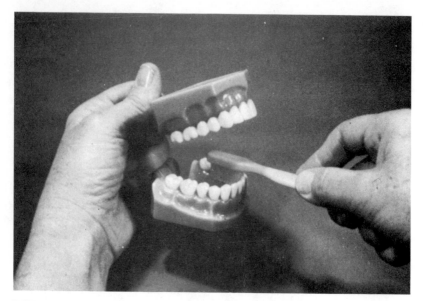

FIGURE 60.1J

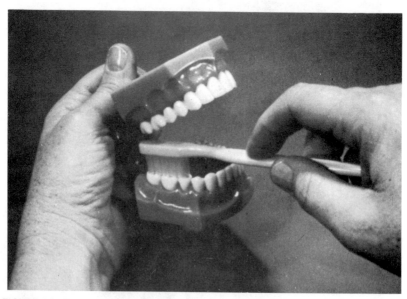

FIGURE 60.1K

8. Care of dentures (See also Technique 41, Dentures, Care of).

   a. Accumulation of food particles or mucous on dentures becomes unsightly and difficult to remove if allowed to remain too long. Dentures may be removed from patient's mouth when cleaned. A stiff brush will facilitate the removal of debris. The dentures should be held over a pan of water during cleaning, so that they will not be broken if dropped. Dentures should be washed in cold water, to prevent their becoming misshapen. A medicated swab or toothbrush may be used to clean the patient's mouth and gums while the dentures are out.

   b. Proper storage of dentures is also important. To prevent damage and patient embarrassment at others seeing the dentures, they should be stored in an opaque container. However, since gum changes can occur if dentures are left out too long, the patient should be encouraged to wear them as much as possible.

   c. To facilitate reinsertion of dentures and to reduce friction, they should be rinsed with cold water before being replaced in the mouth.

B. Communicative Aspects

1. *Observations*

   a. Note condition of teeth and gums.

   b. Assess effectiveness of oral hygiene.

   c. Note signs of infections or irritated areas and the presence of halitosis.

2. *Charting*

DATE	TREATMENT	TIME	OBSERVATIONS	SIGNATURE
5/2	Oral hygiene	1000	Patient assisted with procedure. Gums appear less red and swollen. Teeth appear in good condition.	D. Young, N.T.

3. *Referrals*

   The American Dental Association has many brochures and samples available.

C. Teaching Aspects—Patient and Family

1. If patient's teeth or mouth appear to be in poor condition, the nurse should find out how the patient has been caring for mouth and then make suggestions for improvement.

2. If patient's mouth is in obvious need of attention, recommend that the patient see his dentist and stress the importance of regular dental care.

3. The family can be included, whether teaching consists of normal care or teaching them how to care for a relative unable to care for himself.

IV. EVALUATION PROCESS

A. Have oral hygiene measures been carried out often enough to promote a healthy, fresh mouth?

B. Have mouth or gum problems been detected and treated?

C. Has the patient been taught the correct methods of caring for his teeth and mouth?

D. Does the patient understand the importance of proper dental care?

61

Paracentesis (Abdominal and Thoracic), Assisting With

I. ASSESSMENT OF SITUATION

A. Definition

1. *Abdominal paracentesis:* aspiration of fluid from the peritoneal cavity

2. *Thoracic paracentesis* (thoracentesis): aspiration of fluid or air from the pleural cavity

B. Terminology

1. *Pleural cavity:* a potential space located between the visceral pleura covering the lung and the parietal pleura lining the rib cage

2. *Peritoneal cavity:* a potential space between the visceral peritoneum and the abdominal wall peritoneum

3. *Ascites:* accumulation of serous fluid in the peritoneal cavity

4. *Syncope:* fainting; a transient loss of consciousness

C. Rationale for Action

1. To reduce pressure on vital organs

2. To aid physician in diagnosis

II. NURSING PLAN

A. Objectives

1. To allay the patient's fear and anxiety regarding the procedure by adequate preparation
2. To prevent or reduce infection
3. To observe and record any adverse effects during or after procedure
4. To record site of puncture, characteristics of drainage, and amount of fluid obtained
5. To maintain fluid and electrolyte balances

B. Patient Preparation

1. Since the site of needle insertion is in close proximity to vital organs, it is essential that the patient remain quiet and immobile during the procedure, especially during the insertion phase. A thorough explanation of what will occur and how the nurse will help by physical support may help allay anxiety and promote cooperation.
2. For the legal protection of the patient, nurse, physician, and hospital, a surgical consent form should be signed by the patient and witnessed by two persons of legal age.
3. The urinary bladder is subject to rupture if damaged when distended. The patient should, therefore, void before undergoing paracentesis.
4. Pathogens on the skin and hair could be introduced into the body cavity through the puncture site. The skin should be prepared with an antiseptic solution and shaved if necessary. Instruments must be sterile. Maintenance of aseptic conditions throughout the procedure reduces the possibility of infection.

C. Equipment

1. Thoracentesis or paracentesis tray (with needles, knife handle and blades, trocar and cannula, rubber tubing, syringes, and basins)
2. Procaine hydrochloride (Novocaine), 1%
3. Merthiolate, 1:1,000
4. Large basin
5. Adhesive tape
6. Sterile gloves
7. Laboratory requisition, if indicated
8. Large supercatheter (optional, at physician's request)
9. Intravenous tubing (optional, at physician's request)
10. 3-way stopcock

III. IMPLEMENTING NURSING INTERVENTION

A. Therapeutic Aspects

1. *Abdominal paracentesis:* after the area has been prepared, the physician will apply sterile drapes around the puncture site. He may then inject a small amount of local anesthetic to minimize pain when the cannula and trocar are inserted. The usual site for paracentesis is mid-way between the umbilicus and symphysis pubis, in the center of the abdomen. All equipment used is sterile, and the physician will don sterile gloves prior to beginning the procedure. A small incision is made, through which the cannula and trocar are passed. The trocar, which has previously plugged up the cannula, is removed, allowing the fluid to flow through the cannula. The tubing is connected to the cannula, and the open end is placed in a basin or bottle. The physician may simply wish to aspirate with a 30 to 50 ml syringe and then remove the cannula. If the tubing is to be left in place, it must be adequately secured with adhesive tape and covered with a sterile bandage. The end of the tubing must be secured in the drainage bottle.

2. The patient should be physically supported and reassured while the physician inserts the needle and trocar. A sudden or unexpected movement by the patient can cause trauma to vital organs.

3. *Thoracentesis:* the procedure is the same as for paracentesis, with the following exceptions. The patient should be in an upright postion. He should sit on the bedside, if possible, leaning forward, supported by an overbed table or the nurse (Fig. 61-1). Fluid tends to localize in the base of a body cavity, because of gravity, and the upright posi-

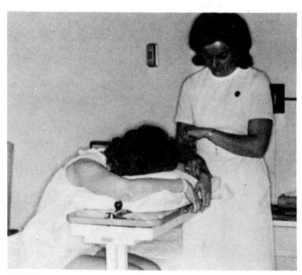

FIGURE 61.1

tion facilitates the removal of fluid. The patient should be warned not to cough or move suddenly during the procedure. Preparation is the same as for paracentesis. The physician determines the site of puncture by percussion and auscultation of the fluid level. The thoracentesis needle is inserted through the intercostal space, into the pleural cavity (Fig. 61-2). The fluid is then withdrawn by direct aspiration with a syringe. A three-way stopcock is used to remove the fluid from the syringe and still keep the system airtight. The needle may be connected to a negative-pressure drainage setup, if desired.

4. Pressure and dressings permit the puncture site to seal itself. After the physician withdraws the needle, pressure and a small dressing or Band-Aid are applied to the puncture site.

5. Place the patient on his unaffected side after thoracentesis. This prevents seepage caused by coughing or gravitational force.

B. Communicative Aspects

1. *Observations*

   a. *Thoracentesis*

      (1) Evaluate at frequent intervals for syncope, vertigo, tightness in chest, uncontrollable cough, blood-tinged frothy mucus, and rapid pulse. Pneumothorax and tension may result from thoracentesis. Pulmonary edema or cardiac distress can be produced by a sudden shift in mediastinal contents when large amounts of fluid are aspirated.

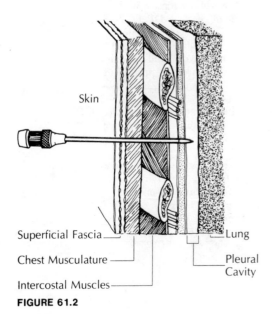

Skin

Superficial Fascia

Chest Musculature

Intercostal Muscles

Lung

Pleural Cavity

FIGURE 61.2

(2) Record the amount of fluid withdrawn, its color, odor, and viscosity.

b. *Abdominal paracentesis*

(1) During the procedure and after, attention should be given to physical status, pulse, respirations, and skin color.

(2) The patient must be observed for untoward reactions associated with electrolyte imbalance.

(3) Record the amount, color, odor, and viscosity of the fluid aspirated.

(4) After the procedure, dressings should be checked frequently. If ascites develops rapidly, the patient will need frequent changes of dressing, clothing, and bedding.

2. *Charting*

DATE	TREATMENT	TIME	OBSERVATIONS	SIGNATURE
5/26	Thora-centesis	0900	Dr. D. visited patient prior to thoracentesis. Procedure explained to patient and wife.	
		0910	Operative permit signed. Demerol 100 mg. IM given as ordered. P 88; R 26. Patient taken to treatment room by way of cart.	
		0930	Left side of chest prepared with merthiolate, 1:1,000. 10 ml 1% procaine hydrochloride (Novocaine) injected into left side of chest by Dr. D. P 88; R 26; color good. Sterile specimen obtained; 250 ml clear, odorless fluid obtained. Pressure dressing applied to puncture site. Specimen sent to lab.	
		0945	Patient placed on right side; patient returned to room 650 by way of cart. P 86; R 22.	
		1000	Patient resting quietly; states he feels much better.	
		1045	Patient remained on right side for 1 hour; no seepage from puncture site. P 84; R 22.	G. Ivers, R.N.

3. *Referrals*

Not applicable

C. Teaching Aspects—Patient and Family

1. Instruct the patient having thoracentesis to stay on the unaffected side for 1 hour after completion of procedure.
2. Instruct patient and family to report any discomfort to the nurse.

IV. EVALUATION PROCESS

A. Did the patient cooperate by remaining immobile or turning as directed?

B. Did the patient's apprehension decrease during or after the procedure?

C. Was there a reduction in the patient's ascites as a result of the procedure?

D. Was coughing or discomfort due to accumulation of pleural fluid decreased after fluid aspiration?

E. Is the environment free from infection hazard?

F. Was the specimen disposed of properly or sent to the laboratory?

G. Is the patient comfortable due to adequate dressing changes?

62

Pediculosis, Nursing Care

I. ASSESSMENT OF SITUATION

A. Definition

An infestation with lice

B. Terminology

1. *Body louse:* a parasite which lives chiefly in the seams of undergarments, to which it clings. Its bite causes characteristic minute hemorrhagic points and a great deal of itching.

2. *Nits:* lice eggs on hair shafts; they are white or light gray and look like dandruff, but they cannot be brushed or shaken off the hair.

3. *Pediculicides:* preparations for the treatment of pediculosis, designed to kill the lice, inactivate nits, and relieve the generalized discomfort

4. *Pediculus humanus, var. capitis:* variety of lice that infests the hair and scalp

5. *Pediculus humanus, var. corporis:* variety of lice that infests the body

6. *Phthirus pubis:* variety of lice that infests the shorter hairs on the body, usually the pubic and axillary hair

C. Rationale for Actions

1. To relieve itching and scratching

2. To destroy lice and their eggs (nits)

3. To sterilize infested clothing

4. To give hygienic care and prevent spread of condition

II. NURSING PLAN

A. Objectives

1. To assure and inform the patient and family in regard to pediculicide applications

2. To relieve the physical and emotional manifestations of the patient's condition

3. To prevent the spread of pediculosis from person to person

B. Patient Preparation

1. The problem of pediculosis can be greatly reduced by patient education. This education should begin during the preparatory phase of treatment with thorough explanations about the spread and prevention of pediculosis. As the equipment is brought to the room, the patient or family member should be told how the procedure is done so that it can be repeated at home if necessary.

2. Chances of spreading the condition can be reduced if all equipment is gathered before the procedure is begun. This will eliminate the need to leave the room or have other personnel enter during the treatment.

C. Equipment

1. Pediculicides, as ordered by the physician

2. Shampoo

3. Comb and brush

4. Bath towels

5. Safety pins

6. Gauze, to protect eyes

7. Gloves and gown

8. Bland ointment for skin, if ordered by physician

III. IMPLEMENTING NURSING INTERVENTION

A. Therapeutic Aspects

1. Hair and scalp

    a. Pediculosis can be spread directly, by contact with infested areas, or indirectly, through clothing, bed linens, combs, brushes, and so on. The nurse must take precautions to minimize the chance of spreading the infestation by wearing a gown, gloves, and cap when treating this patient.

    b. Pediculicides may be irritating to the patient's eyes. For protection, his eyes should be covered with gauze bandages prior to the application of medication. Techniques of application vary for different medications. The nurse should read the directions accompanying the medication which has been ordered. Usually the medicine is applied to the entire scalp area. A clean towel may then be used to cover the head (with face exposed) for the specified length of time (usually 15 minutes). The towel is then removed and discarded in a specially marked linen hamper. All linen for this patient must go in this hamper. The lice and nits should be dead and easily removable at this time. Nits may also be removed by combing the hair with a fine-tooth comb that has been dipped in hot vinegar.

    c. After application of the medication to remove the lice and prevent skin irritation, the patient's head should be washed with shampoo or PhisoHex and warm water, being careful not to get it in the eyes and ears. A brush or comb will help remove the remaining lice.

    d. To prevent the further spread of pediculosis, the patient should put on a clean gown and sit in a clean chair as the nurse changes all bed linen. The linen is removed from the room in isolation bags, which are adequately labeled. The nurse's gown, gloves, and cap are removed similarly.

2. Axillary and pubic areas

    a. These areas receive basically the same treatment as the scalp. Towels are placed under the hips and axillary regions.

    b. The patient's privacy must be protected by screening and draping.

    c. The pediculicide is applied to the axillae and then to the pubic area. If the patient is a male, a male orderly should apply the medicine. The medication should remain on the hair for 15 minutes or as indicated. The medicated areas are then cleansed with soap or PhisoHex and warm water, to prevent skin irritation and remove the lice. The patient may bathe in a tub or shower, unless contraindicated. The tub or shower must then be thoroughly cleaned.

d. To prevent further spread of pediculosis, the patient should don a clean gown. The linen and nurse's apparel are removed as for pediculosis of the scalp.

B. Communicative Aspects

1. *Observations*

a. The nurse must have full cooperation from the patient, and he should be allowed to communicate his feelings about the infestation.

b. Observe and chart what the patient looks like, how the pediculosis and nits look, color of skin, cleanliness, if the patient scratches, any broken skin areas, how the patient reacts to the treatment of pediculosis, and the patient's feelings toward the nurse.

c. Watch for secondary complications, such as impetigo and eczema.

2. *Charting*

DATE	TREATMENT	TIME	OBSERVATIONS	SIGNATURE
4/27	Safety precautions taken to prevent spread of pediculosis. Nurse wearing gown and gloves.	0900	Procedure for treatment of pediculosis explained to patient in detail. Patient seemed nervous and apprehensive and asked about harm in pediculicides. Reassurance given by R.N. that every safety precaution will be taken.	
	Pediculicide applied to head for 15 minutes, and head covered with towel. Gauze over eyes for protection. Hair then shampooed with PhisoHex and warm water.	0930	There are greyish, glistening, oval bodies in the hair and scalp. After medication was applied and left on for the prescribed time, the hair was shampooed and brushed to eliminate the pediculi. Skin is not reddened or irritated.	
		1000	Linens changed. Procedure tolerated well by patient.	F. White, R.N.

3. *Referrals*

A public health referral may be expeditious, especially in eliminating infestation in the home.

C. Teaching Aspects—Patient and Family

1. Instruct family members about cleanliness and how to rid their clothing and home of pediculi.
2. Adequate instruction should be given on how to avoid reinfestation.

IV. EVALUATION PROCESS

A. Has the patient or family member exhibited understanding of health teaching?
B. Has the patient or family member exhibited willingness to comply with home cleanliness instructions?
C. Is the patient comfortable and free from itching?
D. Is the environment cleared of all sources of infestation?

63

Perineal Irrigation

I. ASSESSMENT OF SITUATION

A. Definition

Cleansing of external genitalia

B. Terminology

None

C. Rationale for Action

1. To keep the perineal area clean
2. To minimize offensive odors
3. To prevent infection
4. To decrease discomfort from tenderness and edema due to operative trauma

II. NURSING PLAN

A. Objectives

1. To reduce the patient's anxiety during an embarrassing treatment
2. To provide for the patient's comfort and privacy

3. To observe the condition of the genitoperineal area

4. To report the physical and emotional effects of the treatment

5. To teach the patient self-care

B. Patient Preparation

1. Procedures dealing with the reproductive organs may be a source of embarrassment. The patient should be placed in a dorsal recumbent position, with triangular draping to avoid unnecessary exposure (Fig. 63-1).

2. An explanation of the reason for this procedure as well as a matter-of-fact attitude on the part of the nurse may greatly enhance the patient's comfort and well-being.

C. Equipment

1. Bedpan

2. Drape sheet

3. Tray containing cotton balls, forceps, and solution, as ordered

4. Irrigating can and tubing

III. IMPLEMENTING NURSING INTERVENTION

A. Therapeutic Aspects

1. The solution should be warm (105° F.) but must not be hot enough to injure the delicate perineal tissues.

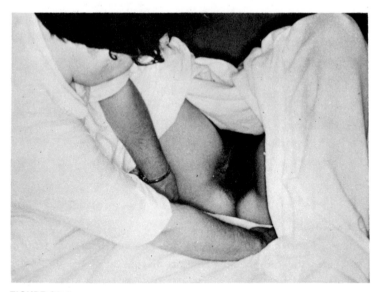

FIGURE 63.1

2. To prevent pathogenic organisms from entering the vagina, a clean field should be maintained and minimum pressure exerted. Air should be expelled from the tubing, and the irrigating can should be held 6 inches above the perineal area. With the nozzle at the level of the anterior labia, the solution should flow downward, over the perineum and into the bedpan.

3. The area above the perineum is considered clean, and the area below is contaminated. With a sterile cotton ball, the right side of the vulvo-perineal area is cleaned with one downward stroke from front to back. The left side and middle are cleaned in a similar manner, with a new sterile cotton ball used each time.

4. The anus and buttocks should be dried with a towel. Wetness causes irritation and bacterial growth.

5. After perineal surgery, the object is to prevent infection. Dressings are usually not applied. The perineum should be irrigated with warm sterile saline several times a day, as well as after each voiding and bowel movement. This should be done gently, to avoid undue stress on the suture line to minimize discomfort. The area may then be gently blotted dry with sterile cotton balls.

B. Communicative Aspects

1. *Observations*

   Note any foul odor or discharge, as well as signs, symptoms, behavior, and complications.

2. *Charting*

   Chart appearance, behavior, and conversation.

DATE	TREATMENT	TIME	OBSERVATIONS	SIGNATURE
4/30	Perineal irrigation	0900	Patient placed in dorsal recumbent position, draped. Solution poured over vulvoperineal area into bedpan. Area dried. Patient made comfortable. Stated, "I feel so much cleaner now." Procedure tolerated well.	F. White, R.N.

3. *Referrals*

   Not applicable

C. Teaching Aspects—Patient and Family

1. If perineal irrigation is ordered for post-hospital care, instruction should be given to patient or family on preparation of solution, height of container, position to assume during irrigation, and care and storage of equipment.

2. This procedure affords an excellent opportunity to emphasize the importance of cleansing from front to back in the perineal area.

IV. EVALUATION PROCESS

A. Was the patient's anxiety reduced?

B. Did the patient understand and cooperate in the treatment?

C. Was a therapeutic nurse–patient relationship maintained, contributing to improved opportunities for communications?

D. Was the patient left comfortable?

E. Did the irrigation tube pass without difficulty?

F. Did the perineal incision heal properly?

64

Phlebotomy, Assisting With

I. ASSESSMENT OF SITUATION

A. Definition

A venisection to reduce the volume of circulating blood

B. Terminology

1. *Syncope:* fainting

2. *Pathogens:* disease-producing organisms

3. *Venisection:* opening a vein for blood extraction (phlebotomy)

C. Rationale for Actions

1. To decrease venous return to the heart, thereby causing a decline in the right ventricular output

2. To decrease volume of circulating red blood cells

II. NURSING PLAN

A. Objectives

1. To make the patient as comfortable as possible

2. To prevent infection

3. To maintain fluid and electrolyte balances

4. To alleviate the patient's apprehension and fears

B. Patient Preparation

1. The patient should understand how and why the phlebotomy is being done. He will be more likely to cooperate with instructions to remain in bed after completion of the procedure if he understands the reason for it.

2. Pathogens are present in the environment, as well as on the patient's skin. Equipment should be prepared using an aseptic technique. The skin at the site of the venipuncture is cleansed with an antiseptic solution.

C. Equipment

1. Phlebotomy tray, including needle, tubing, bag or bottle for blood, and gauze pads

2. Tourniquet or blood pressure cuff

3. Alcohol sponges

4. Labels (if needed)

5. Antiseptic solution

III. IMPLEMENTING NURSING INTERVENTION

A. Therapeutic Aspects

1. The patient's head should be at the same level as his trunk. Constriction of vessels will cause vein enlargement owing to pooling of blood in an extremity; a blood pressure cuff may be applied to the upper arm and inflated to around 100 to 120 mm/Hg. Venipuncture is then done. If the blood is to be saved, it must be labeled accurately.

2. The collection bottle or bag is placed in an upright position lower than the extremity, to use gravity to facilitate blood flow (Fig. 64-1).

3. Opening and closing the hand in a slow, rhythmic fashion will facilitate venous blood accumulation and flow.

4. Adverse effects may result if too much blood is withdrawn. The physician will order the amount of blood to be withdrawn, which is usually 500 ml. The patient must be observed closely during phlebotomy. When the desired amount is drawn, the tubing is clamped and the needle withdrawn. Disposition of blood should be noted on the chart.

5. Bleeding may occur at the puncture site until clotting occurs. The venipuncture site is cleansed with an alcohol sponge, and pressure is applied for 2 minutes.

6. A sudden decrease in circulating blood volume may cause syncope. The patient should remain in bed for at least 1 hour, to allow his circulatory system to adjust to the decreased blood volume.

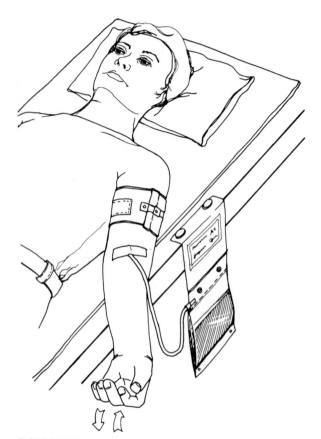

FIGURE 64.1

B. Communicative Aspects

1. *Observations*

   Observe the patient closely during the procedure and for 1 hour afterward for any signs of shock.

2. *Charting*

DATE	TREATMENT	TIME	OBSERVATIONS	SIGNATURE
6/6	Phle- botomy	0900 0915	Dr. D. here. Phlebotomy done; 500 ml blood withdrawn.	
		0930	B.P. 100/70; P 80; R 20. Skin color good. Patient instructed to remain in bed for 1 hour. Blood to lab for studies.	F. White, R.N.

3. *Referrals*

The local blood bank may accept the blood if it meets their standards and there are no contraindications due to the patient's condition.

C. Teaching Aspects—Patient and Family

1. The patient should be offered fluids at frequent intervals, unless contraindicated by his condition, after the phlebotomy is completed.

2. Instruct the patient and family to call for the nurse during the 1-hour period of bed rest after phlebotomy if anything is needed or wrong.

IV. EVALUATION PROCESS

A. Did the patient remain quietly in bed for 1 hour after the procedure?

B. Was the patient cooperative during the procedure?

C. Was aseptic technique carried out?

D. Is the environment clean and free of infectious hazards?

E. Were any adverse reactions noted?

65

Physical Examination, Assisting With

I. ASSESSMENT OF THE SITUATION

A. Definition

A systematic review of the body systems and structures of an adult

B. Terminology

1. *Ophthalmoscope:* instrument used for detailed examination of the eyes

2. *Otoscope:* instrument used to inspect the ears

3. *Sphygmomanometer:* instrument used to measure blood pressure

4. *Stethoscope:* instrument used to transmit sounds from the patient's body to the physician's ears

C. Rationale for Actions

1. To assist physician in physical examination for maximum efficiency and minimal time expenditure

2. To observe patient to aid in deciding nursing priorities in planning care

II. NURSING PLAN

A. Objectives

1. To facilitate the examination by having necessary equipment in readiness
2. To drape and place the patient in a proper position
3. To give the patient prior explanation to ensure cooperation
4. To ensure safety of the patient

B. Patient Preparation

1. For the adult patient, a brief explanation will help alleviate any anxieties aroused by the impending examination.
2. Bladder musculature responds to pressure stimulation by contraction and relaxation, which may result in involuntary emptying of urine. To prevent embarrassment and lessen discomfort, the patient should empty his bladder before the examination.

C. Equipment

1. Face towel
2. Bath blanket or sheet
3. Stethoscope
4. Sphygmomanometer
5. Flashlight
6. Otoscope
7. Ophthalmoscope
8. Percussion hammer
9. Tongue depressor
10. Disposable examining gloves
11. Brown paper bag
12. Gooseneck lamp
13. Vaginal speculum, if needed
14. Rectal scope, if needed
15. Lubricant (K-Y jelly)

III. IMPLEMENTING NURSING INTERVENTION

A. Therapeutic Aspects

1. Consideration must be given to the patient's safety. A patient should not be left alone on a narrow examining table.

2. The patient's privacy and modesty should be respected at all times. He should be screened and draped properly.

3. The male patient should have all clothes removed, a towel over his genitalia, and a sheet over his entire body. The female should be undressed, with a towel over her breasts and a sheet over her entire body. The cover sheets should not be tucked in at the foot of the bed.

4. Equipment should be gathered beforehand, and actions should be smooth, coordinated, and deliberate. The patient may need nonverbal reassurance during the actual examination.

5. The actual examination usually proceeds from head to feet, including a systems review, i. e., a general review of all body systems: respiratory, cardiovascular, genitourinary, etc. The nurse must be ready to assist the patient following the physician's instructions in regard to positioning (Figs. 65-1, 65-2, 65-3, 65-4, 65-5). The physician will usually take the vital signs and examine in the following manner:

   a. Head: for cuts, bumps, and pediculosis

   b. Eyes: check for pupil reaction, cataracts, and hemorrhage (will need ophthalmoscope)

   c. Ears: for excessive wax, foreign objects, lacerations, and intact eardrum (will need otoscope)

   d. Nose: for polyps, blockage, and drainage

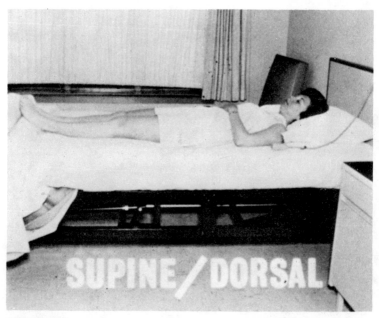

FIGURE 65.1

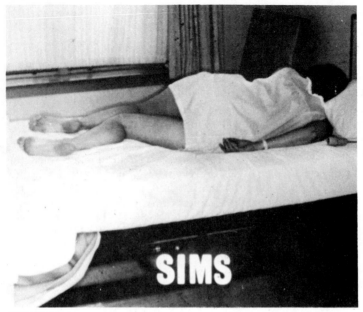

FIGURE 65.2

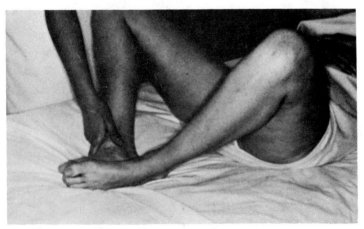

FIGURE 65.3

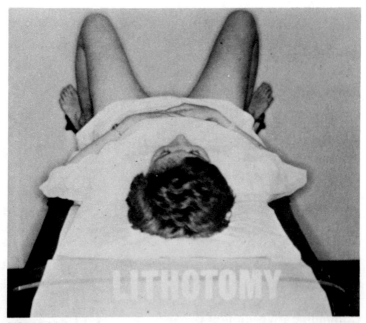

FIGURE 65.4

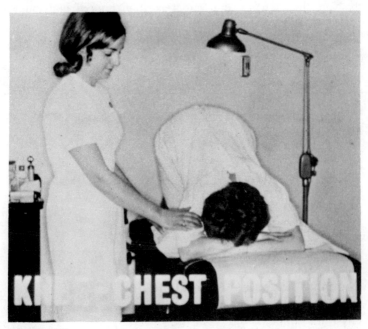

FIGURE 65.5

    e. Mouth: teeth and tongue, lining, tonsils, throat color, and presence of rash (will need flashlight and tongue depressor)

    f. Neck: thyroid gland, lymph nodes, abnormal lumps, swallow reflex

    g. Chest and lungs: rales, breath sounds, congestion, rib abnormalities, and scars (will need stethoscope)

    h. Genitalia: abnormalities, tumors, infection, abnormal drainage, and, in a male, enlarged prostate

    i. Extremities: reflexes, range of motion, dexterity, abnormalities (will need percussion hammer)

    j. Back and spine: alignment, ability to move freely, and abnormalities

    k. Nervous system: equilibrium, and steadiness

    l. Rectum: hemorrhoids, polyps, tumor, bleeding, and fissures (will need glove and lubricant)

6. The physician may also take a written history during the examination, to be dictated later. The patient should be left in a comfortable environment.

B. Communicative Aspects

1. *Observations*

    a. Observe for any abnormal skin eruptions, breaks, and so on.

    b. Note the patient's ability to reposition himself and follow the physician's instructions.

    c. Note the patient's emotional response to the examination.

2. *Charting*

DATE	TREATMENT	TIME	OBSERVATIONS	SIGNATURE
7/27	Physical exam	1000	Dr. J. here. Assisted with physical examination. Patient received full explanation of procedure, seemed relaxed, and willingly assumed positions requested. No evidence of skin eruptions noted. Resumed TV program when procedure complete.	G. Ivers, R.N.

3. *Referrals*

Not applicable

C. Teaching Aspects—Patient and Family

1. Instruct the patient and family about the importance of periodic physical examinations.

2. Instruct the patient and family about the importance of reporting to

the physician new lesions, rashes, or changes in normal elimination habits.

IV. EVALUATION PROCESS

A. Was the examination completed without undue stress on the patient?

B. Did the patient evidence by his compliance that he had an understanding of what was happening? Was he given a full explanation of the procedure?

C. Was the equipment easily available to the physician?

D. Was the equipment in proper working order?

E. Were the findings of the physician recorded in the chart?

66

P.M. Care

I. ASSESSMENT OF SITUATION

A. Definition

Personal care for the patient prior to sleep

B. Terminology

None

C. Rationale for Actions

1. To promote the patient's comfort, personal hygiene, and sleep
2. To provide a clean safe environment for the patient during the night

II. NURSING PLAN

A. Objectives

1. To ensure the patient is clean, safe, and comfortable
2. To observe the patient and evaluate the care given to him during the day; make adjustments and plans for care which will be required during the night
3. To help the patient achieve a comfortable period of sleep, if possible

B. Patient Preparation

Not applicable

C. Equipment

1. Washcloth and towel
2. Basin of warm water, if needed
3. Personal items (cosmetics, toothbrush, toothpaste)
4. Bedpan or urinal
5. Lotion or powder for backrub
6. Other items according to need, *e.g.*, fresh dressings, binders, linens, gowns, and so on.

III. IMPLEMENTING NURSING INTERVENTION

A. Therapeutic Aspects

1. A feeling of comfort will ease the patient's mind and facilitate sleep. The nurse should try to meet all needs during evening care: offer bedpan or urinal; assist with handwashing, brushing teeth, and so on; administer backrub; change dressings; reapply or adjust binders or bandages; tighten and smooth bed linens (change, if necessary); fluff and turn the pillow; administer sleeping medication; turn off light, radio, and television; place call light in easy reach of patient.

2. Particular attention should be paid to safety precautions, especially at night, when medication and fatigue may dull the patient's sensorium. The bed should be in its lowest position, with side rails raised, and a night-light should be turned on. Explain to the patient that he should call the nurse if he wishes to get up, rather than attempt to rise and risk falling.

B. Communicative Aspects

1. *Observations*

   Note the patient's readiness to settle down for the night, effectiveness of P.M. care, and anything significant in regard to his physical or psychological condition or treatments. Record any significant observations in nurses' notes.

2. *Charting*

DATE	TREATMENT	TIME	OBSERVATIONS	SIGNATURE
5/22	P.M. care	2100	Patient appeared very restless. Backrub and other comfort measures did seem to help. Patient stated he was discouraged and wanted to go home. Nurse offered reassurance and remained with patient for longer period of time. Patient quieter at this time.	C. Allen, L.V.N.

3. *Referrals*

Not applicable

C. Teaching Aspects—Patient and Family

1. If the patient will be dependent on others at home, the family needs to be instructed in what constitutes good P.M. care, and to promote patient relaxation and sleep.

2. Specific teaching for the patient depends on what is being done for him. P.M. care provides an opportunity for reinforcement of teaching done previously for particular conditions or treatments.

IV. EVALUATION PROCESS

A. Does patient appear clean, safe, and comfortable?

B. Did the nurse use this time with the patient to make observations pertinent to his care, treatments, and illness?

C. Did the patient rest well?

67

Position, Change of (Manually and Mechanically)

I. ASSESSMENT OF SITUATION

A. Definition

Turning, moving, or lifting the patient in bed, from bed to chair, and from bed to stretcher, either manually or using a mechanical lifting device. (See also Technique 90, CircOlectric Bed and Foster Frame.)

B. Terminology

None

C. Rationale for Actions

1. To prevent complications related to prolonged bed rest

2. To promote optimal comfort

3. To ensure safety of both the patient and the nurse

II. NURSING PLAN

A. Objectives

1. To facilitate safe patient transfer, preventing injury to the patient and personnel
2. To allay the patient's fear and anxiety regarding being moved
3. To assist in determining the reactions and tolerances of patients being moved
4. To teach the patient to help move and lift himself as much as possible, within his limitations
5. To maintain adequate body alignment

B. Patient Preparation

1. If the patient understands what is expected of him and is told how he can help, he is more likely to cooperate.
2. If the patient is helpless, during the bedmaking process a draw sheet or sheepskin is placed under his hips, to be used for turning during the day.
3. If a mechanical lifting device is used, it is checked before the patient is placed in it to be sure it works properly.

C. Equipment

1. Inflatable turning device or sheepskin
2. Hydraulic lift
3. Stretcher
4. Turn sheet and pillows or wheelchair
5. Draw sheet

III. IMPLEMENTING NURSING INTERVENTION

A. Therapeutic Aspects

1. Moving the patient up in bed
   a. Pulling or pushing the patient on a smooth surface requires less force than lifting him. If the patient can help himself, he grasps the top of the bed while the nurse places one arm under the patient's shoulders and the other arm under the hips. Both patient and nurse move at the same time on signal. If the patient is helpless, two nurses join hands under the patient's hips and shoulders, and both pull up at a given signal using proper body mechanics. If the patient can bend his knees and push, two nurses grasp his arms under the axillae and assist (Fig. 67-1).

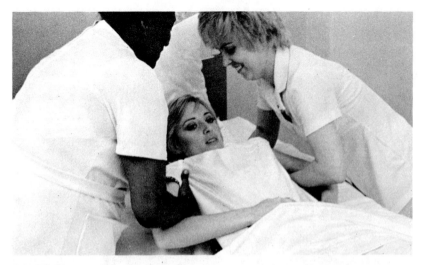

FIGURE 67.1

b. The less friction between the object moved and the stationary object, the less energy is required to make the move. If the patient is helpless, a draw sheet or sheepskin may be used. Two nurses grasp the rolled draw sheet or sheepskin, and both pull together.

2. Turning a patient on his side

    a. A minimum of energy is required to turn an object by rolling it. To turn a patient onto the left side, he is first moved to the right side of the bed, (Fig. 67-2) the right leg is crossed over the left; the left arm is placed in abduction and external rotation with the elbow flexed; and the right arm is placed in abduction and flexion over the chest. The nurse stands on the side of the bed toward which the patient is to be turned, and places one hand on the patient's right hip and the other hand on the right shoulder. The patient is then pulled over onto his side (Fig. 67-3).

    b. Attention should be paid to the safety of both the patient and the nurse. Side rails should be up on the side opposite the nurse if one person is turning the patient. Application of proper body mechanics is essential to avoid injury.

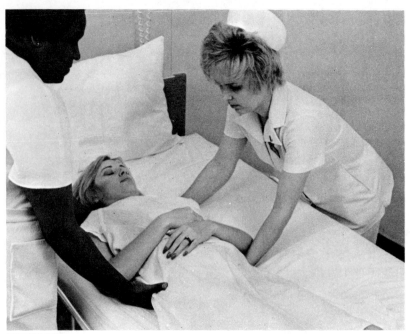

FIGURE 67.2

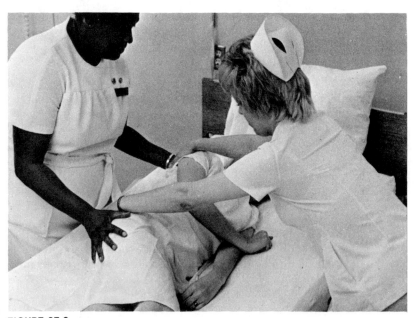

FIGURE 67.3

3. Logrolling
   a. For a patient with a spinal injury, flexion of the back may cause further injury to the spinal column. To turn the patient, the nurse places the patient's arms across his body (Fig. 67-4), and places a pillow between his knees. The patient is told to hold his whole body, except his legs, rigid.
   b. The nurse moves the patient's entire body to the side of the bed keeping the spinal column rigid by keeping the turn sheet taut (Fig. 67-5). The patient is turned in a logrolling manner. Flexion of the uppermost leg may aid comfort (Fig. 67-6). A pillow to the back will help maintain the desired position (Fig. 67-7).

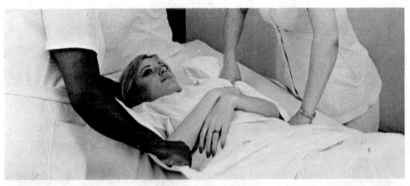

FIGURE 67.4

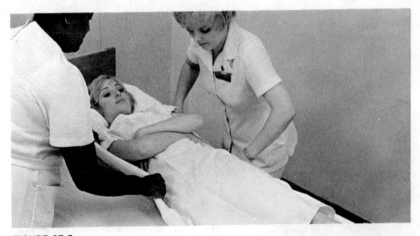

FIGURE 67.5

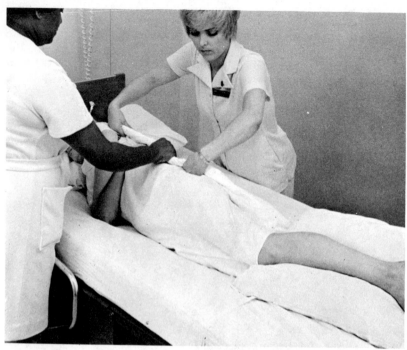

FIGURE 67.6

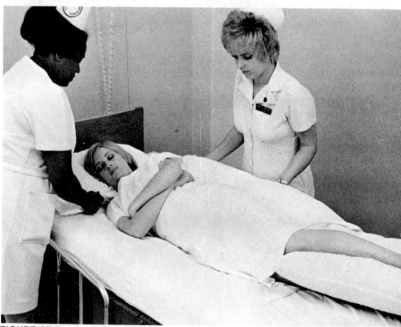

FIGURE 67.7

4. Moving a patient from bed to stretcher

   a. Sliding rather than lifting an object on a flat surface conserves energy and prevents strain. The patient is pulled from the bed to the stretcher by two to six persons, as indicated (Fig. 67-8, 67-9). Patient safety on a stretcher is enhanced by the use of safety belts (Fig. 67-10).

   b. Holding an object closest to its center of gravity will conserve energy. The three-man lift may be used. Three persons standing on the same side of the patient place their arms well under the patient, supporting the heaviest parts (the chest and shoulder area in the man; the hip area in the woman). At a given signal, the three lift the patient to their chests and carry him to the stretcher.

5. Moving the patient from bed to chair

   a. The shorter the distance is for lifting an object, the less energy is required. The chair is placed parallel to the bed at a point near the patient's buttocks.

   b. One person places his arms well under the patient's axillae from behind. One or more persons place their arms under the patient's hips and legs. All simultaneously lift the patient to the chair on a given signal.

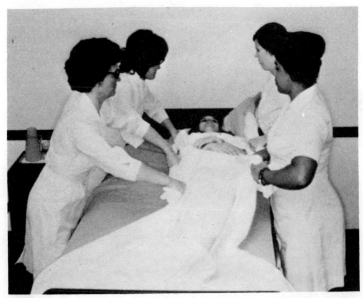

FIGURE 67.8

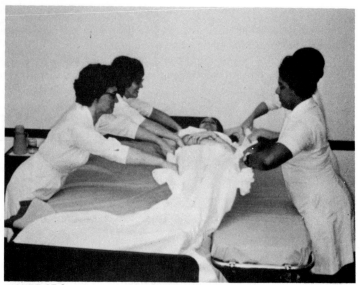

FIGURE 67.9

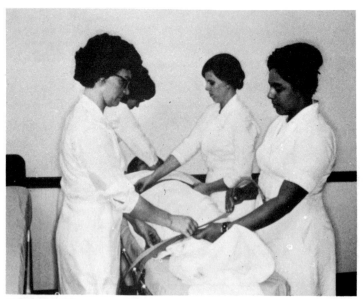

FIGURE 67.10

6. Moving the patient with a hydraulic lift

   a. The use of mechanical lifting devices conserves manpower and reduces the possibility of unnecessary injuries. The sling is placed under the patient by rolling him from side to side. The sling is attached to the lifter and the patient is lifted clear of the bed.

   b. A wheelchair in locked position should be ready. The patient is slowly lowered into the wheelchair, and the lifter is released.

7. Positioning the patient after turning or moving

   a. For the patient in the supine position, attention is paid to the feet to prevent footdrop. A footboard will help alleviate this problem (Fig. 67-11). A firm mattress will provide the back support the patient needs. To prevent neck strain from the unnatural position created by the placement of a pillow under the head, a pillow can be placed under the shoulders as well, to maintain the normal cervical curvature. Hand rolls will help maintain the hands in a position of function and will prevent clawlike contractures. Pillows under the knees should be avoided, as they inhibit circulation and may predispose to clot formation.

   b. For the patient in the lateral recumbent position, a pillow under the head and neck will help maintain normal cervical alignment.

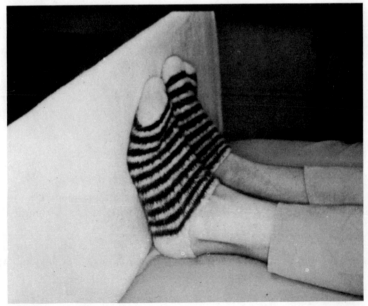

FIGURE 67.11

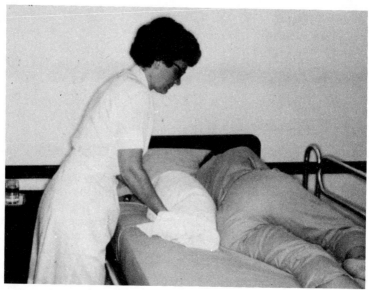

FIGURE 67.12

comfort is enhanced (Fig. 67-13). The upper leg is supported from groin to heel, to prevent its lying against the lower leg and to maintain lumbosacral alignment (Fig. 67-14). The footboard should be placed so that neither foot is dorsiflexed.

c. For the patient in a chair, a pillow behind the lumbosacral area may provide comfort. Any dependent limbs should be supported in a position of function by pillows. Restraints to prevent falling, if indicated, are of primary importance.

B. Communicative Aspects

1. *Observations*

   a. Appearance and vital signs are observed during moving and lifting. They may be contraindications for moving or lifting at this time.

   b. A patient who faints is made to lie flat and protected from injury.

   c. The helpless patient is turned every two hours to prevent the complications or sequelae of immobility.

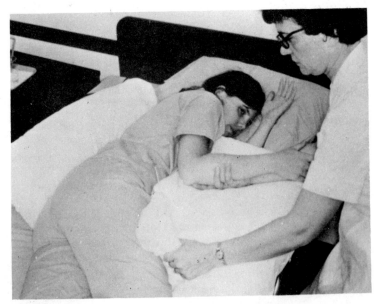

FIGURE 67.13

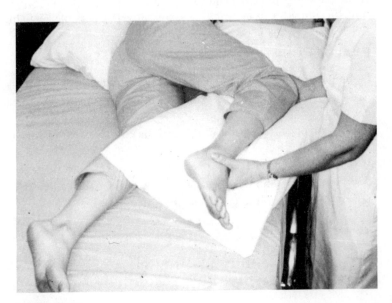

FIGURE 67.14

2. *Charting*

DATE	TREATMENT	TIME	OBSERVATIONS	SIGNATURE
5/20	Wheel-chair	0900	Moved to side of bed with help of the nurse. Sitting position on side of bed for 5 minutes. No complaint of dizziness; good body control. Pivoted on right leg without difficulty. Pleasant and cooperative.	L. Davis, N.T.

3. *Referrals*

a. If the patient is to be referred to an extended care facility, the persons who will be responsible for his care should be fully informed about his usual daily turning schedule and the turning methods that have proven most effective.

b. If the patient will be cared for at home, the family may need visits and support from a health service specializing in home visits.

C. Teaching Aspects—Patient and Family

1. Instruct the family in moving and lifting the patient, detailing all safety precautions for patient and person or persons moving him.

2. If the patient is to be dependent over a long period of time, stress to him the importance of being as cooperative as possible in helping himself and his helpers.

IV. EVALUATION PROCESS

A. Is the patient cooperating and changing positions as necessary?

B. Are safety measures and the principles of proper body mechanics being applied?

C. Is the patient participating in the turning to the extent of his abilities?

D. Is the patient being left in proper body alignment after turning?

E. Are contractures and pressure sores being prevented?

F. Has adequate restraining prevented falls?

68

Postmortem Care

I. ASSESSMENT OF SITUATION

A. Definition

The preparation of the deceased for the mortician

B. Terminology

None

C. Rationale for Actions

1. To show respect for the deceased
2. To aid in preserving the normal appearance of the deceased
3. To safeguard all belongings of the deceased

II. NURSING PLAN

A. Objectives

1. To meet legal requirements accurately and quickly
2. To aid in keeping the body tissue in the best possible condition, so that problems in preparing the body for viewing are minimized
3. To offer support to the bereaved family

B. Patient Preparation

Not applicable

C. Equipment

1. Shroud
2. Bath equipment
3. Dressing tray, if necessary
4. Clean linens, if necessary

III. IMPLEMENTING NURSING INTERVENTION

A. Therapeutic Aspects

1. Care of the family
   a. The verbalization of feelings permits an outlet of emotion, which helps to reduce mental anguish. When death occurs, the nurse should direct her attention toward supportive care of nearby pa-

tients and of the relatives and friends of the deceased patient. A clergyman may offer immeasurable support, if requested by the family.

b. The impact of death on the family will show itself in various forms of stress or shock. If members of the family are extremely emotional or have physical manifestations, such as fainting, the physician should be notified.

2. Care of the deceased

a. Raising the head and shoulders of the deceased with a pillow or backrest will prevent blood from settling in the face and discoloring it.

b. Maintaining normal position is desirable (Fig. 68-1). To prevent distortion of the face and body, the body is arranged in straight alignment. The dentures are placed in position as soon as possible and the mouth closed. To maintain the appearance of normal sleep, the eyes are closed naturally by applying gentle pressure with the fingertips for a moment. If the eyes will not stay closed, a moist cotton ball may be placed on each eyelid for a few moments. A folded towel is placed under the chin.

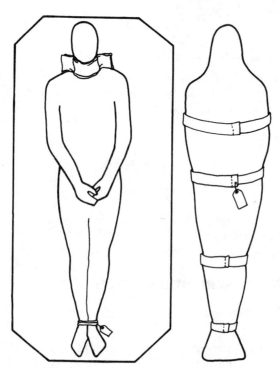

FIGURE 68.1

c. The nurse has a responsibility to prevent the loss of personal items. Clothing and valuables are gathered, labeled, and given to the next of kin. This should be noted on the chart, along with notation of any jewelry that remains with the deceased.

d. The dignity of the deceased should be maintained by preventing unnecessary exposure as the nurse applies the shroud, assures proper identification, and removes drains, tubes, and other equipment. Cleansing wounds, applying fresh dressings, and bathing the body will reduce the possibility of odor caused by microorganisms.

e. After the family leaves, the body is transported to the morgue by stretcher. It should be covered completely with a sheet and blanket. The body should be transported as quietly and inconspicuously as possible, to avoid upsetting other patients and visitors. Service elevators and seldom-used corridors should be used. The body should be stored in a refrigerated area until it can be picked up by the funeral home.

B. Communicative Aspects

1. After the patient is pronounced dead by the physician, the charge nurse may call the mortician, or a member of the family may do so.

2. If the deceased's hair had been shaved for surgery, send the hair with the body.

3. Avoid discussing the death of a patient with other patients or visitors.

4. Have permission for removal of the body signed by the next of kin and witnessed.

5. If there is a delay in the arrival of the mortician or if the deceased is in a room with another patient, have the body prepared and removed to the morgue.

6. Autopsy consent

a. The physician is responsible for discussing and obtaining permission for an autopsy from members of the immediate family.

b. The nearest of kin must sign the autopsy permit (wife or husband, even if separated, but not if divorced).

c. The attending physician should witness the signing of the autopsy permit, but if the physician does not, it is the responsibility of the nurse in charge. The signatures of two witnesses are required. If permission is given by telephone, it must be witnessed by two hospital employees, and the relatives must be instructed to come to the hospital and sign the permit or, if they are out of town, to send a telegram giving permission.

7. Charting

a. The time the vital signs apparently ceased, and anything unusual connected with the death of the patient

b. The time the doctor was notified, and who pronounced the patient dead

c. The name of funeral home notified, and the name and relationship of the person requesting the funeral home

d. That the permit for removal of body was signed and by whom

e. That the autopsy permit was signed and witnessed and by whom

f. Disposition and inventory of personal belongings and valuables

g. Disposition of the body; time and name of the funeral home

DATE	TREATMENT	TIME	OBSERVATIONS	SIGNATURE
4/20		1110	Large amount of projectile emesis. Vital signs apparently ceased.	
		1112	Dr. B. notified.	
		1125	Pronounced dead by Dr. B.	
		1130	Permit for removal of body to C. Funeral Home and autopsy permit signed by wife, Mrs. J. Witnessed by Dr. B. and by G. Ivers, R.N.	
		1140	Mrs. D., Supervisor, R.N., notified.	
		1145	C. Funeral Home notified by Dr. B.	
		1145	Pathologist notified by Dr. B.	
		1150	Clothes, watch, and gold wedding band given to wife.	
		1155	Body removed to morgue. Hair sent with body.	G. Ivers, R.N.

C. Teaching Aspects—Family

Keep the family informed of actions when appropriate and the reasons for them.

IV. EVALUATION PROCESS

A. Were legal requirements met?

B. Were the family and nearby patients given emotional support?

C. Was normal body alignment maintained?

D. Was normal facial appearance preserved?

E. Was proper respect shown for the body?

69

Preoperative, Intraoperative, and Postoperative Care of the Patient

I. ASSESSMENT OF SITUATION

A. Definition

1. *Preoperative:* the period of psychological and physical preparation, determined by the needs of the individual patient, from the time of hospital admission to actual surgical operation

2. *Intraoperative:* the period of time in the surgical cycle during which the surgical operation takes place

3. *Postoperative:* the incorporation of a series of activities that minister to the patient's psychological and physical needs after surgery, beginning when the patient is removed from the surgical table to a stretcher

B. Terminology

1. *Preoperative*

   a. *Allay:* to subdue or reduce in intensity; to make quiet or calm

   b. *Fluid and electrolyte balances:* an electrolyte (sometimes called a salt or mineral) is a substance in the body capable of developing electrical charges when dissolved in water. Fluids are present in two body spaces, outside the cells (extracellular fluid, such as plasma), and inside the cells (intracellular [interstitial] fluid, in which tissues and cells are bathed). The fluid and electrolyte balances must be in equilibrium to promote homeostasis in the body.

   c. *Metabolic rate:* metabolic activity described in terms of the basal metabolic rate, that is, the amount of heat produced by the body cells when they are as close to being at rest as possible.

   d. *Nonverbal fear:* a fear that is not expressed verbally but may be expressed overtly by some action or behavior, such as a facial grimace or clenched fists

   e. *Operative permit:* written permission, witnessed by the physician, nurse, or other authorized person, that protects the surgeon and the hospital against claims of an unauthorized operation

f. *Pathogen:* an organism or material capable of producing disease

g. *Rapport:* a relationship marked by accord or affinity

h. *Surgical preparation:* preoperative preparation of the skin at the surgical site to render it as free as possible of microorganisms without damage to its physical and physiological integrity

2. *Intraoperative*

a. *Anesthesia:* loss of sensation or feeling. The various types are:

(1) Block: anesthesia produced by blocking the transmission of impulses through a nerve

(2) Caudal: anesthesia produced by injection of an anesthetic into the caudal (sacral) canal lying below the cord; affects the nerve trunks that supply the perineal area; used to relieve childbirth pain

(3) Central: lack of sensation caused by disease of nerve centers

(4) Endotracheal: anesthesia produced by introducing an anesthetic agent through a tube inserted into the trachea

(5) General: a state of unconsciousness and insusceptibility to pain produced by an anesthetic agent

(6) Infiltration: anesthesia produced by the injection of the anesthetic solution directly into the tissues

(7) Inhalation: anesthesia produced by the respiration of a volatile liquid or gaseous anesthetic agent

(8) Local: anesthesia confined to a limited or localized area of the body

(9) Rectal: anesthesia produced by introduction of an anesthetic agent into the rectum

(10) Refrigeration: the loss of feeling or sensation of a limited area caused by chilling the part to near-freezing temperature

(11) Regional: insensibility caused by interrupting the sensory nerve conductivity of any region of the body

(12) Spinal: anesthesia produced by injection of the agent beneath the membrane of the spinal cord

(13) Surgical anesthesia: the degree of anesthesia at which the operation may safely be performed

(14) Topical: application of a local anesthetic directly to the involved area

b. *Hypothermia (induced):* a deliberate reduction of temperature of part or all of the body; sometimes used as an adjunct to anesthesia in surgical cases involving a limb. Induced hypothermia is also used as a protective measure in cardiac and neurologic surgery. Local hypothermia refers to lowering of the temperature of only a part of the body, such as a limb. General hypothermia refers to the reduction of body temperature below normal to reduce oxygen and metabolic requirements; however, general hypothermia is used very little today.

c. *Positions used for surgery*

(1) Lateral positions: several versions of the side-lying position are used for surgery on the kidney and the chest. The kidney position places pressure on the lower leg and arm, and pools blood in these areas.

(2) Lithotomy position: the patient lies on his back with his buttocks at the break in the operating room table; the thighs and legs are flexed at right angles and the feet are in stirrups. After the patient is properly positioned, the bottom section of the table is lowered. This position is used in perineal, rectal, and vaginal surgery.

(3) Prone position: the patient lies on his abdomen with his face to one side and arms at his side; the palms are pronated and the fingers extended. This position is used for back, spinal, and some rectal surgery.

(4) Reverse Trendelenburg position: the patient lies on his back, the head is elevated, and the feet are lowered. This position permits better visualization of the biliary tract in surgery.

(5) Supine position: the patient lies flat on his back with arms at his side; palms are down, with fingers extended and free to rest on the table; legs are straight, with feet slightly separated. This is one of the most commonly used operative positions.

(6) Trendelenburg position: the patient lies on his back; the head and body are lowered into a head-down position; and the knees are flexed by breaking the table. This position is used for lower abdominal and pelvic surgery. Since the upward position of the viscera decreases diaphragmatic movement and thus interferes with breathing, this position is not maintained any longer than necessary.

d. *Stages of anesthesia*

(1) Stage I: extends from the beginning of the administration of an anesthetic to the beginning of the loss of consciousness

(2) Stage II (stage of excitement or delirium): extends from the loss of consciousness to the loss of eyelid reflexes

(3) Stage III (stage of surgical anesthesia): extends from the loss of the lid reflex to cessation of respiratory effort. At this stage, the patient is unconscious, his muscles are relaxed, and most of his reflexes have been abolished

(4) Stage IV (stage of danger or stage of overdose): an undesired stage that is complicated by respiratory and circulatory failure, whereupon death will follow unless the anesthetic is immediately discontinued and artificial respiration performed

3. *Postoperative*

　　a. *Dehiscence:* literally means "bursting forth"; after surgery, refers to the spontaneous release of sutures or suture line after healing has begun

　　b. *Evisceration:* the spontaneous protrusion of viscera through a surgical incision

　　c. *Pathogen:* an organism or material that is capable of producing disease

　　d. *Positions used frequently after surgery:*

　　　　(1) Dorsal position: the patient lies on his back, without elevation of the head. The head is turned to one side, to facilitate the evacuation of secretions.

　　　　(2) Fowler's position: the patient sits in bed; the head of the bed is raised at least 45°

　　　　(3) Sims's or lateral position *(semiprone position)*: the patient lies on either side, with the upper arm forward, the under leg slightly flexed at the thigh, and the head turned to one side to facilitate the evacuation of secretions and prevent aspiration. A pillow is placed at the back for support.

　　e. *Pulmonary embolus:* a blood clot that becomes dislodged from its original site, is carried to the heart, and forced into the pulmonary artery, where it plugs the main artery or its branches. Symptoms are sharp stabbing pain in the chest, dilated pupils, and rapid, irregular pulse. It can lead to death.

　　f. *Surgical aseptic technique:* the practices that aim at eliminating pathogenic agents during surgery

C. Rationale for Actions

1. *Preoperative*

　　a. To obtain optimal emotional and physical condition for the patient before surgery

　　b. To lessen the danger of infection by eliminating infectious sources

　　c. To prevent avoidable complications

2. *Intraoperative*

　　a. To prevent complications during the introduction of an anesthetic agent

　　b. To ensure safe, proper positioning of the patient before, during, and after the surgery

　　c. To observe diligently and provide intensive physical and psychological support (if a local anesthetic is used)

3. *Postoperative*

　　a. To restore patient to his optimal capacity of functioning

b. To meet the individual needs of the patient upon his return to his unit, and thereafter until his discharge from the hospital

c. To protect, support, and comfort the patient and his family

II. NURSING PLAN

A. Objectives

1. *Preoperative*

a. To promote early assessment of the psychological and physical preparatory needs of the preoperative patient

b. To implement a plan of nursing care that meets the individual needs of the preoperative patient by using a series of activities that prepare the patient (and family) for surgery

2. *Intraoperative*

a. To maintain the safety of the patient during surgery

b. To assist with preoperative procedures or techniques for surgery

3. *Postoperative*

a. To assess the psychological and physical needs of the postoperative patient

b. To implement a plan of personalized nursing care that relates to individual patient needs

c. To comprehend and participate in achieving the objectives of the surgeon

B. Patient Preparation

1. *Preoperative*

a. The preoperative patient is subject to many emotions regarding preoperative procedures. A clear and calm explanation of what to expect is absolutely necessary. The patient's level of education should be determined and considered before explanations are given or reinforced.

b. Families need reassurance and support, and will be less disturbed if they know what to expect. They should understand preoperative procedures, hospital routines, and visiting privileges.

c. The patient or his representative signs an operative permit (consent) form, to protect his rights, as well as those of the physician and the health care facility. To ensure clarity of interpretation of the operative procedure to be performed, neither abbreviations nor initials should be used on the consent form.

d. Diagnostic studies will be prescribed as part of the physical preparation of the patient. The nurse has the responsibility to know normal values and to detect significant deviations.

2. *Intraoperative*

If the patient is having a procedure under local anesthesia, he will need constant reassurance from those around him. The nurse must answer his questions slowly, clearly, and loudly enough to be heard.

3. *Postoperative*

Knowledge that the surgery is completed may help reduce anxiety and enhance cooperation. As the patient regains consciousness, the nurse should explain that the operation is over, tell him where he is, and indicate the presence of tubes and catheters. Repetition and clarification may be necessary.

C. Equipment

1. *Preoperative*
   a. Operative permit (consent) forms
   b. Preoperative checklist
   c. Patient gown
   d. Personal hygiene requisites
   e. Denture cup, if needed
   f. Special equipment, as needed
   g. Preparation tray

2. *Intraoperative*

Operating room supplies used as indicated.

3. *Postoperative*
   a. Side rails
   b. IV standard
   c. Emesis basin
   d. Tissue wipes
   e. Blanket
   f. Stethoscope
   g. Sphygmomanometer
   h. Special equipment, as needed

III. IMPLEMENTING NURSING INTERVENTION

A. Therapeutic Aspects

1. *Preoperative*
   a. Surgical skin preparation is done to remove as many microorganisms as possible without injuring the natural barrier. This involves shaving the operative area (Figs. 69-1, 69-2, 69-3, 69-4, 69-5). The skin is moistened and lathered with soap or cream. The razor must be very sharp, to remove all hair on and around the operative site. Care should be taken to avoid scratches, since

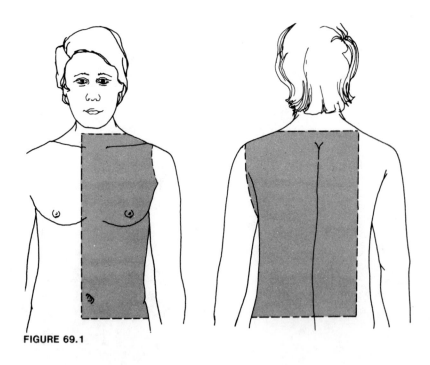

FIGURE 69.1

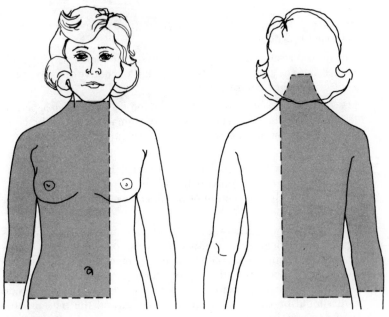

FIGURE 69.2

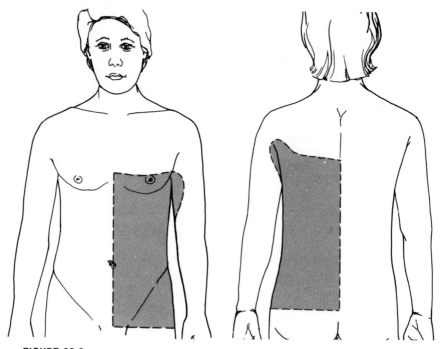

FIGURE 69.3

these are potential sources of infection. The area is then rinsed and dried thoroughly.

b. A calm and rested patient takes an anesthetic more easily, which in turn lessens the possibility of shock. A sedative may be prescribed the night before surgery.

c. The patient may be refused fluids or food by mouth for a period designated by the physician. An empty stomach reduces the danger of distention and aspiration during the anesthesia or postanesthesia stage.

d. An enema may be ordered before surgery. Emptying the intestines will prevent the contents from being discharged involuntarily and aid in the prevention of postoperative distention, gas, and impaction.

e. Preoperative medication may be given to reduce reflex irritabilities caused by fear and pain, to assist in smooth induction of anesthesia, to minimize secretions, and to protect the cardiovascular system by depressing the vagus nerve. Proper identification should be ascertained before the medication is administered. Side rails should be raised after administration, and the patient cautioned to remain in bed.

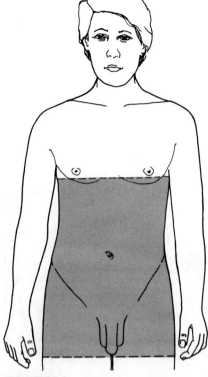

FIGURE 69.4

f. Personal articles should be protected from loss. These may be given to the family or placed in the hospital safe. Adequate safety measures will help prevent injury to the patient. Hairpins, hairpieces, prostheses, and jewelry should be removed before surgery. Removal of partial plates is essential.

g. Vital signs aid in the determination of the physical status of the patient undergoing surgery. The vital signs should be measured before the administration of preoperative medication and before surgery.

h. Effective preoperative teaching promotes more rapid recuperation, less frequent need of drugs, fewer complications, and a shortened term of hospitalization. A plan of care in regard to preoperative teaching should be begun on admission.

i. A surgical procedure is a time of apprehension for the family as well as for the patient. Every consideration should be shown the family members. Relatives should know where to wait and should be kept informed of the patient's progress.

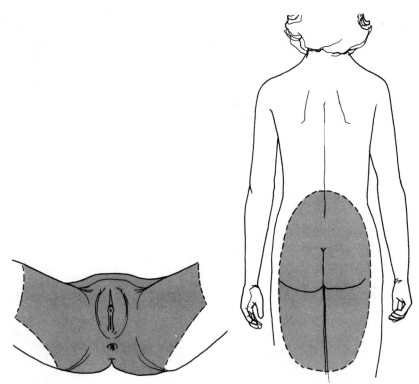

FIGURE 69.5

2. *Intraoperative*

    a. The proper anesthetic is administered to the patient in the operating room by authorized personnel.

    b. The position of the patient on the operating table is maintained during the operative procedure.

    c. Vital signs are carefully monitored during the surgery. Early signs of complications, such as shock and hemorrhage, are noticed and recorded on operating room form.

3. *Postoperative*

    a. The patient is transferred as quickly and safely as possible. A bed should be ready to receive the patient, with the sheets fanfolded (see Technique 29, Bedmaking). All necessary equipment should be available: IV pole, emesis basin, side rails, vital sign monitoring equipment, suction, and so on.

    b. Many wounds are closed under considerable suture tension. The patient is moved gently and carefully from the cart to the bed. The wheels of the cart are locked during each transfer.

    c. Maintenance of a patent airway is of primary importance in the immediate postoperative period. The most common cause of obstruction is the tongue falling back against the throat because of relaxation induced by anesthesia. This is usually prevented by insertion of an airway (Fig. 69-6). Secretions may be removed from the throat by suction. If permissible, the patient's head should be turned to one side. As the patient begins to regain consciousness, he should be encouraged to turn, cough up secretions, and breathe deeply.

d. Vital signs include temperature, pulse, respiration, blood pressure, and level of consciousness. Temperature elevation may indicate infection or brain damage. Pulse rate changes may indicate inadequate oxygenation of the blood. The level of consciousness should change, progressing from unconsciousness to alertness. Any lapse (*i.e.*, from a waking to a disoriented state) may be cause for alarm and must be evaluated. During the time the patient is emerging from anesthesia, his vital signs must be monitored every 15 min until they are stable.

e. Accurate recording of intake and output is essential in the early postoperative period. Most patients will receive IV fluids, and these must be carefully watched to ensure that they are running at the right rate, are not infiltrated, and are not allowed to run out unless ordered. The urinary output is very important in the postoperative period; the first voiding is especially important, because some forms of anesthesia can cause urinary suppression or retention. All intake and output must be recorded. All drains and tubes should be scrutinized immediately after surgery to ensure patency and relief of the tension that may occur if fluid is allowed to build up near the suture line. All drainage must be accurately recorded as output.

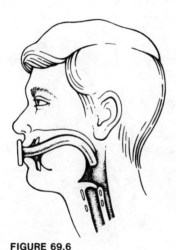

FIGURE 69.6

f. The nurse must be alert to early signs of complications, such as hemorrhage or abnormal wound drainage, and therefore watches for increased pulse rate and inspects dressings frequently. To prevent contamination of surgical sites by pathogens, surgical aseptic technique is used.

g. Frequent position changes help relieve general discomfort, increase circulation, and aid in the prevention of pulmonary congestion. To further prevent complications, deep breathing at frequent intervals should be encouraged. The operative area should be splinted with a pillow or hand to prevent undue strain and discomfort (Fig. 69-7). The patient should fully expand his lungs, hold his breath for a second or two, then release. Coughing may be ordered to help relieve lung congestion, although the routine use of this procedure is diminishing in frequency. The same principles apply: splinting and deep breathing; then the patient is instructed to cough as deeply as possible and to cough up any phlegm or obstructive materials.

h. Feelings of comfort and safety are reinforced by including the family in the plan of care. They should be allowed to visit the patient as soon as he is fully reactive. As the patient begins to respond, he will frequently lapse back into sleep. He should be al-

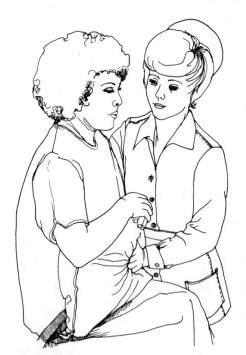

FIGURE 69.7

lowed to awaken at his own rate. He should not be shaken or shouted at in an effort to awaken him more quickly.

i. The patient should be made to walk as soon as the physician prescribes. The patient will need at least two persons, one on each side, to assist him. Ambulation should begin slowly. If the patient feels dizzy or light-headed, he should be allowed to rest for a few seconds and to breathe deeply. The patient should not look down at his feet, since this may produce dizziness.

j. During the postoperative period, certain discomforts are expected. A certain amount of pain is common and is usually relieved by narcotics and analgesics. The nurse must assess the pain, to be sure it is due to the operation and not indicative of some complication, such as pulmonary embolus or pneumothorax. Often the pain may be a manifestation of emotional feelings, and this, too, must be explored. Gas pains are common and are usually relieved by ambulation or a rectal tube (see appropriate techniques). Some medications and anesthetics cause nausea; antiemetics should give relief.

k. Legal aspects

(1) The patient's chart accompanies him to the operating room and to the recovery room after the operation. Orders for immediate postoperative treatment may be written in the operating room and sent to the recovery room with the patient.

(2) All orders for medication and treatment are automatically cancelled when the patient goes to the operating room.

(3) Hot water bottles are in no instance to be left in the bed of a postoperative patient; because of his depressed state, he may receive severe burns without feeling them.

(4) A person from the operating room is responsible for going to the unit with the patient and providing the following information: name, room number, and physician's name. After the patient is placed on the cart, he is strapped securely and never left alone.

(5) Charts should include the anesthetic record (completed by the anesthetist) and the operative sheet (completed by the circulating nurse) indicating accurate procedures.

B. Communicative Aspects

1. *Observations*

a. *Preoperative:*

(1) The nurse notes signs, symptoms, behavior, and complications.

(2) Preoperative diagnostic test reports are read by the nurse, and any significant deviations from normal are reported to the physician.

(3) The aging process may affect reactions to injury (*i.e.,* the reactions are less pronounced and slower to appear); also, certain drugs (*i.e.,* scopolamine, morphine, and barbiturates) may be poorly tolerated in the older patient and may cause confusion and disorientation.

(4) The observation of vital signs is important in evaluating the patient's physical condition before surgery. The nurse observes and reports temperature elevation, pulse irregularities, respiratory difficulties, or blood pressure discrepancies. Any undue cough or congestion of which the physician is unaware should be reported, as it may indicate postoperative complications.

(5) The nurse should try to encourage the preoperative patient to have a positive attitude toward his surgery, and should provide opportunities for him to express any fears he might have. How the patient regards the surgical procedure to be performed and its possible effects influences his chances for survival and recovery. Report any patient concern to the physician.

(6) Observation of renal function is important, not only because it influences the operative risk, but also because it affects the capacity of the patient to handle the parenteral fluids and electrolytes administered during the postoperative period. Although output should be compared with intake for all patients, in patients with limited renal reserve, *this measurement is essential.*

(7) Dehydration and malnutrition are common conditions that can seriously affect the preoperative patient. The nurse must observe and record intake and output.

b. *Intraoperative*

(1) The nurse should learn the interactions of the drugs used in the preanesthetic preparation of the patient and also know the effects (desired and undesired) of the anesthetic agents given during the operative phase so that safe, effective care may be given to the patient in the postoperative period.

(2) The nurse must be aware of the positioning of the patient required for every surgical procedure.

c. *Postoperative*

(1) The nurse should be able to describe and recognize complications, and report and institute nursing measures, as necessary, until medical treatment is obtained.

(*a*) The nurse must ensure the maintenance of the patient's airway. Respiratory depression may occur in the form of shallow respirations, due to anesthesia, sedatives, or opiates given for pain.

(*b*) Surgical shock is indicated by the character of the pulse, respirations, and blood pressure. The nurse reports a weak, thready pulse, shallow respirations, falling or low blood pressure. There may also be symptoms of sighing respirations, air hunger, ringing in the ears, cold, pallor, and restlessness.

(2) Pulmonary embolism may be evidenced by sharp pain in the chest area.

(3) The nurse must evaluate the condition of the wound site and drainage: is it intact? is there wound dehiscence or evisceration?

(4) In ensuring fluid and electrolyte balance, the nurse notes the patient's ability to take fluids orally. If fluids are administered by infusion, the nurse observes how the infusion is tolerated and the condition of the infusion site and tubing. Any vomiting and its character are noted. The patient's ability to void and the character and amount of urine are also important. If the patient has a catheter, its patency and the condition of perineal area are evaluated.

(5) The nurse watches for abdominal distention, which may indicate intestinal obstruction, gas, and other problems.

(6) The condition of the skin is observed as it can indicate adequate nutritional status or dehydration.

(7) The nurse observes whether nutrition is being maintained adequately. The patient's behavior during mealtime and interest in food are good indicators.

(8) The nurse notes any circulatory complications, and watches for symptoms of clot formation in the veins. Obesity, debility, old age, and muscular inactivity may precipitate this. A temperature accompanying inflammation of the veins may indicate thrombophlebitis.

(9) The character of the patient's ambulation is observed.

(10) The character and occurrence of defecation are important; the patient's ability to defecate should be noted.

(11) The patient's response and adherence to postoperative teaching and rehabilitation measures should be noted.

(12) Laboratory tests aid in determining patient status. Any significant deviations (*e.g.,* in blood gas values or CBC) should be reported immediately.

(13) Central venous pressure (CVP), if instituted, indicates cardiac output, blood volume, and electrolyte balance. The nurse must watch for abnormal alterations.

(14) The nurse must observe the patient's response to postoperative care and treatment and note his behavior.

(15) Infection (respiratory, wound, or other) may be indicated by increased temperature or erythema. Respiratory infection

may also be manifested by difficult breathing, pain in the chest, and coughing.

(16) Continued observation of vital signs, to aid in the determination of the patient's physiological status, is essential.

2. *Charting*

a. *Preoperative*

(1) The charting should be complete and should include the patient's appearance, behavior, and conversation, as well as the following additional items in this list:

(a) Current temperature, pulse, respiration, and blood pressure

(b) Dentures (*e.g.,* if full set is in place)

(c) Preoperative medications, chart pulse, and respirations (usually, a preoperative narcotic is given)

(d) Any significant observation that relates to the patient's psychosocial and physiological status

(e) Patient voiding before surgery

(f) Time of departure and mode of transportation to operating suite

DATE	TREATMENT	TIME	OBSERVATIONS	SIGNATURE
3/29	Preop	0730	Patient has bathed and is gowned.	
		0800	Preoperative IM medication given. P 84; R 20. Patient instructed not to get out of bed. Side rails up. Appears to be calm. States "I feel very rested." Wife with patient.	F. White, R.N.
		0900	Patient has voided. Partial plate removed. Watch given to wife.	
		0915	To surgery per cart.	F. White, R.N.

b. *Intraoperative*

(1) Each operating room has its own specific charting forms and procedures. The floor nurse should be acquainted with these procedures and forms to enhance the care given to the patient upon return to his unit.

(2) The patient usually goes to the recovery room following surgery until he has fully regained consciousness.

c. *Postoperative*

(1) Chart the patient's appearance, behavior, and conversation.

(2) Immediate postoperative charting, up to the time of the patient's arrival on the floor, should be complete and cover the aforementioned areas.

DATE	TREATMENT	TIME	OBSERVATIONS	SIGNATURE
4/1	Placed in Sims's position	1100	Patient returned from surgery. Responding to verbal stimuli. Dressing checked on rt. lower quadrant of abdomen. Small amount of sanguineous drainage. Color of skin is pink. Vital signs taken. BP 138/60; P 92; R 24. Pulse is strong and regular. Respirations appear shallow. Encouraged to breathe deeply and cough. Supported with pillow. Patient asking for ice chips. States he isn't nauseated. Ice chips given. IV running well. Side rails up. Wife is with patient. Patient instructed to keep head to side. No complaints of pain.	F. White, R.N.

3. *Referrals*

Not applicable

C. Teaching Aspects—Patient and Family

1. *Preoperative*

a. The physician should give a clear explanation to the patient and family regarding the operative procedure and the early and late postoperative periods. Reinforce the explanation as necessary.

b. Preoperative instruction in breathing and coughing is essential. Perform demonstration and return demonstration, as necessary. The patient should know that he may be uncomfortable doing this in the postoperative period, but that deep breathing and coughing aid in the prevention of pneumonia.

c. Explain the oxygen, drainage tubes, intravenous fluids, and specific reasons for having these.

d. Inform the patient how often and for what reasons blood pressure, pulse, and temperature will be taken.

e. Inform the patient about what will take place the night before surgery (enema, bath, preparation, sleeping pill, and so on).

f. When applicable, explain the intensive care unit, visiting hours, and privileges in a matter-of-fact manner, so as not to cause alarm.

g. Before abdominal surgery, show the patient how to turn from side to side, to assume Sims's position. Encourage a turning routine of every two hr for the first 24 hr (or longer) after surgery, to stimulate circulation, maintain muscle tone, and prevent respiratory and circulatory complications. Preferably, encourage the patient to move himself, depending on the nature of surgery.

h. Show the patient how to move his foot in a circle and how to flex his leg, which he should do slowly but frequently. Flexing the legs is done for a number of reasons: to lessen abdominal gas pain; to facilitate moving from side to side; to adjust more easily to sitting, standing, and walking; and to increase circulation in the legs and minimize thrombus formation.

i. Explain the preoperative medication, which will relax the patient, pointing out that the patient may become thirsty and that following surgery, medications will keep him comfortable.

j. Explain the "nothing by mouth" order, which is usually in effect after midnight the night before early surgery.

k. Teach the patient how to record intake and output and the purpose and value of maintaining electrolyte and fluid balances.

l. Give specific information to relatives about where to wait and when and where to see the physician. The patient and family should know that they will be informed of the patient's various phases throughout the surgical and postsurgical period.

m. Explain the recovery room period, and notify the family of the patient's arrival in the recovery room.

2. *Intraoperative*

a. If the patient is to be awake during surgery, explain the preoperative medication that will have a relaxing effect; mention that the patient may become thirsty and that after the operation, medications will keep him comfortable.

b. If the patient appears apprehensive under local anesthesia, talk to him in a calm, quiet manner.

3. *Postoperative*

a. A clear explanation should be given to the patient and family by the physician regarding the operative procedure and the early and late postoperative periods. Reinforce the physician's explanation.

b. For other instructions (*e.g.*, exercise), see "Teaching Aspects, Preoperative."

c. Institute a plan of teaching for the patient's particular needs in relation to the surgery performed and his condition, and give these instructions to the patient before discharge.

IV. EVALUATION PROCESS

A. Were the nursing actions carried out expeditiously?

B. Were comfort and understanding promoted in the patient?

C. Were the communicative aspects of observation and charting proficiently done, in order to provide relevant information for the physician and hence promote comfort for the patient?

D. Was health teaching provided for the patient and family?

E. Were complications prevented or reported early in the postoperative period?

F. Was wound integrity maintained?

G. Was fluid and electrolyte balance monitored?

H. Was proper position in operating room maintained?

70

Pressure Sore (Decubitus Ulcer), Prevention and Treatment

I. ASSESSMENT OF SITUATION

A. Definition

A circumscribed area in which cutaneous tissue has been destroyed because of the restriction of blood flow from excessive or prolonged pressure, with progressive destruction of the underlying tissue. Pressure sores may occur in many areas (Fig. 70-1).

1. Over bony prominences

   a. Coccyx

   b. Hip (greater trochanter and ischial prominences)

   c. Elbow

   d. Heel

   e. Shoulder blade (scapula)

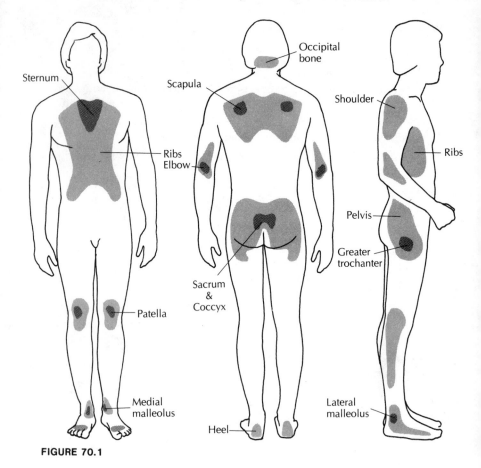

FIGURE 70.1

     f. Knee (patella)

     g. Ankle prominence (malleolus)

     h. Back of head (occiput)

     i. Ear

  2. Between folds of flesh in obese patients

     a. Under breast

     b. Under buttock

     c. On abdomen

B. Terminology

None

C. Rationale for Actions

1. To prevent pressure on any one area of the body

2. To ensure patient's comfort
3. To prevent spread of pathogenic microorganisms
4. To alleviate patient's fear and anxiety regarding his pressure sore
5. To promote healing of tissue and integument

II. NURSING PLAN

A. Objectives

1. To maintain clean, dry skin
2. To examine bony prominences and skin folds regularly
3. To observe and note factors that may interfere with the healing process
4. To prevent or reduce infection and promote healing

B. Patient Preparation

Many patients who are susceptible to pressure sores are severely debilitated and unable to turn themselves. It is, therefore, desirable that the patient understand why frequent turning is necessary. Even when careful preparation does not elicit acceptance and cooperation, strict adherence to a regular turning schedule is vital for the prevention of pressure sores.

C. Equipment

1. Hydrogen peroxide
2. Normal saline solution
3. Heat lamp
4. Medicated ointment, as ordered
5. Disinfectant solution, as ordered
6. Dressings, as necessary

III. IMPLEMENTING NURSING INTERVENTION

A. Therapeutic Aspects

1. Pressure sores are caused by prolonged pressure, which restricts blood flow to the area, resulting in tissue breakdown (Fig. 70-2). The desirable aspect in the treatment of pressure sores is prevention. Frequent turning, relief of pressure, and encouragement of circulation to skin overlying bony prominences are essential to prevention and early detection. The patient should be turned at least every hour or as ordered. Each time the patient is turned, his skin should be closely observed for any signs of pressure areas. Bony prominences should be gently massaged with lotion to promote circulation. The patient should be turned in as many positions as he is physically able to assume. Lying prone is an excellent means of relieving pressure on the skeletal frame of the back. Care must be taken to ensure that

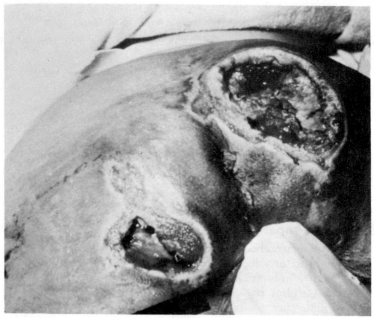

FIGURE 70.2

breathing is not restricted and that comfort is attained in the prone position. Sitting is also a desirable means of shifting weight and pressure, if the patient is able. Rolled pads are useful to keep body parts in alignment, but they themselves may cause pressure. They should be used judiciously.

2. Since pathogenic microorganisms can be transferred by direct contact, proper handwashing technique, both before and after care of the pressure sore, is essential. The pressure sore area should be cleansed thoroughly with hydrogen peroxide, followed by normal saline solution. A heat lamp may be applied for 20 min, placed at a distance of 45 to 50 cm (18 to 20 in) from the patient.

3. The use of rubber or other protective materials may cause the patient to perspire. This buildup of moisture predisposes to further tissue breakdown. A more desirable bed covering is a sheepskin, air mattress, or flotation pad, which causes less pressure and enhances circulation. The use of these devices does not eliminate the need for turning the patient or massaging pressure points, however (Fig. 70-3).

4. Moisture from incontinence causes maceration of the skin. The nurse must encourage bowel and bladder control if the patient can cooperate; offer the bedpan and urinal frequently, and change linens and give skin care as indicated. An indwelling catheter may be necessary.

5. Congestion of blood reduces the activity of the cells. This can be pre-

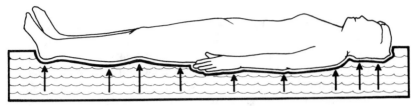

FIGURE 70.3

vented or lessened by gentle massage of unbroken pressure areas with alcohol or lotion.

6. An optimal nutritional status is essential to the healing process. A high-protein diet promotes healing. Between-meal feedings may help ensure adequate intake.

7. The patient should be left in a comfortable position, with bony prominences supported for minimal pressure.

B. Communicative Aspects

1. *Observations*

   a. Any reddened or irritated skin should be reported promptly and given special attention to prevent further irritation.

   b. If circulation is impaired, if fever is present, or if the function of the cells is altered, destruction of tissues may be relatively easy.

   c. Predisposing factors in the formation of a pressure sore are wrinkled bedclothes and crumbs or other objects in the bed; top linen applied so that it restricts freedom of movement; and pressure and irritation from casts, adhesive, tubing, and armboards.

   d. Drainage that appears at the site of an open pressure sore should be observed for type and amount. If persistent, the physician may wish to order a culture and sensitivity test.

   e. When a pressure sore develops, the plan of treatment is the physician's responsibility. *Preventive* measures should be planned, implemented, and evaluated by the nurse.

2. *Charting*

DATE	TREATMENT	TIME	OBSERVATIONS	SIGNATURE
4/20	Pressure sore care	0900	Small reddened area 5 cm (2 in) in diameter, located on coccyx.	
		0930	Reddened area cleansed with peroxide and saline. Heat lamp applied for 20 min. Explanation given to the patient of the importance of turning frequently.	G. Ivers, R.N.

3. *Referrals*

   a. If the patient is to be cared for at home by a family member, referral to a visiting nurse agency might provide the family with the encouragement and assistance they need to accomplish this difficult task. The knowledge that they will not be completely severed from professional counsel and advice after the patient is discharged can be a great comfort to families.

   b. Referral to an extended care facility should include the written plan of care, including the turning schedule to which the patient is accustomed.

C. Teaching Aspects—Patient and Family

1. Instruct the patient and family on the importance of frequent turning in bed.

2. Instruct the patient and family in methods to avoid pressure, early signs of impending tissue breakdown, and the most likely sites of breakdown.

3. Tell family to keep the patient clean and dry, and the bed free from wrinkles and crumbs.

4. If bandages are used, teach proper application to the patient and family.

IV. EVALUATION PROCESS

A. Is the patient willing to cooperate in the turning process?

B. Have patient and family been included in care of the pressure sore?

C. Is adequate nutrition being maintained?

D. Is pressure being alleviated in the affected or susceptible area?

E. Is the patient placed in proper body alignment each time he is turned?

F. Has gentle massage of bony prominences been done regularly?

71

Radiation Therapy, Nursing Care

I. ASSESSMENT OF SITUATION

A. Definition

The therapeutic use of radium, radon, radioactive gold, and other radioactive substances to kill malignant cells, requiring special nursing care and consideration

B. Terminology

1. *Radioactive:* the ability of a substance to emit alpha, beta, or gamma rays from its nucleus
2. *Radium:* a metallic radioactive element found in pitchblende that exists in a continuous state of disintegration; useful in treating disease, because it kills cells, especially young, immature, actively growing, abnormal cells (*e.g.,* cancer cells, leukemia cells)
3. *Radon:* a radioactive gas, which is a by-product of radium disintegration
4. *Shielding:* sealing off radioactive materials

C. Rationale for Actions

1. To prolong life by destroying malignant cells
2. To aid in the patient's comfort
3. To cause partial or complete remission of the malignant process

II. NURSING PLAN

A. Objectives

1. To maintain a calm and reassuring manner
2. To prepare the patient adequately for the impressive size of the machinery used in cobalt therapy and for possible side effects
3. To maintain an optimistic outlook
4. To treat side effects and minimize discomfort
5. To take adequate precautions to protect staff, visitors, and other patients from the harmful effects of radiation

B. Patient Preparation

1. The machinery used to administer cobalt-60 is massive and may frighten the patient (Fig. 71-1). For their own protection, the personnel stand behind a lead screen or wall during the treatment. For these reasons, the patient could find his first cobalt-60 treatment a terrifying experience. He must be adequately prepared in advance for the first sight of the equipment and for the fact that he will be left alone. The nurse should explain that there is no pain or sensation involved. Prior positive preparation can do much to help the patient accept these treatments.

2. The patient should understand the reason for and expected effects of the therapy before instigation. Before receiving the radioactive materials, he should fully understand the care he will receive, visitor limitations, and restrictions on himself.

3. The patient should be told that he will not feel the radiation itself. He may have some discomfort from the surgical implantation site; however, there is no sensation in radiation treatments.

C. Equipment

"Radiation Area" sign

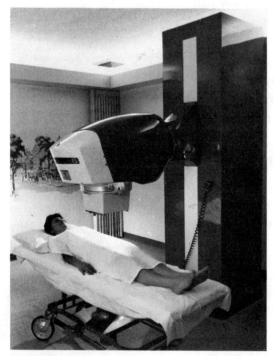

FIGURE 71.1

III. IMPLEMENTING NURSING INTERVENTION

A. Therapeutic Aspects

1. *Cobalt-60 therapy*

   a. The cobalt-60 equipment is very large. There is no pain or sensation involved in the actual treatment, however, and after the initial treatment, the patient will feel more secure about the prospect of future treatments. He should be prepared for the side effects, which may occur after the first few treatments, so that these will not be viewed as setbacks.

   b. Knowledge that he has cancer can be overwhelming to a patient. Many people view radiation therapy as the "last resort" and associate it with terminal care. The patient needs a thorough understanding of what radiation therapy is and how it works.

2. *Radium and radon*

   a. Nursing staff should be aware of the three methods of self-protection against radiation.

      (1) *Time.* Personnel should spend the least amount of time possible in one span with a radioactive patient. It is desirable to work quickly and return at intervals to check on the patient.

      (2) *Distance.* The farther away personnel stand from the implant patient, the better. It is also desirable to keep as far away from the radiation source as possible and to keep as much bulk between the radiation source and the nurse as possible. Thus, the nurse should stand near the head of the bed and avoid the foot of the bed of a patient who has a vaginal radium implant.

      (3) *Shielding.* Personnel should wear lead aprons or screen the patient with lead screens (Fig. 71-2). If a lead-lined room is not available, the patient should be in a room by himself, with the area of radiation facing an outside window.

   b. Visiting time should be minimized, and visitors must have adequate instruction before visiting. Young children and any adult female who might possibly be pregnant should not visit. Visitors should remain at least 3 ft away from the patient. A sign stating "Radiation Area" must be given to the patient to prevent feelings of hostility and neglect. Personnel should stop by the patient's room and check on him from the door to help the patient overcome feelings of loneliness.

   c. Radium and radon implants can become dislodged from the body. If any unusual metallic-appearing needles, seeds, capsules, or tubes are ever found in a radiation patient's room, the staff must not touch them. They should be moved with long-handled lead forceps, by a radiologist or by trained personnel only. All dressings and linen must be checked before leaving the room. If the implant is in the bladder, all urine must be collect-

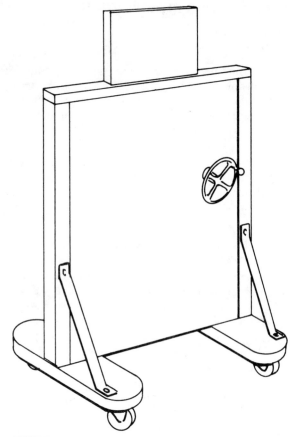

FIGURE 71.2

ed and visually examined for radioactive material. If systemic radioactive isotope therapy is being carried out, the nurse should save all body waste, including emesis, until it is positively deemed nonradioactive. Body waste is saved in a metal emesis basin or bedpan and should not be touched by the nurse. Radioactivity is determined with a Geiger counter by an experienced radiologic technician or radiologist.

d. When radium is in place, extreme care must be taken to ensure that it remains in the exact location desired by the radiologist. Several measures taken to guard against dislodging it are bed rest, use of an indwelling catheter, minimal movement in bed, and the administration of sedatives and antiemetics.

3. Side effects in all types of radiation therapy are varied and common. The patient should be told that some side effects may occur; however,

the nurse should avoid such statements as "people always get nause-ated from radiation therapy." The goal is to decrease the patient's fear and anxiety if side effects do occur, not to increase his chances of having them by the power of suggestion. Usual side effects include nausea, vomiting, anorexia, skin reaction, malaise, and alopecia. If skin reactions occur, they must *never* be referred to as "radiation burns," as this implies carelessness. They should be called dermatitis or skin reactions.

B. Communicative Aspects

1. *Observations*
   a. Observe for any reaction to therapy, and treat early. A bland cream may help local skin reaction; vigorous rubbing should be discouraged. Antiemetics help curb nausea.
   b. Observe the patient's reactions to the treatment for signs of ac-ceptance of the clinical diagnosis.
   c. Observe the patient's environment (*e.g.,* linens, floor) for any signs of dislodged radioactive materials.

2. *Charting*

DATE	TREATMENT	TIME	OBSERVATIONS	SIGNATURE
5/1	Returned from O.R. p̄ radium implant in cervix	0945	Flat in bed. Foley patent. Cautioned to remain in bed. Fruit juice offered. No N&V at this time.	G. Ivers, R.N.

3. *Referrals*
   a. The American Cancer Society may assist the patient in obtaining supplies for posthospital care (*e.g.,* wheelchairs, dressings, ambu-latory assistance equipment).
   b. If transportation assistance is needed to and from the radiation treatment facility, volunteer organizations such as service clubs, Sunday school classes, and others are often willing to provide rides.

C. Teaching Aspects—Patient and Family

1. Help the patient's family and friends understand the restrictions they face when visiting the patient. They will usually be more compliant if they know the reasons for these restrictions. However, avoid un-duly alarming the patient or his visitors.
2. Familiarize other personnel with the radioactivity sign and symbol and the precautions to be taken.

IV. EVALUATION PROCESS

A. Did the patient face initiation of therapy calmly or with fear and apprehension?

B. If side effects occurred, was the patient prepared and did he react positively?

C. Did side effects occur? Were they handled promptly and effectively?

D. Were proper safety measures carried out by everyone who came in contact with the patient?

E. Was all radium or radon present and accounted for at the completion of treatment?

72

Range of Motion Exercises

I. ASSESSMENT OF SITUATION

A. Definition

Range of motion is the maximum amount of movement that is possible in any particular joint.

B. Terminology

1. *Abduction:* movement away from the body midline

2. *Active exercise:* exercise performed by the individual

3. *Adduction:* movement toward the body midline

4. *Ankylosis:* fixation or immobilization of a joint from disease, injury, or surgery

5. *Atony:* absence of muscle tone

6. *Atrophy:* wasting of muscle

7. *Circumduction:* movement that combines flexion, extension, abduction, and adduction in which the distal end of the limb forms a circle and the shaft of the limb describes the surface of a cone (Fig. 72-1)

8. *Contractures:* conditions of fixed, high resistance to passive stretch of muscles resulting from fibrosis of the tissues supporting the muscles or joints, or from disorders of the muscle fibers

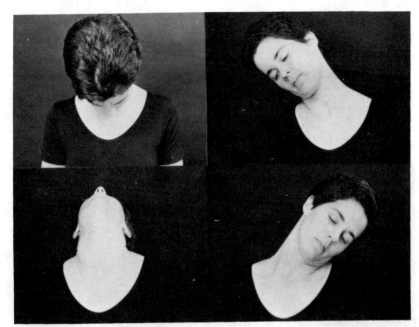

FIGURE 72.1

9. *Extension:* movement increasing the angle of a joint
10. *Flexion:* movement decreasing the angle of a joint
    a. Dorsiflexion is backward flexion or bending of the hand or foot (Fig. 72-2A)
    b. Plantar flexion is bending or stretching of the foot in the direction of the sole (Fig. 72-2B)
11. *Hyperextension:* state of exaggerated extension (Fig 72-3)
12. *Isometric exercise:* movement involving a muscular contraction
13. *Isotonic exercise:* rhythmic movement, involving muscle contractions, resulting in a change in muscle length, such as extension of a limb
14. *Lateral rotation:* away from the midline
15. *Medial rotation:* toward the midline
16. *Osteoporosis:* loss of calcium, nitrogen, and phosphorus from the bone
17. *Passive exercise:* movement of the patient's body by another person
18. *Resistive exercise:* external resistive force used in active exercise
19. *Rotation:* the twisting of a part of the body around the longitudinal axis of that area (Fig 72-4)
20. *Supination:* movement that places forearm in anatomic position

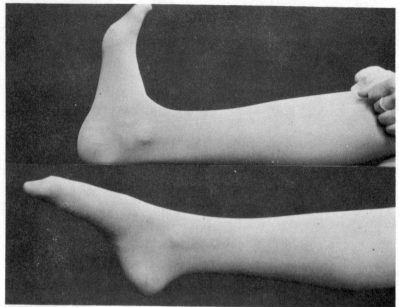

FIGURE 72.2 A & B

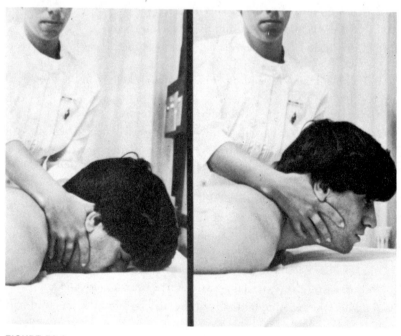

FIGURE 72.3

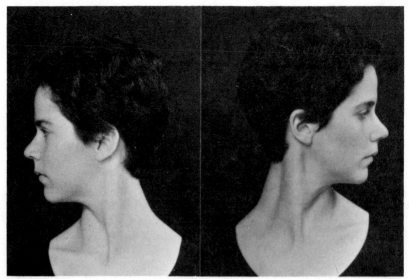

FIGURE 72.4

C. Rationale for Actions

1. To provide optimal activity and functioning of the musculoskeletal system throughout all stages of life
2. To prevent loss of function that can result from prolonged inactivity of any joint or muscle
3. To provide regular exercise, which is essential to optimal functioning and affects all systems of the body
4. To promote optimal "body quality" by effective exercise
5. To prevent complications during periods of illness when regular body movement and function are limited, since every body area may be subject to dysfunction in cases of prolonged immobilization
6. To provide maintenance regimens for degenerative and rheumatoid arthritis

II. NURSING PLAN

A. Objectives

1. To promote optimal motor function by establishing proper body alignment and a regular exercise regime
2. To prevent disability and deformity
3. To initiate active and passive exercise as soon as possible
4. To use mechanical aids as indicated: walker, crutches, cane, Foster frame, CircOlectric bed, trapeze

B. Patient Preparation

1. The patient must fully comprehend the importance of and need for exercise. This is the basis for treatment. Therefore, instructions must be clear and easily understood.

2. The partially or totally immobilized patient must have a complete acceptance of his own part in the restoration of function. Nurses and therapists are teachers and helpers—not healers.

3. Instructions and interpretations must emphasize the responsibility of the patient. This is a key to effective results.

4. Some individuals are much more capable of assuming this responsibility than others. It may be a slow process in some situations.

C. Equipment

1. Cervical traction
2. Ankle traction
3. Bar
4. Ball
5. Stryker frame
6. Cane
7. Walker
8. Crutches
9. CircOlectric bed

III. IMPLEMENTING NURSING INTERVENTION

A. Therapeutic Aspects

1. Musculoskeletal disorders can lead to immobilization of one part of the body, of several parts, or of the entire body.

2. Musculoskeletal disorders are characterized by pain, stiffness, weakness, and spasms.

3. Myofascial pain is pain that originates in muscles, ligaments, and tendon tissues. Names for soft tissue disorders are *bursitis, myositis,* and *tendinitis.*

4. Exercise is the essential element in musculoskeletal maintenance and rehabilitation. Some basic principles may be summarized as follows:

   a. Active exercise is preferable to passive exercise.

   b. Each joint of the body has a normal range of motion.

   c. Range of motion exercises are planned for each patient according to age group, body build, and condition.

   d. Range of motion exercises are important when there is physical inactivity, depending on the patient's condition and prognosis.

e. A patient's range of motion is affected by his genetic makeup, physical condition, and disease process.

f. Range of motion assessment and testing are done by a physician or qualified physical therapist.

g. There are several positions for range of motion for a particular part of body; for example, neck: flexion, extension, and hyperextension (Fig. 72-5).

5. Techniques of range of motion exercise are as follows:

a. Place the patient in supine position, arms to side, and the knees extended (Fig. 72-6).

b. Always hold the extremity at the joint. Move the extremity slowly and gently.

c. Move one joint through the range of motion at least three times.

d. Avoid forcing movement; discontinue movement if pain is severe.

e. During painful muscle spasm, move the limb slowly and steadily until the muscle relaxes.

6. Techniques to treat or reverse each condition must be planned individually, *e.g.,* external hip rotation, footdrop, pressure sores, ambulation, crutch walking, and cane use. (Note: For rehabilitation concepts see L.S. Brunner and D.S. Suddarth, *The Lippincott Manual of Nursing Practice,* 3rd ed, Rehabilitation concepts, p. 51, Philadelphia, JB Lippincott, 1982.)

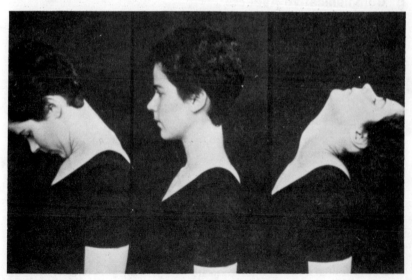

FIGURE 72.5

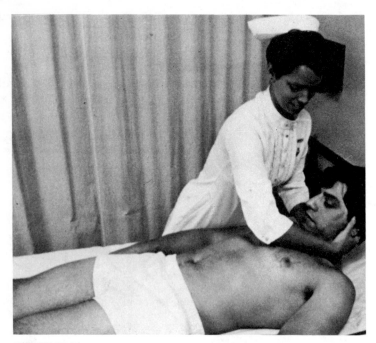

FIGURE 72.6

B. Communicative Aspects

1. *Observations*

   a. Assess the patient's physical condition and range of motion on admission.

   b. Observe closely for signs of immobility in any part of the body. Implement preventive and corrective measures immediately.

   c. Observe for signs of poor nutrition as factors predisposing to changes in the bone and muscle structures.

   d. Observe for edema, which may interfere with the supply of nutrients to the body.

   e. Observe for any break in the skin, redness, or gray-blue color indicating subcutaneous weakening.

2. *Charting*

   a. The patient's record should contain observations, preventive measures, and intervention methods used to alleviate immobilization of any part of the body.

   b. Nursing notes should indicate progress or the effectiveness of treatment.

3. *Referrals*

   Referral to a resource in the community or a state vocational rehabilitation agency should be considered if the patient will need long-
   term care.

C. Teaching Aspects—Patient

1. A major aspect of physical mobilization is the motivation and desire
   of the individual. A planned teaching program will provide the
   knowledge and methodology, but the patient must be willing to participate and follow through.

2. The teaching program should be planned according to the patient's
   level of understanding.

3. Teaching in this area requires patience and constant reinforcement.

IV. EVALUATION PROCESS

A. Were the problems of immobilization recognized early, and were corrective measures taken?

B. Did the patient respond to the need for regular movement and appropriate exercise?

C. Was the plan of exercise individually developed, and were the patient's needs met?

D. Were suitable rehabilitation measures considered in the initial assessment and plan of care?

73

Rectal (Digital) Examination, Assisting With

I. ASSESSMENT OF SITUATION

A. Definition

A diagnostic procedure whereby the physician or nurse uses a gloved
finger to examine the rectum

B. Terminology

1. *Rectum:* the lower part of the large intestine, about 12 cm (5 in) long, located between the sigmoid flexure and the anal canal

2. *Sims's position:* a semiprone position, in which the patient lies on his left side; right knee and thigh are drawn well up above the left; left arm is behind the patient and hanging over the edge of the table; chest is inclined forward so that the patient rests on it

3. *Knee-chest position:* the patient is on his knees, thighs vertical; head and upper part of chest are resting on the table; arms are crossed above the head

4. *Anus:* the outlet of the rectum, lying in the fold between the buttocks

5. *Sphincter:* circular muscle constricting an orifice or opening

C. Rationale for Actions

1. To detect changes in the anatomy of the rectum or of organs or tissues palpable through the wall of the rectum

2. To detect presence of pathology in surrounding organs (some 50% of lesions in the large bowel are within reach of the examiner's finger)

3. To determine the presence of a fecal impaction

II. NURSING PLAN

A. Objectives

1. To allay fear and anxiety of the patient regarding pain, discomfort, and the findings of the examination

2. To provide comfort

3. To maintain the patient's dignity by minimizing embarrassment caused by unnecessary exposure

4. To assist in obtaining tissue specimen, if indicated

5. To teach the patient and his family the importance of early detection and treatment

6. To assist the physician in adequate preparation of the patient and of the equipment

B. Patient Preparation

1. The patient should void prior to the examination, as emptying the bladder reduces the pressure within the abdominal and pelvic cavities and allows the rectum to be examined in its usual anatomic position.

2. It is essential that the patient understand not only what will take place during the rectal examination but also why the examination is being done. A matter-of-fact attitude may greatly reduce the patient's anxiety.

C. Equipment

1. Clean glove
2. Lubricating jelly
3. Drape sheet
4. Specimen container, if indicated

III. IMPLEMENTING NURSING INTERVENTION

A. Therapeutic Aspects

1. Modesty and training inhibit relaxation of the voluntary muscles. The contracted external anal sphincter will cause the patient discomfort when it is mechanically irritated during examination. Privacy may be provided by proper screening and draping. The patient should breathe deeply to aid in relaxation. A lubricating jelly reduces friction and lessens discomfort of digital insertion.

2. The area to be examined must be easily reached and readily viewed for more accurate determination of findings. The patient should be placed in the Sims's or the knee-chest position.

3. Warmth and privacy facilitate relaxation and cooperation from the patient. The top linens should be fanfolded to the foot of the bed. The patient's legs should be draped and another sheet or a gown used to cover the trunk (Fig. 73-1).

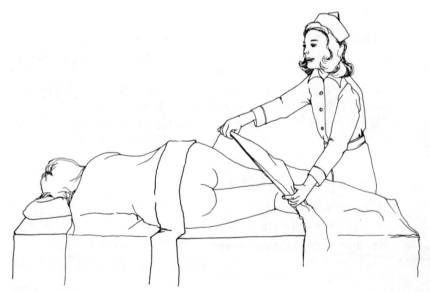

FIGURE 73.1

4. After examination, the rectal area should be cleaned with a warm, moist cloth. The patient should be left in a clean and comfortable environment.

B. Communicative Aspects

1. *Observations*

   a. Observe for the appearance of any abnormal structures (*e.g.,* hemorrhoids, skin lesions, or irritation).

   b. Observe the drainage that appears following the examination and determine whether it is sanguineous, serosanguineous, mucopurulent, or mucous.

   c. Observe the characteristics of fecal material on examining glove.

2. *Charting*

DATE	TREATMENT	TIME	OBSERVATIONS	SIGNATURE
7/27	Rectal exam	1000	Digital rectal examination by Dr. T.; no significant findings reported. Explanation of report communicated to patient. Patient stated his fear of having cancer and relief he now felt.	G. Ivers, R.N.

3. *Referrals*

   Not applicable

C. Teaching Aspects—Patient and Family

1. Discuss positive aspects of early detection of abnormalities, which often results in a cure.

2. Stress yearly physical examination, especially for the high-risk group, (*i.e.,* women over 30 and men over 40).

3. Inform the patient and family that rectal bleeding at any time warrants immediate attention and should be checked by a physician.

4. Stress good bowel and nutritional habits.

IV. EVALUATION PROCESS

A. Is the patient relieved of fear and anxiety?

B. Is the patient comfortable?

C. Are lines of communication open and being effectively utilized?

D. Are patient and family being taught the importance of proper diet and early detection of abnormalities?

E. Has a proper bowel regimen been established?

74
Respiratory Therapy

I. ASSESSMENT OF SITUATION

A. Definition
The administration of medication and therapeutic gases by the respiratory tract

B. Terminology
1. *Alveoli:* minute air sacs in the lungs in which the gaseous exchange of oxygen and carbon dioxide takes place
2. *Anoxia:* oxygen deprivation, which, if severe enough, may cause cell death in as short a time as 30 sec
3. *Atomization:* production of large droplets from a solution
4. *Bronchodilators:* drugs that enlarge the passageways of the lungs
5. *Mucolytics:* drugs that liquefy secretions and facilitate expectoration
6. *Nebulization:* production of a fine mist from a solution

C. Rationale for Actions
1. To assist in oxygenation of the patient's blood by providing a readily usable source of pure oxygen
2. To improve breathing by the administration of bronchodilators, mucolytics, or other drugs directly into the lungs by means of aerosol instillation
3. To increase vital capacity by forcing gases under pressure into the patient's lungs in a controlled situation
4. To assist the patient in critical condition in the maintenance of the basic life function of breathing until he is physically able to breathe for himself
5. To maintain an atmosphere of high humidity in an effort to break up secretions and aid the patient in coughing them up

II. NURSING PLAN

A. Objectives
1. To be sure the patient gets the right gases at the right rate
2. To observe for signs of inadequate oxygenation, such as cyanosis, confusion, restlessness, and dyspnea

3. To evaluate the patient's reaction and tolerance to positive pressure treatments, and notify the physician if changes are needed

4. To maintain patency of breathing equipment

5. To assist the family in dealing with their feelings when assisted ventilation is being used to prolong life

6. To maintain continuous high humidity by keeping vaporizers filled with water and the room closed

B. Patient Preparation

1. When an externally applied device will be utilized to administer oxygen, the patient should be shown the device and told its purpose and method of application, if feasible. This is especially true of the face mask, since it covers such a large area and can be very frightening.

2. Positive pressure treatments can be very frightening to the patient who is unprepared for the sudden influx of air. Many think their lungs are going to "burst." An explanation will allow the patient to be prepared for this so that he can offer greater compliance with the breathing equipment.

3. The success of a high-humidity atmosphere is greatly dependent upon keeping the system closed to the greatest degree possible. If the patient and family understand the reasons, they will be more cooperative about keeping doors and windows closed.

C. Equipment

1. Oxygen tank (or O_2 outlet, if piped in)

2. Cannula, catheter, or mask

3. Medication and nebulizer

4. Positive pressure machine

5. Steam inhalator or vaporizer

III. IMPLEMENTING NURSING INTERVENTION

A. Therapeutic Aspects

1. Oxygen is a basic necessity of life. Without it, cells die, and life cannot be sustained. When oxygen is being administered, the nurse must remember that it is highly combustible. For this reason, extra care must be taken to prevent fire when oxygen is in use. "No Smoking" signs must be plainly visible and readily enforced. Electrical equipment must be used with extreme caution (or not at all) in oxygen-rich environments.

2. Though oxygen is vital to life, it is not stored in large reserves in the body. Therefore, a continuous supply is necessary. Oxygen may be administered by several means, as follows:

   a. Catheter: a small plastic tube, which is inserted through the nose into the oropharynx. To approximate the distance of insertion, the nurse measures in a horizontal line from the tip of the nose to the earlobe (Fig. 74-1). This is how far the catheter should be inserted. After insertion the tip of the catheter should be visible behind the uvula. If it is inserted too far, it may cause gagging or pass into the esophagus, causing inflation of the stomach. The end of the catheter is connected to the oxygen tubing and the rate adjusted as ordered, usually between 5 and 8 liter/min. The catheter should be taped in place (Fig. 74-2) and changed every 8 hr.

    b. Cannula: a plastic tube with two protruding outlets that fit into the nose; it is held in place by an elastic band around the head (Fig. 74-3). The patient must be able to breathe through his nose to get any benefit from this method. Mouth breathing renders this method useless.

    c. Face mask: a means of administering oxygen when the percentage must be very high (near 100%). The face mask usually covers the nose and mouth (Fig. 74-4) and may cause a suffocating sensation. The patient with a face mask needs much reassurance.

3. Oxygen administered alone causes a drying effect on the delicate mucous membranes. For this reason, to prevent drying it is usually administered after being run through distilled water, and thus it enters the patient with some degree of humidity. The bottle should be kept two-thirds full of distilled water. A flow meter measures the amount of oxygen in liters per minute; it is set at the level ordered. Frequent oral hygiene lessens discomfort to mucous membranes. Semi-

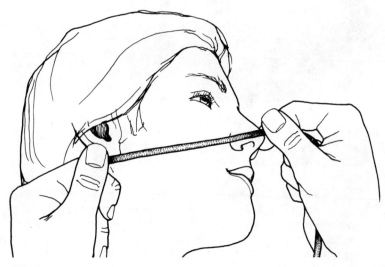

FIGURE 74.1

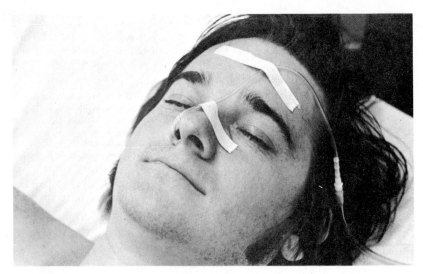

FIGURE 74.2

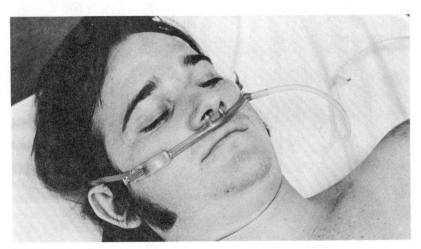

FIGURE 74.3

Fowler's position is usually most comfortable to patients receiving oxygen.

4. Positive pressure treatments help inflate the lungs, expand vital capacity, and administer medications by direct inhalation. These treatments require a special machine and administer the gases under pressure (usually 10 to 20 psi). Due to hazards involved, these treatments should be administered by someone with considerable knowledge and training in the use of this specialized equipment. However,

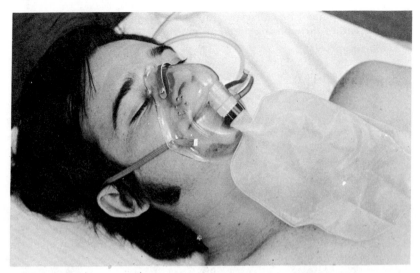

FIGURE 74.4

the nurse should be alert to signs indicating that the patient needs a treatment or the effectiveness of a treatment. The nurse should also know the expected therapeutic result of the treatment to ensure the patient is receiving maximum benefit. Changes in vital signs are early indications of untoward reactions to medications.

5. Highly humidified atmospheres are considered desirable in the presence of conditions causing considerable pulmonary congestion. The humidity helps liquefy this mucus, so it can be expectorated. It also alleviates discomfort caused by dry mucous membranes. The humidity may be warm (steam) or cool (cool mist). It is necessary to keep the doors and windows closed to maintain constant high humidity.

B. Communicative Aspects

1. *Observations*
   a. Watch all patients for signs of inadequate oxygenation of blood, such as cyanosis, restlessness, and dyspnea.
   b. Watch humidifier bottles to make certain that they do not run dry, resulting in nonhumidified oxygen being administered, which can cause great discomfort.
   c. Evaluate patency of oxygen tubing. Kinks will stop oxygen flow.
   d. During positive pressure treatments, observe the patient for gastric distention, which means air is being forced into the stomach rather than into the lungs.
   e. Observe for severe chest pain and dyspnea, which may indicate pneumothorax.

f. If the patient has a nasal cannula, observe him to ensure that he breathes through the nose and not through the mouth.

2. *Charting*

DATE	TREATMENT	TIME	OBSERVATIONS	SIGNATURE
4/19	O₂ by cannula	0815	Patient relaxed and breathing through nose. O₂ at 4 L/min P 76, R 14.	F. White, R.N.

3. *Referrals*

   a. If the patient must use respiratory appliances after dismissal, he may qualify for assistance from the American Lung Association.

   b. If the patient must receive positive pressure treatments at home, a visiting nurse should make periodic visits to ensure that equipment is in proper order and treatments are being administered properly.

C. Teaching Aspects—Patient and Family

1. Assure the patient that there is no pain involved in oxygen administration. Prepare him for some drying of the nares and oropharynx, and encourage him to take plenty of fluids, if this is not contraindicated.

2. If the patient is to be dismissed to utilize positive pressure breathing treatments at home, instruct him and his family in the use and care of the equipment as well as in precautions to be observed.

IV. EVALUATION PROCESS

A. Did equipment function properly?

B. Did the patient and family accept the inhalation therapy regimen?

C. Did humidity remain constant and above 70% to 80%?

D. Did the patient and family understand home care instructions?

E. Did the patient receive the ordered gases and medications?

F. Was adequate oxygenation of tissue achieved?

G. Did positive pressure treatments help breathing? Were there any untoward effects?

75

Restraints

I. ASSESSMENT OF SITUATION

A. Definition

A physical method of restricting movement or confining an adult patient to bed

B. Terminology

None

C. Rationale for Actions

1. To prevent the patient from falling out of bed
2. To prevent the patient from injuring himself or others
3. To immobilize the patient to promote the healing process or aid in therapy

II. NURSING PLAN

A. Objectives

1. To attempt to gain compliance by giving the patient a careful explanation before applying restraints
2. To use restraints only when absolutely necessary
3. To prevent complications that might arise from falls

B. Patient Preparation

The use of restraints may have negative connotations for the patient. Give a careful and adequate explanation in a kind and nonjudgmental way before the restraints are applied.

C. Equipment

1. Posey belt, to prevent patient from falling from chair or out of bed. The three types of Posey belts are *a*) locked chest, *b*) unlocked chest, *c*) unlocked waist.
2. Wrist and ankle restraints, may be made of cloth, stockinette, or leather

III. IMPLEMENTING NURSING INTERVENTION

A. Therapeutic Aspects

1. Posey belt
   a. Since these belts can be obtained in small, medium, and large sizes, use the one that fits best.
   b. Place the belt under the patient's waist. If the chest style is used, slip the arms of the patient through the shoulder straps.
   c. Position the buckles on top of the patient.
   d. Secure the belt by placing the end of the belt through the buckle so that it is snug but not too tight.
   e. Secure the long straps of the belt to the chair or bed frame.
   f. If the locked Posey belt is used, fasten the buckles with a key. Center the belt with the padded side under the patient's back. Secure the long straps to the bed frame; buckle the short straps around the patient's waist, and lock. The key should be kept in a definite place, usually at the nurses' station.

2. Wrist and ankle cloth restraints
   a. Place the patient in a comfortable, proper position.
   b. Use a clove-hitch knot to apply a wrist-type restraint to an extremity. Such a knot will not cut off circulation to the extremity, while permitting the patient some mobility.
   c. If leather restraints are used, pad the extremity well.
   d. Check the immobilized extremity every 15 min for sensation and circulation.
   e. Do not place restraints on both extremities on the same side of the patient, if possible.
   f. Remove the restraint at specific intervals, and give skin care and range of motion exercises, unless contraindicated.
   g. Use a square knot to secure long strap ends to bed frame or wheelchair.

B. Communicative Aspects

1. *Observations*
   a. Restraints that are too tight will impair circulation. Restraints improperly applied may cause irritation to the skin and impair circulation. Check restraints and extremities every 15 min. To prevent skin irritation, place sufficient padding over bony prominences such as ankles and wrists.
   b. Remove the restraint at specified intervals to allow movement of the extremity. When restraints are removed, observe the extremity carefully for any signs of redness, edema, or bruising.

2. *Charting*

DATE	TREATMENT	TIME	OBSERVATIONS	SIGNATURE
4/8	Posey belt to waist	0700	Attempting to climb over side rails. Appears confused. Locked nylon Posey waist restraint applied. Appears relaxed and comfortable.	J. Davis, R.N.

3. *Referrals*

Not applicable

C. Teaching Aspects—Patient and Family

1. Instruct patient and family on the purpose and necessity of restraints.
2. Ask the patient and family to alert the nurse if a restraint is causing discomfort.
3. Explain to the patient that his position may be changed and restraints applied as often as necessary for his comfort, or as indicated by physician.

IV. EVALUATION PROCESS

A. Is the patient comfortable?
B. Has the communication aspect been completed?
C. Have the restraints been checked every 15 minutes?
D. Are the patient's extremities normal in appearance and mobile?
E. Has the patient been restrained safely?

76

Shaving the Patient

I. ASSESSMENT OF SITUATION

A. Definition

Removal of facial hair (whiskers) from a male patient

B. Terminology

None

C. Rationale for Actions

1. Whiskers tend to itch and irritate the skin after 2 to 3 days growth.

2. If he is not shaved at least every other day, the unshaved patient has an unkempt appearance, which is not conducive to general well-being.

II. NURSING PLAN

A. Objectives

1. To promote optimal physical comfort by keeping the patient clean-shaven

2. To prevent trauma to facial tissue by keeping the patient clean-shaven and by using good shaving technique

3. To reassure the family by having them see the patient as they are accustomed to seeing him, that is, well-groomed

B. Patient Preparation

1. The patient should understand before beginning the procedure what will happen. Even the comatose patient should receive an explanation, since the actual depth of perception cannot be measured.

2. All equipment should be gathered and brought to the room before beginning to avoid chilling the patient.

C. Equipment

1. Razor and blade

2. Shaving lather or soap, if available

3. Basin with hot water

4. One bath towel, two face towels, one washcloth

5. After-shave lotion, powder, or benzalkonium chloride (Zephiran)

6. Electric razor, if patient prefers

III. IMPLEMENTING NURSING INTERVENTION

A. Therapeutic Aspects

1. Inability to shave himself may be interpreted by the patient as a loss of independence. The patient should be allowed to assist as much as he is able and to offer suggestions to facilitate the procedure.

2. Wet or soiled linens may produce chilling and discomfort. The patient's linen should be protected by placing a dry towel over his shoulders.

3. Heat, moisture, and lather help reduce surface tension and soften the beard. The face may be steamed with a hot towel for 5 to 10 min to soften the beard before applying lather.

4. For facial hair that grows in a downward direction, shaving is begun

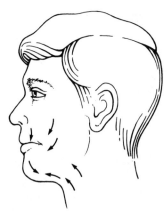

FIGURE 76.1

along the sideburns with short downward strokes of about 1 in. Shaving in the direction of growth minimizes nicks. There are many irregular surfaces on the face. Around the nose, mouth, and neck areas, the nurse pulls the skin taut and is especially gentle, taking very short strokes. (Fig. 76-1)

5. After-shave lotion or Zephiran acts as an astringent and closes facial pores. After washing off remaining lather and drying the face, the lotion is applied with the palms of the hands. The patient is left dry and comfortable.

B. Communicative Aspects

1. *Observations*
   a. Note the patient's tolerance of the procedure.
   b. Observe for any nicks or cuts inflicted with the razor.
   c. Observe the nature of the beard to determine if the patient is being shaved often enough.

2. *Charting*

DATE	TREATMENT	TIME	OBSERVATIONS	SIGNATURE
4/26	Shaved	0800	Shaved by nurse without difficulty. One very small cut on chin; slight bleeding has stopped. Patient did not appear to tire during the procedure.	C. Allen, L.V.N.

3. *Referrals*
   Not applicable

C. Teaching Aspects—Patient and Family

If patient will not be able to resume care of himself, instruct the family in correct shaving technique.

IV. EVALUATION PROCESS

A. Has shaving helped patient feel more comfortable?

B. Were communicative aspects completed?

C. Does the family seem pleased to see the patient clean and well-groomed?

D. If the underarms or legs of a female patient have been shaved, was the patient adequately draped?

E. Was shaving accomplished with minimal trauma to patient?

77

Suction, Oral and Nasal

I. ASSESSMENT OF SITUATION

A. Definition

Aspiration of secretions by a rubber or polyethylene catheter (14 to 18 F.) connected to a suction machine

B. Terminology

1. *Hypoxia:* varying degrees of lack of oxygen

2. *Patent:* open; unobstructed

C. Rationale for Actions

1. To maintain patent airway through mouth or nose or both to trachea

2. To obtain secretions for diagnostic purposes

II. NURSING PLAN

A. Objectives

1. To maintain patent airway to facilitate exchange of gases

2. To relieve patient's anxiety

3. To prevent infection

B. Patient Preparation

1. The patient should be told what will occur even if he is semiconscious or does not seem to comprehend. The patient and family should understand that the purpose of suctioning is to keep the airway from becoming obstructed.

2. The patient should be positioned to facilitate drainage of secretions from the pharynx and to prevent aspiration (*i.e.*, head elevated and turned to one side).

C. Equipment

1. Portable suction machine or gauge attached to wall suction
2. Y connector
3. Rubber or polyethylene suction catheter (14 to 18 F.)
4. Cup of tap water
5. Paper bag (to hold contaminated catheters)
6. Clean gloves

III. IMPLEMENTING NURSING INTERVENTION

A. Therapeutic Aspects

1. Microorganisms can be transmitted by direct contact, so the nurse should scrub her hands before suctioning and wear rubber gloves.

2. The catheter tip should be dipped in water before insertion to reduce friction and facilitate insertion (Fig. 77-1).

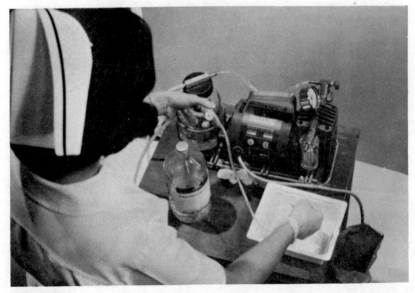

FIGURE 77.1

3. The catheter may be inserted through the mouth or a nostril. Insertion into the mouth may stimulate the gag or cough reflex and aid the patient in bringing up secretions. To prevent trauma to the delicate mucous membranes, the catheter should never be forced, nor should suction be applied as the catheter is inserted (Fig. 77-2).

4. A partial vacuum is created by continuous suction. The catheter should be withdrawn with a gentle rotating motion while suction is accomplished by placing one finger over the Y tubing. Rotating the catheter and keeping it patent prevents tissue trauma from occurring when the mucosa is drawn into the catheter during prolonged suction in one area.

5. Suction should not be applied for more than 15 sec at one time, as the airway is obstructed during suctioning, and hypoxia is thus intensified.

6. Pathogens can be destroyed by proper sterilization procedures. Rubber catheters should be placed in a paper sack and labeled. Disposable polyethylene catheters may be discarded in lined waste containers.

7. Extreme caution should be used in suctioning patients who have had nasopharyngeal surgery. The thoracic cavity should not be suctioned in a postoperative tonsillectomy patient, as this may dislodge clots that have formed.

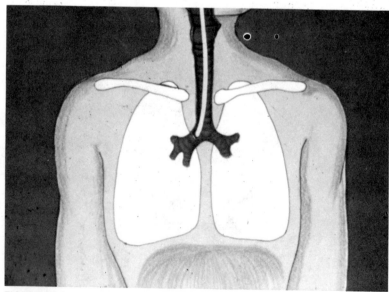

FIGURE 77.2

B. Communicative Aspects

1. *Observations*

    a. Note the amount of secretion and its consistency, color, and odor.

    b. Approximate the length of time for the procedure.

    c. Observe the reaction of the patient during the procedure.

2. *Charting*

DATE	TREATMENT	TIME	OBSERVATIONS	SIGNATURE
4/24	Oral and nasal suctioning	0900	Patient positioned on left side; head elevated about 30°. Lg amount, thick, purulent, yellowish secretion obtained. Patient became very apprehensive during procedure; stated she felt like she was choking. Procedure explained to patient again. Patient appeared to understand explanation.	
		0905	Patient appears to be comfortable; voices no complaints when questioned.	G. Ivers, R.N.

3. *Referrals*

Not applicable

C. Teaching Aspects—Patient and Family

1. Instruct the patient to expectorate secretions when possible.

2. Explain to the patient and family that the purpose of using a sterile catheter and clean rubber gloves is to prevent cross-contamination.

3. Instruct the patient and family to call for assistance if patient experiences any respiratory difficulty, and instruct them how to use call light.

IV. EVALUATION PROCESS

A. Is the patient comfortable?

B. Is the environment free of infections and hazards?

C. Have communication aspects been completed?

D. Has the procedure helped the patient to expectorate more secretions?

E. Is the airway patent?

78

Sutures, Removal of

I. ASSESSMENT OF SITUATION

A. Definition

The process of removing material used to secure wound edges or body parts together.

B. Terminology

1. *Continuous:* sutures formed by one continuous thread, alternating from one lip of the wound to the other
2. *Interrupted:* suture formed by single stitches, inserted separately
3. *Staples:* metal fasteners that penetrate the skin vertically to hold the incision closed

C. Rationale for Actions

1. To discontinue support no longer needed
2. To remove substance that may act as a foreign body in the tissues
3. To promote continuation of the healing process

II. NURSING PLAN

A. Objectives

1. To allay patient's fear and anxiety regarding wound rupture and pain
2. To provide physical comfort
3. To maintain asepsis
4. To observe the healing process

B. Patient Preparation

1. An adequate explanation is essential to gain the patient's trust and compliance. The nurse should emphasize that the wound has healed sufficiently so it no longer requires the support of sutures; that the patient will experience some tickling discomfort during removal but pain will be minimal; and that after the sutures are removed, he may feel less incisional support, but this in no way indicates weakness of the incision.
2. A position of comfort without undue tension on the suture line is desirable for suture removal. Since the patient may feel a slight sense of

nausea or dizziness, it is usually best to have him recline during suture removal.

C. Equipment

1. Sterile suture removal set, including scissors, forceps, and hemostat, or staple remover
2. Skin antiseptic (benzalkonium chloride [Zephiran] or alcohol)
3. Sterile dressings, as indicated

III. IMPLEMENTING NURSING INTERVENTION

A. Therapeutic Aspects

1. Suture removal is a delegated medical function; a physician's order is necessary before sutures may be removed.
2. The use of a disinfectant on and around the wound decreases the number of microorganisms and thus lessens the danger of infection. Cleansing should begin with the suture line and extend outward for an area of 2 in. (5 cm). A sterile cotton ball and forceps should be used, a new cotton ball used for each stroke.
3. Direct visualization aids in accurate removal of thread sutures. The knot of the first suture should be grasped with a sterile hemostat or forceps and elevated so that the portion below the knot is clearly visible.
4. Using sterile scissors, the nurse cuts one side of the suture *below the knot,* close to the skin (Fig. 78-1), avoiding cutting the knot. Cutting the suture near the skin prevents drawing the exposed contaminated portion of the suture through the tissues.
5. Each suture should be removed smoothly and in one continuous motion to minimize pain. All should be removed in sequence from one end of the incision to the other to prevent accidental loss of a suture.

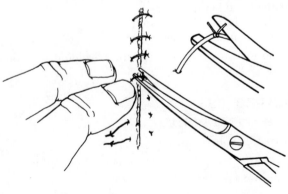

FIGURE 78.1

Succeeding interrupted sutures are removed by repeating this process for each suture. Succeeding continuous sutures are removed in the same manner, except that each portion to be cut is grasped by the suture itself, as there is no knot for each stitch.

6. Skin staple is removed in one motion with the staple remover.

7. To reduce chances of infection, the incision should be cleansed with a disinfectant and covered with a sterile dressing.

B. Communicative Aspects

1. *Observations*

  a. Observe the wound for approximation of the edges, signs of inflammation and infection, and amount of drainage.

  b. Observe the sutures for tissue reaction, continuity of suture line, and the possibility of embedded sutures.

2. *Charting*

DATE	TREATMENT	TIME	OBSERVATIONS	SIGNATURE
5/19	Suture removal	1500	Dr. S. here; examined incision.	
		1515	Sutures removed from abdominal incision by R.N. Wound edges in close approximation. No drainage or signs of inflammation. Patient tolerated procedure with minimal discomfort.	G. Ivers, R.N.

3. *Referrals*

Not applicable

C. Teaching Aspects—Patient and Family

1. Instruct the patient to keep his fingers away from the wound.

2. Instruct the patient and family to report any abnormal changes in the appearance of the incision. (The incision should become less red, and only a line should remain after several weeks.)

3. Reinforce the doctor's instructions regarding avoiding strain on the incision.

IV. EVALUATION PROCESS

A. Is the patient relaxed and informed?

B. Is the patient comfortable?

C. Was sterile technique maintained throughout the procedure?

D. Was the healing process observed and noted?

E. Is the suture line intact?

79

Teaching the Patient

I. ASSESSMENT OF SITUATION

A. Definition

A system of actions intended to produce learning by the patient; any interpersonal influence aimed at changing the ways in which patient can or will behave

B. Terminology

1. *Learning:* the discovery of meaning through the acquisition of new experiences and information
2. *Learner objectives:* goals that identify the degree of competency that the patient demonstrates by changes in behavior as a result of the teaching
3. *Teaching:* activities by which the nurse helps the patient to learn
4. *Teaching plan:* a plan developed by the nurse with assistance from the patient for use in implementing the basic concepts of teaching

C. Rationale for Actions

1. To promote knowledge of health maintenance and prevention of disease
2. To involve patient in his nursing care in the hospital
3. To expand the patient's information and knowledge about his condition
4. To help the patient adjust to stress during illness
5. To prepare the patient for discharge from the hospital

II. PLANNING PATIENT TEACHING

A. Objectives

1. To assess the extent to which patient teaching should be incorporated in providing patient care
2. To incorporate the principles of the teaching-learning process in the teaching situation
3. To identify the elements involved in assessing patient's readiness for learning
4. To develop a well-organized plan for patient teaching based on his needs

5. To use appropriate teaching techniques or strategies for the patient

6. To implement the teaching plan for the patient

7. To evaluate the effects or results of the implementation of the teaching plan

8. To learn basic assumptions about the teaching-learning process

   a. The patient as a learner

      (1) Knowledge is meaning, and since the person is an integrated whole, to be meaningful knowledge must be viewed as integrated.

      (2) The process of learning is the process of becoming, through perceiving and behaving, based on one's field of perception.

      (3) Meaningful learning is more likely to occur when patients select or help select goals of real need or interest, and even more likely when they relate these goals to individual purposes.

      (4) When patients choose goals, they are more likely to assume the responsibility for the fulfillment of these goals.

      (5) Patients learn best when they are challenged within the range of their abilities and interests.

      (6) The more individual needs and purpose become the focus of learning, the greater the depth of patient involvement and commitment becomes

      (7) The most desirable form of learner discipline is self-discipline.

      (8) Freedom of choice in learning must be accompanied by the realization of responsibility for the behavior that ensues.

      (9) Learning experiences become most desirable and meaningful when they enable patients to fulfill present needs, interests, and goals. Learning experiences are not something apart from the student but an integral part of his daily life.

      (10) The rate, depth, and intensity of learning vary according to individual abilities, drives, purposes, attitudes, and values, in relation to felt needs and that which is to be learned.

      (11) People respond to learning experiences when there is a relevant relationship between the learning experiences and problems of daily life.

      (12) With diagnostic help and a clear understanding of purposes, individual learners will select and organize learning experiences relevant to objectives.

      (13) The discovery of new knowledge and new meanings is more likely to occur when learners have the opportunity to identify and explore problems that interest them and for which no obvious solution is foreseeable at the time.

(14) Transfer of knowledge to behavior takes place when patients are given the opportunity to act on that which they value; that is, knowledge that is meaningful to the patient will automatically transfer to his behavior.

(15) The process of transferring knowledge and meaning to behavior is best achieved when patients have opportunities to relate knowledge and meaning to unique situations, to unknown problems, and to areas of living.

(16) Each person has his own learning style, his own preferences for study, his own rate of learning, and his own degree of involvement in the learning process.

b. The nurse as a teacher

(1) The nurse has at her disposal many teaching techniques: the art of questioning, the lecture, the small group discussion, the one-to-one relationship, and others.

(2) Both nurse and patient analyze learning errors, diagnose learner problems, and then attempt to help the learner meet his needs.

(3) The nurse must know the patient—his strengths, areas for improvement, needs, and goals.

(4) Learning experiences should be planned by the patient and nurse together in order to provide satisfying and meaningful experiences for the patient.

(5) These planned learning experiences should promise a certain degree of achievement to the nurse and the patient.

(6) When teaching techniques are varied and are directed to the total development of the patient, personal responsibility for effective learning will more likely be realized.

(7) People learn best through concrete, relevant, and predominantly first-hand experiences that elicit critical thinking, discovery, and total involvement.

(8) The more intense the motivation of patient and nurse, the greater is the possibility for the patient's involvement, commitment, and responsibility for choice.

(9) The nurse is responsible for applying knowledge about learners and learning so as to establish the best possible learning environment for the patient.

9. Principles on which patient teaching is based may be stated as follows:

a. The teaching-learning process is a cooperative effort, in which trust plays an important part.

b. Teaching what the learner already knows is a waste of time and lowers the learner's self-esteem.

c. A favorable environment facilitates learning.

(1) Anxiety reactions, such as denial, fear, or frustration, reduce the motivation to learn.

(2) Physical discomfort or a distracting environment impairs the learner's perception.

(3) An important criterion of readiness for learning is the patient's acceptance of his condition.

d. Reinforcement and repetition are necessary steps in learning.

e. Ways of accomplishing goals must vary according to the needs of the learner.

(1) The process of trial and error is a way of learning.

(2) Individuals interact differently, depending on age, culture, custom, education, environment, and language.

f. Starting at the patient's level provides for continuity of learning and promotes teacher-learner interaction, rather than a teacher's monologue.

g. Effective learning requires active participation.

h. Conceptualization occurs in the learner's mind. It involves perception, ideas, emotions, facts, and symbols.

i. Accomplishment reinforces learning, and near-accomplishment motivates the learner.

B. Patient Preparation

1. After the need for patient teaching has been identified, the nurse evaluates the patient's ability and readiness to learn. The patient is then prepared for the teaching by cooperatively establishing with the nurse satisfactory learning objectives.

2. After careful study, the nurse and patient decide on the most appropriate teaching method for the particular learning-teaching situation.

C. Equipment

Depending on the information to be taught, teaching materials such as treatment equipment, teaching plan charts, brochures, etc., should be brought to the teaching-learning situation.

III. IMPLEMENTING NURSING INTERVENTION

A. Therapeutic Aspects

1. *Steps in Teaching*

a. Demonstrate interest in the needs of the patient as an individual and in those of the family as a group.

b. Establish the extent of the patient's need for learning, using observation, physician's prescriptions, and direct communication with the patient and family.

c. Plan the content, time span, and sequence (from simple to complex) of the learning experience.

d. Evaluate the readiness for learning of the patient and family.

e. Enlist the aid of a supporting or reinforcing person whom the patient knows and trusts.

f. Have well-defined objectives and a clear outline for the sessions, but avoid a stereotyped approach to individuals and groups.

g. Begin teaching at the patient's level, using terminology he will understand and explaining terms that are new.

h. Begin teaching at the bedside by deliberate ritualization of single phases of care, with simple explanations, and by encouraging early participation by the patient.

i. Teach concepts rather than procedures, and encourage the learners to express these concepts in their own ways.

j. Provide learning experiences in such a way that the patient can have satisfying or nearly satisfying accomplishments.

2. *Summary of Teaching Process*

a. Assessment of need to learn

b. Assessment of readiness

c. Setting of objectives

d. Teaching–learning situation

e. Evaluation

IV. EVALUATION PROCESS

A. Any evaluation of behavioral change or patient progress is based on an ongoing diagnosis of patient needs, and ability to make choices.

B. Self-selected goals are the meaningful standards of behavioral change or progress.

C. Self-evaluation is the most meaningful of all forms of patient evaluation.

D. Self-analysis by the nurse is the most valid form of evaluation and the first prerequisite for behavior change. Evaluation is continuous; behavior is reinforced or modified; or new behavior is developed.

E. Nurse behavior is multidimensional and is interdependent with the outcomes of instruction.

F. The nurse must determine how well the patient is progressing in the process of teaching.

G. Both the nurse and the patient must have an understanding of what the achievement criteria are, and both must be able to secure evidence of progress toward these criteria.

80

Traction, Nursing Care

I. ASSESSMENT OF SITUATION

A. Definition

1. A process of exerting a pulling force on portions of the body by means of pulleys and weights or both or support to a bone by means of a strut

   a. *Skin traction:* a weight that pulls on tape, sponge, rubber, or plastic materials attached to the skin; traction on the skin transmits traction to the musculoskeletal structures. Types of skin traction are the following:

      (1) *Buck's extension:* traction applied to the lateral and medial aspects of an extremity with moleskin or adhesive (Fig. 80-1, A, B)

      (2) *Russell traction:* traction composed of Buck's extension on the foreleg, three pulleys at the foot, and a sling under the knee, which is attached to a rope and pulley above the knee (Fig. 80-2)

      (3) *Cervical traction:* traction applied to the neck by use of a head halter (Fig. 80-3)

      (4) *Pelvic traction:* traction applied to the lumbosacral region by means of a pelvic belt (Fig. 80-4A) or a pelvic sling (Fig. 80-4B)

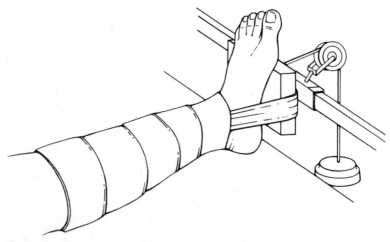

FIGURE 80.1A

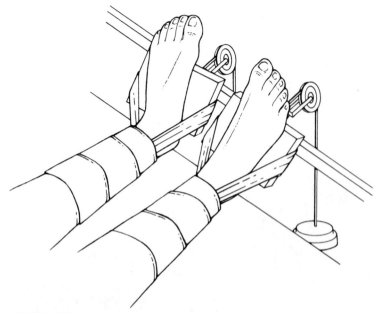

FIGURE 80.1B

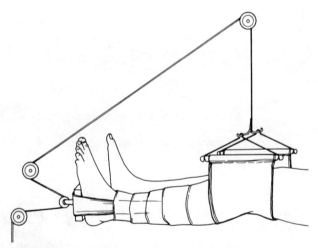

FIGURE 80.2

(5) *Thomas' splint:* a full leg splint used in emergency transport situations or after amputation; keeps the leg fully extended and long bones in alignment. Pressure is on the ischium and perineal area, not on the knee (Fig. 80-5)

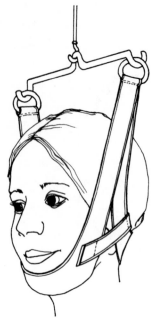

FIGURE 80.3

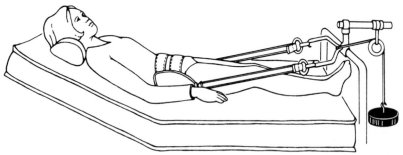

FIGURE 80.4A

      (6) *Side-arm traction:* similar to Buck's extension but placed on
the arm (Fig. 80-6)

  b. *Skeletal traction:* immobilization by means of a pin surgically inserted through a bone

B. Terminology

None

C. Rationale for Actions

1. To reduce and immobilize a fracture

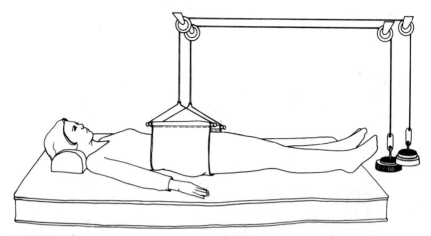

FIGURE 80.4B

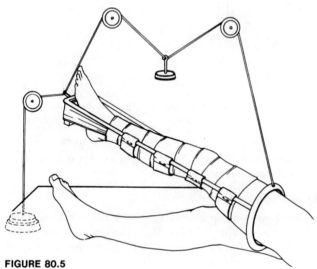

FIGURE 80.5

2. To decrease or eliminate muscle spasm
3. To prevent fracture deformity or flexion contractures
4. To relieve pressure on nerve roots

II. NURSING PLAN

A. Objectives

1. To maintain proper support to the musculoskeletal area until healing has occurred

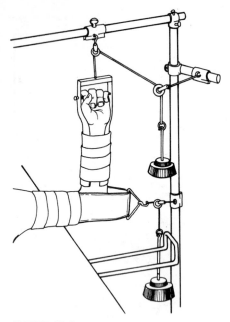

FIGURE 80.6

2. To prevent infection and complications of other body systems that may occur as a result of immobilization

3. To maintain the patient's mental and physical capabilities

4. To teach the patient exercises and other procedures that will assist in rapid recovery to the highest possible level

B. Patient Preparation

1. Even when muscle tension is appropriate, as with the use of traction, it adds to the fatigue and pain of illness. Back pain may be prevented by placing bed boards under the mattress. A regular schedule should be maintained for changing positions of and exercising arms and legs.

2. Immobility fosters feelings of helplessness and dependence. The patient should be encouraged to participate in his care. A clear explanation of why the traction is being applied and the expected results may encourage the patient to cooperate more actively in his care.

3. Shaving the affected part and applying tincture of benzoin disinfects the skin and causes the traction strip to adhere better and more comfortably.

C. Equipment

1. Adhesive, moleskin, or adhesive foam

2. Razor and tincture of benzoin

3. Specific traction equipment necessary to achieve the traction system prescribed by the physician

4. Sheepskin

5. Bed boards

6. Pillows

7. Trochanter rolls

8. Sandbags

III. IMPLEMENTING NURSING INTERVENTION

A. Therapeutic Aspects

1. The injured part should be maintained in the position as placed or prescribed by the physician. *Traction must not be removed if the object is immobilization or reduction.*

2. Pressure on the skin constricts circulation and causes pressure areas leading to pressure sores (decubitus ulcers). The heel of the extremity in traction should be free of pressure, and a sheepskin should be used as a hip protector. Bandages should be checked frequently and rewrapped as indicated to correct constriction of circulation. Pressure areas under the traction may be discerned by gently rubbing the hand over skin surfaces, observing skin irritation and odor, and listening to the patient's complaints.

3. The line of traction should remain constant. Traction should be checked often to ascertain that weights are freely swinging, alignment is straight, pulleys are separated with ropes intact and free of knots, and the linens are not obstructing the pulley.

4. The main complication resulting from skeletal traction is infection in or around the pin tract. Microorganisms gain entrance through breaks in the skin. The site must be inspected and cleaned daily to clear the tract and the pin of the slight drainage that occurs. The nurse should be alert to the odor, appearance, and amount of drainage, as well as to changes in the vital signs. The area of pin insertion should be covered with a sterile dressing.

5. Fat embolism may occur following fractures of the long bones. The patient should be observed for respiratory and circulatory distress.

6. Prolonged periods of immobilization predispose the patient to the development of hypostatic pneumonia and constipation. Deep breathing at regular intervals should be encouraged. Constipation is to be prevented or relieved by dietary modifications.

7. Suitable diversion should be provided to relieve boredom.

B. Communicative Aspects

1. *Observations*
   a. Monitor vital signs
   b. Check circulation

    c. Observe condition of skin

    d. Check position and alignment

    e. Note the amount, odor, and appearance of drainage

    f. Be watchful for neuromuscular spasms or other pain

  2. *Charting*

DATE	TREATMENT	TIME	OBSERVATION	SIGNATURE
4/21	Applica-tion of bilateral Buck's traction. 7 lb (3.1 kg.)	1700	Traction in correct alignment. States that traction has not lessened pain in lower back.	
	weights to	1715	Oral analgesic given.	
	each leg	1900	Complaining of tingling in right foot. Foot slightly edematous. Ace bandage reapplied.	F. White, R.N.

  3. *Referrals*

    After prolonged immobilization of an extremity, the patient may need assistance when he again begins ambulation. A physical therapy referral may provide the guidance necessary for his successful and rapid return to full ambulation.

C. Teaching Aspects—Patient and Family

  1. Teach the appropriate exercises to maintain muscle tone and prevent muscle atrophy or circulatory and respiratory complications.

  2. Teach the principles and purposes of traction to the patient and family to ensure cooperation and therapeutic involvement in the treatment regimen.

  3. Teach the patient and family the observations that are essential to a successful outcome of the treatment regimen.

IV. EVALUATION PROCESS

  A. Was the patient cooperative during treatment?

  B. Was adequate diversion provided to reduce boredom?

  C. Was correct alignment maintained during the healing process?

  D. Were complications prevented?

  E. Did the patient maintain muscle tone in his unaffected limbs?

81

Urinal and Bedpan, Placing and Receiving

I. ASSESSMENT OF SITUATION

A. Definition

Assisting the patient with the processes of elimination through use of a bedpan or urinal

B. Terminology

1. *Bedpan:* a metal or plastic receptacle for receiving fecal and urinary discharges from a patient confined to the bed
2. *Urinal:* a receptacle used by male patients for the voiding of urine

C. Rationale for Actions

1. To promote healthful habits of regular bowel and urinary elimination
2. To provide for accurate observation and measurement of patient's urine and stool

II. NURSING PLAN

A. Objectives

1. To establish a routine of elimination by offering the bedpan or urinal at regularly scheduled times or at the patient's request
2. To allay the embarrassment and guilt that occur when a patient is dependent on others for fulfillment of this private, basic need

B. Patient Preparation

1. If the patient cannot assist himself, adequate explanation of how the bedpan will be placed and what will be expected of the patient should be given.
2. Proper elimination may be hampered because the patient cannot assume a normal physiological position. The bedpan or urinal may be unfamiliar and uncomfortable. Elimination will be enhanced if the head of the bed is elevated to as near a natural position as possible, if this is not contraindicated by the patient's condition. The bedpan should be warmed by running warm water over it (Fig. 81-1). (Metal retains heat, so the nurse must ensure that it is not hot enough to

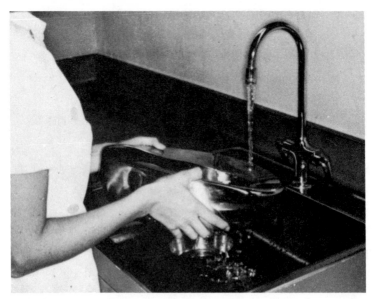

FIGURE 81.1

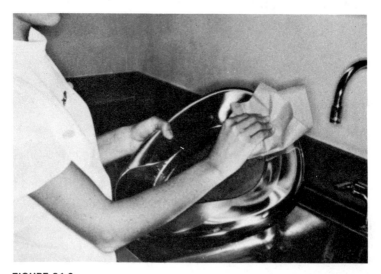

FIGURE 81.2

burn the patient.) The bedpan is then dried (Fig. 81-2) and pow-
dered to facilitate insertion and removal by reducing friction.

3. A position of comfort will facilitate elimination. The patient should
raise his hips and assist in placing the bedpan as much as he is able.
He may need padding beneath the lumbosacral area to enhance com-

fort and reduce pressure. If the patient is unable to place the urinal, it should be slipped gently in place with minimal exposure.

C. Equipment
1. Clean, labeled bedpan
2. Toilet tissue
3. Washcloth, towel, soap and water, if indicated
4. Clean, labeled urinal
5. Cover, if necessary
6. Aerosol air freshener

III. IMPLEMENTING NURSING INTERVENTION

A. Therapeutic Aspects
1. Since normal functions of elimination may be inhibited by dependence on others, respect the patient's desire for modesty and privacy. If possible, have a person of the same sex assist the patient with elimination needs. Relieve feelings of embarrassment by spraying an air freshener after elimination is completed.

2. Prolonged bed rest may adversely alter normal patterns of elimination. Explain to the patient that these changes are usually temporary and related to lack of activity, changes in diet, and medications. Normal regularity usually resumes when the patient's health improves and normal activities are resumed.

3. A rolling motion creates less strain and exertion for the patient and the nurse than a pushing or lifting motion. If the patient cannot raise his buttocks for placement of the bedpan, turn him to one side, place the bedpan against him in proper position, and hold it in place while he is rolled back onto it (Figs. 81-3–81-6).

4. Place the signal light within easy reach of the patient and answer it promptly to prevent unnecessary time on the bedpan. If the patient is confused, weak, or anxious, remain with him.

5. Perineal irritation or infection may occur if proper cleansing following the use of the bedpan is not carried out. In an effort to preserve independence, allow the patient to clean himself after elimination. If he is unable, clean the patient in a matter-of-fact way, with the least exposure. In the female, the perineum is always cleaned from front to back. If the skin does not clean thoroughly with toilet paper, the patient may be washed with soap and warm water and dried thoroughly. The patient should wash his hands after each elimination (Fig. 81-7) and should be left in a comfortable position. After noting contents and collecting a specimen, if needed, empty the bedpan into the toilet, clean it thoroughly, and store it properly.

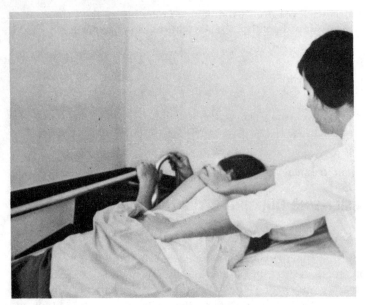

FIGURE 81.3

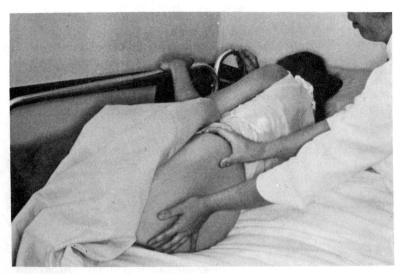

FIGURE 81.4

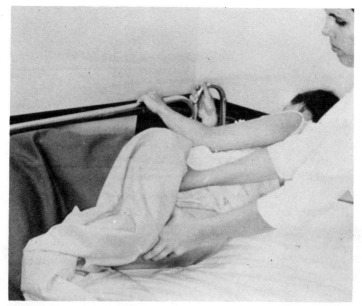

FIGURE 81.5

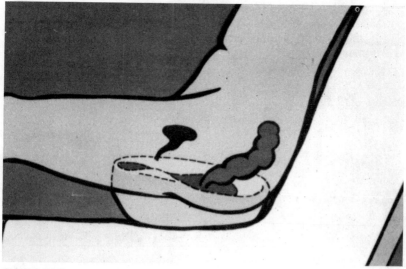

FIGURE 81.6

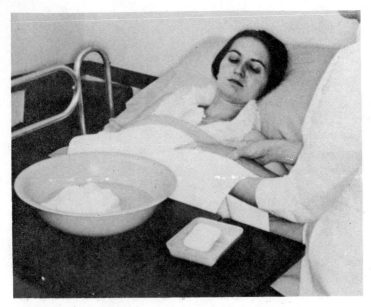

FIGURE 81.7

B. Communicative Aspects

1. *Observations*

    a. If intake and output must be recorded, measure the urine accurately and chart the amount on a worksheet. Also observe the color, odor, and consistency of the urine.

    b. If the patient has passed feces, note the color, consistency, odor, and amount, if applicable. Report observations. Note any abnormal stools.

2. *Charting*

DATE	TREATMENT	TIME	OBSERVATION	SIGNATURE
5/1	Bedpan	1000	Patient had large, softly formed brown stool. States he feels much better now and that added roughage in the diet seems to have helped elimination.	G. Ivers, R.N.
5/1	Urinal	1215	Patient voided 750 ml cloudy, dark yellow urine with stale odor; voiced no difficulties with voiding.	C. Allen, L.V.N.

3. *Referrals*

    Not applicable

C. Teaching Aspects—Patient and Family

1. Instruct patient concerning factors that maintain normal elimination patterns, such as adequate fluid intake, roughage in diet, and laxative juices (*e.g.,* prune, apricot).

2. Tell the patient to inform the physician when serious problems with elimination arise, so medication or treatment to correct the problem can be prescribed to prevent severe complications.

3. Some patients are not aware of what constitutes regularity and feel that if they do not have a daily bowel movement, something is wrong. Teach the patient and family that the normal pattern of elimination varies greatly among individuals. For one person, two or three stools daily may be normal, while for another, a stool every other day is normal.

4. Instruct the patient about how variations from the normal pattern of living, such as hospitalization, vacations, and emotional stress, can temporarily affect elimination.

5. Teach the family the techniques of using the bedpan and urinal if the patient will not be able to resume normal activities when discharged.

6. Emphasize to all female patients the great importance of cleansing the female perineum from front to back.

IV. EVALUATION PROCESS

A. Was the patient able to accept the idea of assistance with basic elimination processes? Did he request the bedpan or urinal without hesitation?

B. Was the patient able to assume a position of comfort during elimination?

C. Were the patient's needs for elimination met immediately?

D. Do the intake and output and nursing records reflect attention to and adequacy of elimination function?

82

Vaginal Examination, Assisting With

I. ASSESSMENT OF SITUATION

A. Definition

A vaginal examination of the patient undergoing obstetric or gynecologic care; an examination to ascertain possible pathologic or abnormal gynecologic conditions. Types of examinations include the following:

1. An examination performed by a physician for diagnosis and evaluation of an obstetric or gynecologic condition, which necessitates the presence of a nurse as a supporting assistant
2. An examination of the condition of the internal genitals as one indicator of the progress of labor

B. Terminology

1. *Meconium:* first feces of a newborn infant, greenish black and tarry in appearance. Intrauterine release of meconium may indicate fetal distress.

C. Rationale for Actions

1. To examine internal structures of the female pelvis
2. To obtain specimens for diagnostic purposes
3. To remove a vaginal pack
4. To evaluate the progress of labor

II. NURSING PLAN

A. Objectives

1. To allay patient fear and embarrassment
2. To assist the patient and physician
3. To record any unusual discharge
4. To send specimens to the laboratory
5. To record the effects of the examination and the information obtained
6. To note and record the progress of labor

B. Patient Preparation

1. The female patient may face an impending vaginal examination with embarrassment. The nurse should explain the exam and provide adequate draping.

2. The examination should be carried out as quickly and efficiently as possible. All equipment should be assembled ahead of time to avoid unnecessary delay.

3. A full bladder may displace the uterus and cause discomfort during the examination. The patient should void before the examination. Correct positioning will further facilitate comfort. The patient should be assisted into the lithotomy position.

C. Equipment

1. A vaginal examination tray, containing vaginal speculum, sponge forceps, tenaculum forceps, and sponges

2. Sterile gloves

3. Sterile lubricant, if needed

4. Gooseneck lamp or headlight

5. Specimen slides, containers, and fixative from the lab

6. Lab requisitions

7. Gauze packing, if needed

III. IMPLEMENTING NURSING INTERVENTION

A. Therapeutic Aspects

1. During the vaginal examination the nurse should serve as a reassuring interpreter, helping the patient to understand what the physician says in terms that are familiar to her. The nurse should remain in the room with the physician and patient at all times while the examination is in progress.

2. Visualization of the vagina and cervix requires direct light. A stool and lamp or headlight should be provided.

3. Organisms from external genitalia may be transferred into the internal canal. For this reason, the external genitalia should be prepared, according to physician's wishes, with an antiseptic agent.

4. Lubricants may impair the quality of the desired specimen and should be used only if requested by the physician. When necessary, the lubricant should be water-soluble, such as K-Y jelly.

5. A vaginal pack is usually inserted in conjunction with surgery. Therefore, its removal must be accomplished under sterile conditions. Using sterile technique, the nurse dons gloves, cleans the labia with cotton balls and disinfectant, and, with sterile-gloved hand, gently removes vaginal pack. A sanitary pad may be necessary.

6. Mouth breathing promotes relaxation. During the internal examination, the patient should be encouraged to breathe slowly and evenly through the mouth. If the patient is in labor, the examination should be done between contractions.

7. The nurse should have the patient in the lithotomy position with feet in stirrups (Fig. 82-1). The drapes should be in a triangular fashion with one corner around each leg. Equipment should be ready when the physician arrives to avoid prolonging the patient's discomfort and embarrassment. The physician will don sterile gloves, and will lubricate the speculum (unless contraindicated) and gently insert it (Fig. 82-2). The light should be positioned to offer maximum visualization of vaginal canal. The nurse should be at the patient's side to remind her to relax and breathe regularly. The physician may request a slide and swab to take a smear. After removal of the speculum, he will usually insert two fingers into the vagina and, with the other hand, palpate the lower abdomen to detect cysts, tumors, or other abnormalities. On completion of the examination, the patient's perineum should be wiped clean of excess lubricant, and she should be assisted back to her room.

8. If a patient in labor is to be examined by a nurse

   a. The position and identity of the presenting part may be determined by abdominal palpation. This should be done before the

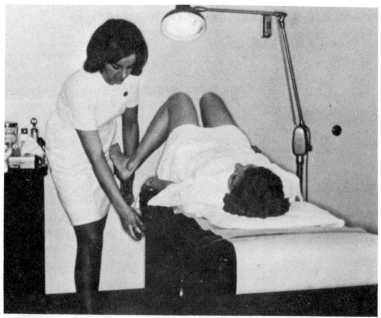

FIGURE 82.1

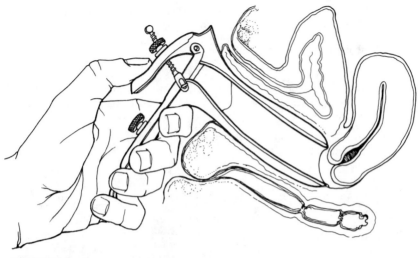

FIGURE 82.2

vaginal exam is undertaken, because of the danger of massive hemorrhage in the case of placenta previa. (A patient with vaginal bleeding should be examined only by a physician.)

b. The patient should be given a few seconds to relax at the end of a contraction. The genital area is cleansed with a disinfecting solution. The second and third fingers of a sterile-gloved hand are gently introduced into the introitus. The nurse should pause before advancing the examining fingers.

c. The ischial spines are located, as they indicate station 0 of the presenting part of the fetus. Station 0 is a measurement guide, and the progress of the fetus below this level is referred to as Station 1, 2, and so on.

d. A characteristic of normal labor is the progressive dilation of the cervix. The extent of dilatation is determined by examination of the internal os.

e. Effacement is the incorporation of the cervix into the lower uterine segment, during which thinning and softening occur. This can also be determined by digital examination.

f. Incidence of intrauterine infection and newborn infection are highest when prolonged rupture of the membranes occurs. After the membranes are ruptured, vaginal examinations should be limited to reduce the risk of infection.

g. In early labor, the mucus show is thin and pale pink. In the transitional phase, it is heavy and dark. At no time will this discharge clot, unless there is frank bleeding.

h. Meconium-stained amniotic fluid indicates fetal distress and should be reported to physician immediately.

B. Communicative Aspects

1. *Observations*

a. Note any deviations from normal in the patient's appearance and temperature, and in the odor and color of the mucus that would indicate the need for medical intervention.

b. Note cervical dilation and effacement, and the station of the presenting part.

2. *Charting*

DATE	TREATMENT	TIME	OBSERVATIONS	SIGNATURE
7/27	Vaginal exam	0900	Patient taken to treatment room for vaginal exam by Dr. T. Large cystocele noted. Smear taken for pap exam and sent to lab. Culture of vaginal discharge taken and sent to lab. No vaginal bleeding noted. Patient appeared to be slightly uncomfortable; instructed in relaxation techniques. The patient was able to relax.	F. White, R.N.
		0930	Returned to room, patient asked numerous questions about tests being sent to lab. Nurse gave answers at patient's level of understanding.	F. White, R.N.

3. *Referrals*

Not applicable

C. Teaching Aspects—Patient and Family

1. Cervical cancer is the most common cancer of the reproductive system in women. The disease is almost always curable in its preinvasive state. Therefore, to discover the disease early, every adult female should have a thorough gynecologic examination yearly.

2. A woman should never douche before a gynecologic examination, as such a treatment will wash away cellular deposits used in diagnostic procedures.

3. Danger signals that every woman should report to her physician are spotting, irregular or excessive bleeding, any bleeding after menopause, persistent painful menstruation, leukorrhea, urinary disturbances, or pelvic discomfort.

4. In cleansing the external genitals, particularly after elimination, the female begins at the urethral meatus and wipes downward to the rectum. Otherwise, bacteria may be carried over the introitus and urethral meatus, which may predispose to vaginal and urinary tract infections.

IV. EVALUATION PROCESS

A. Were the patient's fears and anxieties reduced?

B. Was a therapeutic nurse-patient-physician relationship maintained?

C. Does the chart show pertinent information?

D. Were medical instructions carried out effectively?

E. Was sterile technique maintained?

F. Was the progress of labor accurately assessed to allow adequate time to prepare for the delivery?

G. Was the vaginal pack successfully removed?

83

Vital Signs

I. ASSESSMENT OF SITUATION

A. Definition

1. Signs reflecting the physiological state that are governed by the body's vital organs (brain, heart, lungs) and are necessary to sustaining life.

   a. Temperature, measured as

   (1) Oral

   (2) Rectal

   (3) Axillary

   b. Pulse, measured at pulse points

   (1) Radial, femoral, temporal, brachial

   (2) Apical (auscultated)

   (3) Pedal

   c. Respiration

d. Blood pressure, measured by

(1) Auscultation

(2) Palpation (fingertips used instead of stethoscope; only systolic pressure can be determined accurately)

B. Terminology

1. *Blood pressure:* the force of blood exerted against the arterial wall

   a. *Systolic pressure:* greatest pressure exerted against the arterial wall (during contraction of ventricles)

   b. *Diastolic pressure:* lowest pressure exerted against the arterial wall (during relaxation of ventricles)

   c. Common sites for measurement

   (1) Arm: antecubital fossa (brachial artery)

   (2) Leg: popliteal fossa (popliteal artery)

2. *Pulse:* the rhythmic throbbing caused by regular expansion (rise) and contraction (fall) on an artery, as blood is forced into it by the contraction of the left ventricle of the heart

3. *Respiration:* the exchange of gases between an organism and its environment. The respiratory cycle includes inspiration (breathing in) and expiration (breathing out). Rate can be obtained by palpating, seeing, and listening.

4. *Temperature:* heat maintained by a living body expressed in degrees; the balance between heat produced and heat lost

C. Rationale for Actions

1. To assess the patient's condition on admission

2. To determine the baseline values for future comparisons

3. To detect as early as possible any deviation in patient's status

4. To communicate with other members of the health team any observations relative to the patient's well-being

II. NURSING PLAN

A. Objectives

1. To recognize the interrelationships between vital signs, physiological activity, and pathophysiological change

2. To recognize the periodic nature of physiological activity as a basis for evaluating measurement of vital signs

3. To use the information offered by measurement of vital signs as a determinant of patient progress, response to therapy, and nursing intervention

4. To recognize and evaluate the response of the individual patient to environmental factors, internal and external, as indicated by the measurement of vital signs

5. To recognize the necessity to measure vital signs above and beyond an ordered period of time if the patient's condition warrants

6. To communicate the measurement of vital signs to health team members in correct terminology and on correct records

7. To recognize the changes in vital signs that require urgent medical or nursing intervention

B. Patient Preparation

1. The patient should be notified in advance if he will be awakened during the night for vital sign measurement. Knowing the reason for this action may make the procedure less unpleasant.

2. The patient should be at rest or normally active when vital signs are measured for a routine status check. Thus signs should not be measured right after a hot or cold drink, smoking, or unusual exertion. These activities can give false readings of normal vital signs.

C. Equipment

1. Thermometer (oral or rectal)

2. Watch with second hand

3. Sphygmomanometer

4. Stethoscope

5. Lubricant

6. Alcohol sponge

7. Tissue

III. IMPLEMENTING NURSING INTERVENTION

A. Therapeutic Aspects

1. Temperature

   a. The thermometer should be wiped clean of solution before being used, because chemical solutions may irritate mucous membranes and skin and have an objectionable odor or taste. The thermometer should be placed as indicated by the patient's condition. Oral temperatures are taken on all adult patients except those who are unconscious; confused; subject to seizures; or receiving oxygen; and those who have a nasogastric tube in place, have a pathologic condition of the nose, mouth, or throat or have physician instructions otherwise. In an oral reading, the thermometer is placed for 2 min under the tongue, with the lips together (Figs. 83-1, 83-2). The normal oral temperature is 37.0C (98.6F). A rectal temperature is taken by lubricating the rounded tip of the thermometer, inserting it gently 1 to 1½ in (2.5 to 3.8 cm) into the adult rectum and holding it in place for 2 to 5 min. The normal rectal reading is 37.5C (99.6F). The patient's rectum should be cleaned afterward (Figs. 83-3–83-6). Axillary readings are taken by holding a

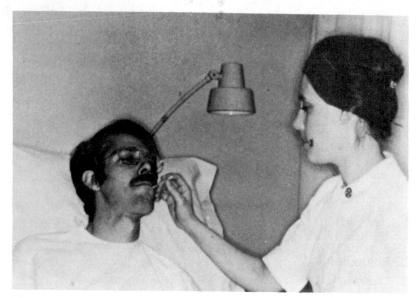

FIGURE 83.1

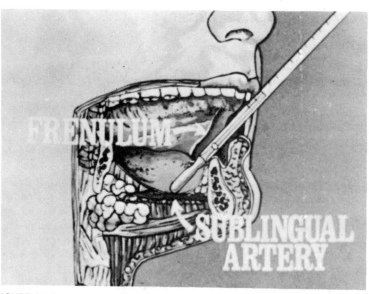

FIGURE 83.2

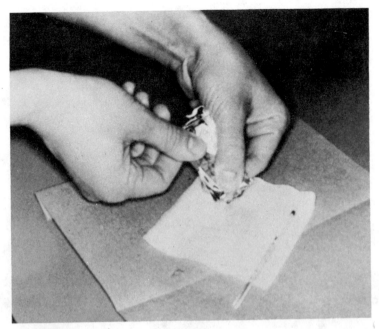

FIGURE 83.3

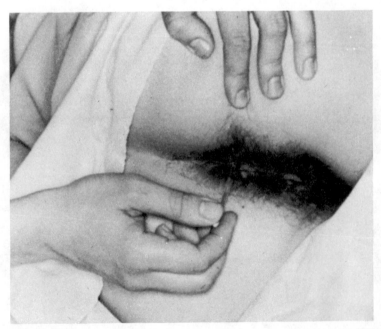

FIGURE 83.4

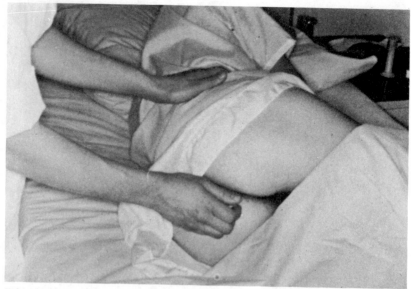

FIGURE 83.5

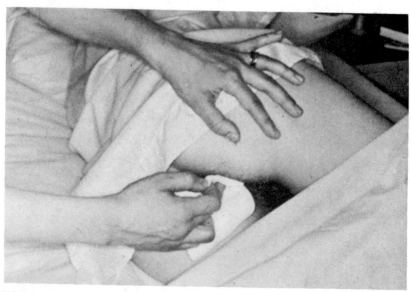

FIGURE 83.6

thermometer in a dry axilla for 5 min. The normal reading is 36.1C (97.5F) (Fig. 83-7). The mouth, rectum, or axillae are used generally, because they most closely simulate the inside of the body, because of their abundant blood supply and the relation of the vascular system to heat regulation.

b. Mercury expands when heated. A constriction in the mercury line near the bulb of the thermometer prevents the mercury from receding to the lowest reading. Before each use, the thermometer should be shaken down vigorously and, using a firm twisting motion, dried.

c. Holding the thermometer horizontally at eye level will facilitate reading. It should be rotated between fingers until the mercury line can be clearly seen.

d. Any remaining fecal material, lubricant, or mucus, should be wiped from the thermometer immediately after use to prevent the growth and spread of microorganisms. Friction with a tissue will help loosen matter from the surface.

2. Pulse

a. The fingertips are very sensitive to touch and are thus used to feel the patient's pulse. The thumb and forefinger have pulses that can be mistaken for that of the patient; therefore, it is better to place the second and third fingers along the appropriate artery

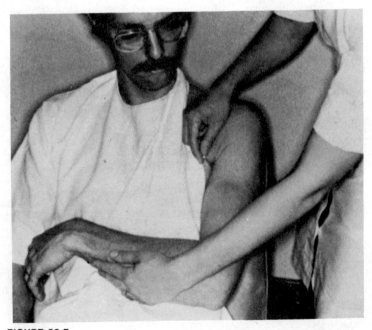

FIGURE 83.7

and press gently. Too much pressure will obliterate the patient's pulse, and too little will make it imperceptible.

b. Sufficient time is needed to detect irregularities and other defects. The pulse should be counted for 30 to 60 sec. If it is irregular, it should be counted for at least 60 sec. The normal ranges are 68 to 72 beats/min for men and 72 to 84 beats/min for women. Auscultation of the apical pulse is accomplished by placing the diaphragm of the stethoscope over the apex of the heart and counting for 1 min. The radial pulse is noted on the inner wrist area (Fig. 83-8A, B). The pedal pulse is located on top of the foot, over the instep (Fig. 83-9A, B). The popliteal pulse is located behind the knee (Fig. 83-10A, B). The femoral pulse is located in the groin area. (Fig. 83-11A, B).

3. Respiration

a. A complete cycle of inspiration and expiration constitutes one act of respiration. This may be noted by the rise and fall of the patient's chest.

b. It may be helpful to count the respirations immediately after counting the pulse, with the fingertips still on the patient's artery. If he is conscious of your counting his respirations, he may inadvertently alter his usual breathing rate.

c. In order to sufficiently observe the rate, depth, and other characteristics of respirations, the nurse should count them for 30 secs. If an abnormality is noted, they should be counted for a full minute. The normal adult range is 16 to 20 respirations/min.

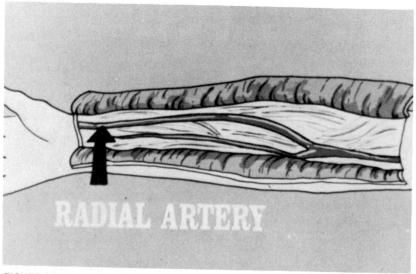

FIGURE 83.8A

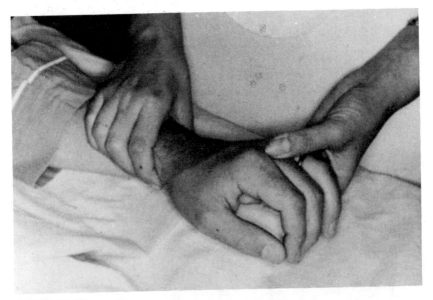

FIGURE 83.8B

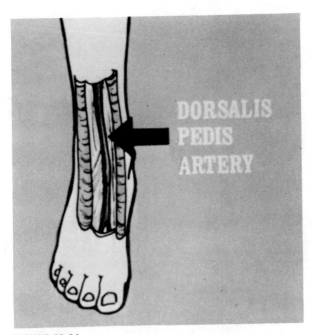

DORSALIS PEDIS ARTERY

FIGURE 83.9A

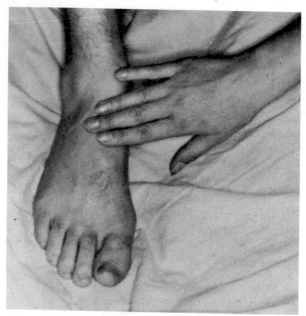

FIGURE 83.9B

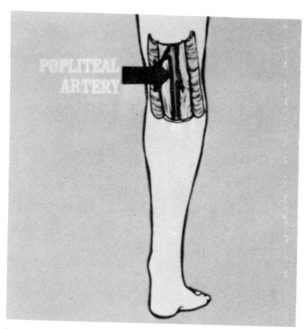

FIGURE 83.10A

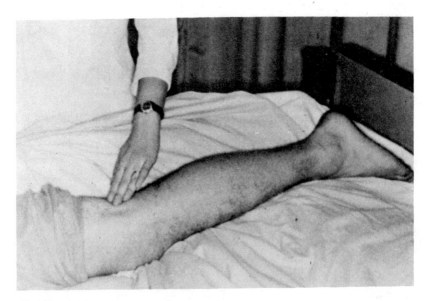

FIGURE 83.10B

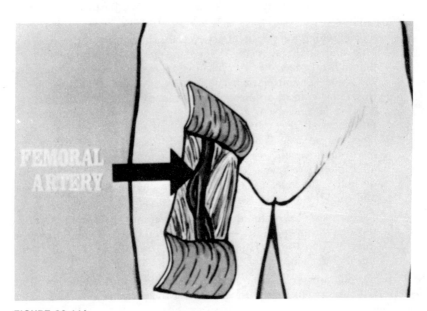

FIGURE 83.11A

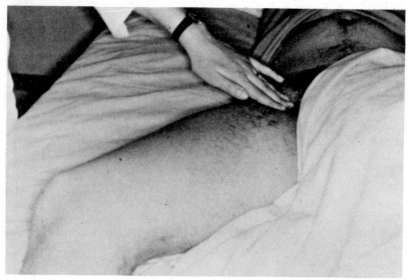

FIGURE 83.11B

4. Blood pressure

   a. The cuff of the sphygmomanometer is applied to the arm above the antecubital fossa or to the leg above the popliteal fossa. The extremity should be positioned for maximum patient comfort and examiner accessibility. The leg is usually used for blood pressure readings only as a last resort, if both arms are inaccessible.

   b. The brachial and popliteal arteries are superficial in the antecubital and popliteal fossae. When the bell of the stethoscope is placed firmly over the artery, sound will be transmitted with little distortion. The artery may be located by palpation with fingertips. The cuff is applied around the extremity (Figs. 83-12–83-14). The meniscus of mercury on mercury-type manometers must be read at eye level, no more than 3 ft (0.9 meters) away. The aneroid type also has a cuff, but it is attached to an instrument that gives the pressure reading on a dial indicator. Normal adult blood pressure is considered to be 120/80 (120 systolic, 80 diastolic), but may vary greatly depending on the patient's age and condition.

   c. Pressure exerted by the inflated cuff prevents blood from flowing through the artery. The cuff should be inflated to a point approximately 20 to 30 mm Hg above the last reading or until pulsation can no longer be felt or heard.

   d. Systolic pressure is the point at which blood in the artery is first able to force its way through against the pressure exerted by the

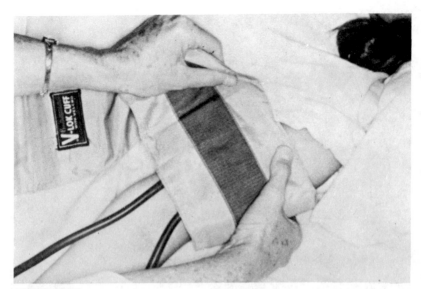

FIGURE 83.12

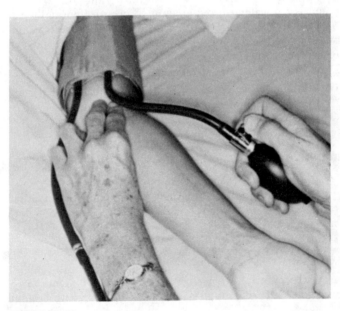

FIGURE 83.13

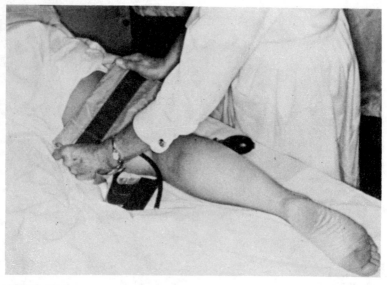

FIGURE 83.14

inflated cuff. It is found by slowly releasing the pressure valve. The point at which the first beat is heard is the systolic reading.

e. Diastolic pressure is the point at which blood flows freely in the artery and is equivalent to the amount of pressure normally exerted on the wall of the arteries when the heart is at rest. While continuing to release the cuff pressure slowly and evenly, the examiner will note the point at which the last distinct sound is heard and record it as the diastolic reading.

f. The patient should be left in a clean and comfortable environment. Proper cleaning of equipment will retard spread of infection. The earpieces of the stethoscope should be cleaned with a disinfectant solution before and after use.

B. Communicative Aspects

1. *Observations*

a. Times for observations are determined by the patient's condition or the physician's instructions. The following routine observations are suggested:

   (1) All new admissions

   (2) Twice daily (8 AM and 4 PM) on all patients

   (3) Every 4 hr or more often on all postoperative patients for 3 days; and on all critically ill patients and patients with deviant vital signs

b. Pulse and respiration should be taken each time the temperature or blood pressure is taken, to assist in assessment of patient's total status. (The pulse usually increases ten beats per degree of temperature increase.)

   c. The rhythm, tension, and volume, as well as rate, should be carefully observed when taking pulse and respiration to detect signs of irregularity.

   d. The interval between systolic and diastolic pressures should be noted regularly, and a steady decrease should be reported to the team leader.

   e. Steady or sudden decreases or increases in one or all vital signs should be reported to the team leader, and more frequent readings should be taken for evaluation of patient status.

2. *Charting*

   a. Record vital signs on the floor temperature worksheet, patient's chart, and bedside vital signs sheet, if applicable (see Technique 37, Charting Guidelines).

   b. Record observations of vital signs in the nurses' notes to assist in continued assessment of patient condition.

DATE	TREATMENT	TIME	OBSERVATIONS	SIGNATURE
5/5		0900	Pulse appears thready, rapid and irregular. Rate 120. Stated, "My heart is pounding and feels as if it's going to explode." Respirations are very short and shallow, with rate of 28. 190/120. Dr. D. notified.	F. White, R.N.

3. *Referrals*

Not applicable

C. Teaching Aspects—Patient

1. Instruct the patient concerning scheduled times for readings of vital signs.
2. Instruct the patient concerning oral restrictions before readings.
3. Inform the patient of any change in schedule and the reason for it.

IV. EVALUATION PROCESS

A. Was the patient cooperative and relaxed during the procedure?

B. Were all significant data noted?

C. Were significant deviations from previous vital sign measurements checked and reported to the appropriate person?

D. Were vital signs effectively interpreted to ensure patient safety?

E. Was medical asepsis maintained?

84

Wheelchair and Walker

I. ASSESSMENT OF SITUATION

A. Definition

Aids in patient mobility. A wheelchair is a chair suspended between two large wheels in back and 2 smaller wheels in front. A walker is a support that accompanies the patient during ambulation.

B. Terminology

None

C. Rationale for Actions

1. To transport the patient who is unable to walk or to walk unsupported
2. To offer a means of mobility to an otherwise bedridden patient
3. To enhance patient safety

II. NURSING PLAN

A. Objectives

1. To maintain optimal safety standards by locking wheelchair, teaching good body mechanics, and giving sufficient assistance during transfer from bed
2. To minimize patient discomfort during transfer
3. To make the patient as comfortable as possible
4. To support dependent body parts adequately

B. Patient Preparation

1. If the patient is informed of the ways in which he can facilitate the lifting technique, he is more likely to cooperate. The assurance that the nurses know what they are doing will also bolster the patient's confidence that he is secure and will not fall.
2. The patient may be bathed before getting up in the wheelchair, and the bed can be made while he is up to lessen exertion.

C. Equipment

1. Wheelchair or walker
2. Pillows, if needed
3. Sheet, if needed

III. IMPLEMENTING NURSING INTERVENTION

A. Therapeutic Aspects

1. Generally, the patient must use a wheelchair because he cannot walk on his own. For this reason, he also usually needs support and assistance in transferring to a wheelchair. The wheelchair should be locked by pushing forward on the lever on the side of the chair that locks the large wheels (Fig. 84-1). The foot and leg supports should be moved out of the way (Fig. 84-2). The chair should still be held when the patient is getting into it, to prevent it from accidentally slipping.

2. The patient may be transferred to the wheelchair in two ways.

    a. *Lifting technique:* to minimize distance, the wheelchair is placed next to the bed at a right angle. The brake must be locked into position. The patient is assisted into a sitting position manually or by raising the head of the bed. The patient is turned to sit parallel to the length of the bed, with his back to the chair. One nurse stands on each side and places her hands under the patient's axillae. Both nurses lift simultaneously, moving the patient backward into the chair. (See Technique 67, Position, Change of [manually and mechanically].)

    b. *Pivot technique:* to minimize distance and exertion, the wheelchair should be placed near and parallel to the bed (Fig. 84-3). The wheels must be locked. The patient is helped into a sitting position on the side of the bed (Fig. 84-4). While one person holds the chair, the other, with hands under his axillae, helps the

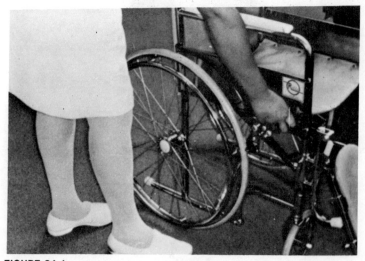

FIGURE 84.1

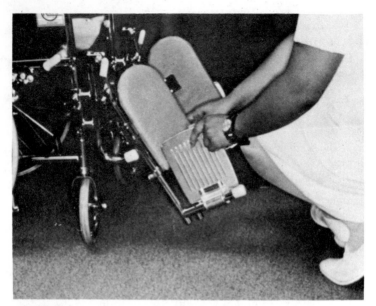

FIGURE 84.2

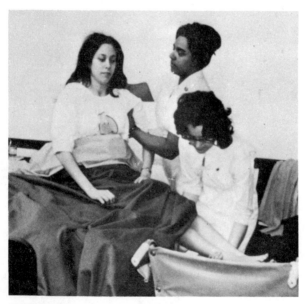

FIGURE 84.3

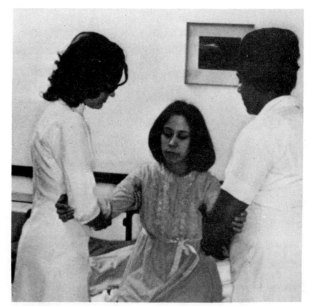

FIGURE 84.4

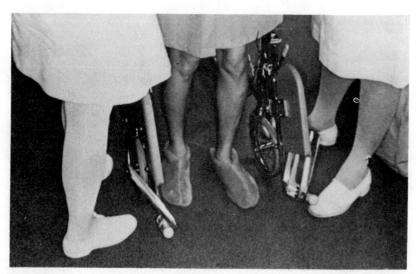

FIGURE 84.5

patient into a standing position. When the patient is upright and stable, he slowly pivots to the side, with his back toward the chair. He then lowers himself, with the nurse's help, into the chair (Figs. 84-5, 84-6).

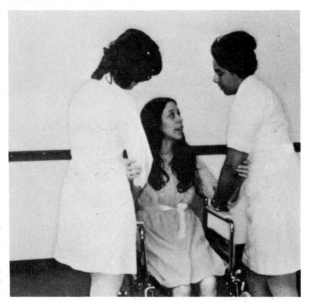

FIGURE 84.6

3. To return to bed, the patient may pivot, if he is able, or he is lifted with one person supporting his shoulders, one person supporting his trunk, and one person supporting his feet and legs (three-man lift). For pivoting, the steps in getting the patient up are done in reverse (Figs. 84-7–84-11).

4. Because of weakness, the patient may be prone to falls from the chair. If this is a possibility, a safety belt or restraint must be secured around the patient's waist. If his condition indicates, a second belt may be placed around his chest, with care not to restrict his breathing.

5. The patient's body should be in proper alignment when in the wheelchair, and dependent parts must be supported. Any limb with a cast should be elevated and not left to dangle. A pillow in the lap will support an arm cast. The leg cast should be secured with restraining straps to ensure that it does not fall off the support.

6. The patient's modesty and warmth may be provided for by placing a sheet over his lap and knees.

7. In lieu of a wheelchair, the patient may be able to use a walker. The walker is a device to assist in ambulation when the patient requires more balance than can be provided with a cane but is able to ambulate without another person assisting. The walker may have wheels or may have four legs so that the patient must lift it with each step. It encircles the front of the patient and has hand grips. To take a step, the patient lifts or rolls the walker approximately 6 to 10 in (14 to 25 cm) in front of him. Then, using the hand grips to balance and sup-

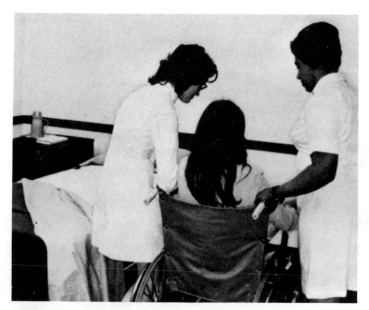

FIGURE 84.7

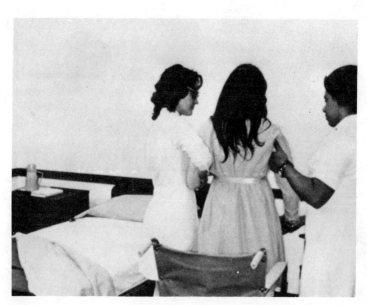

FIGURE 84.8

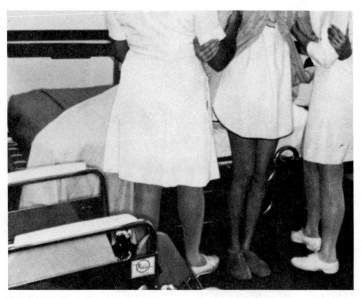

FIGURE 84.9

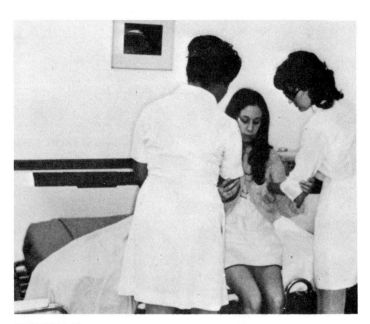

FIGURE 84.10

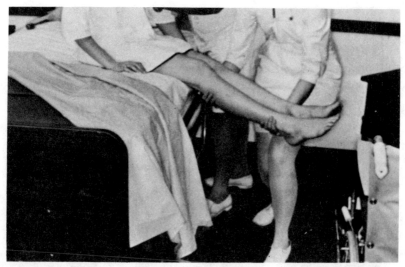

FIGURE 84.11

port himself, he brings himself up to the walker by taking a step (Fig. 84-12). This same process is repeated for each step. The nurse should assist the patient the first few times he walks with a walker to be sure he can balance and support himself and will not fall.

B. Communicative Aspects

1. *Observations*

   a. Check the patient's general condition before getting him up. Unusual fatigue, unstable vital signs, or recent reception of a narcotic, hypnotic, or sedative may be contraindications.

   b. Check the patient frequently while he is up for signs of fatigue or weakness that would mandate a return to bed.

   c. Observe body alignment and position. Use pillows to prop the patient into proper position and support dependent parts. Do not allow the patient to slip downward or to one side, resulting in unnatural curvature of the spine.

2. *Charting*

DATE	TREATMENT	TIME	OBSERVATIONS	SIGNATURE
5/9	Up in wheel-chair	0730	Ate breakfast and sat up for 20 min with right arm cast supported by pillow in elevated position. No swelling of fingers. No sign of discomfort. Seemed to tolerate the procedure better than yesterday. No dizziness.	B. Smith, L.V.N.

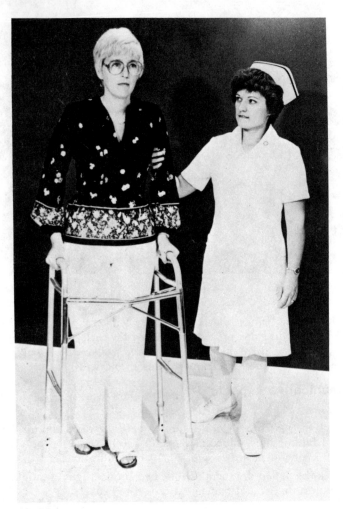

FIGURE 84.12

3. *Referrals*

    a. If the patient will require an ambulatory aid after dismissal, such items may be purchased or rented from a surgical supply house.

    b. A periodic check by a physical therapist may offer confidence and security to the patient who will need ambulatory assistance for an extended period after hospitalization.

C. Teaching Aspects—Patient and Family

1. If the patient is able, encourage and teach him to assist himself as much as possible. Reassure him that he will not fall.

2. If the patient will need a wheelchair at home, teach the family proper

techniques, safety measures, and body mechanics. The patient may be taught to transfer himself, depending on the extent of incapacitation and his own strength and determination.

IV. EVALUATION PROCESS

A. Did the patient actively participate in the ambulation or wheelchair procedure?

B. Was patient comfort maintained before, during, and after transfer?

C. Were dependent parts supported?

D. Was proper body alignment maintained?

3

Techniques for Critically Ill Patients

85

Blakemore-Sengstaken Tube, Assisting With Insertion

I. ASSESSMENT OF SITUATION

A. Definition

1. An intragastric and esophageal tamponade used as a temporary measure to control esophageal hemorrhage; a nasogastric tube with three lumina (Fig. 85-1)

   a. One lumen traverses the entire length of the tube and is used for irrigation, aspiration, and gavage.

   b. One lumen inflates the balloon distal to the cardiac sphincter.

   c. The third lumen inflates the elongated balloon proximal to the cardiac sphincter.

B. Terminology

1. *Cardia:* the upper orifice of the stomach, connecting the stomach with the esophagus.

2. *Gavage:* a method of artificial feeding by means of intubation

3. *Sphincter:* circular muscle constricting an orifice

4. *Tamponade:* a plug used to stop hemorrhage

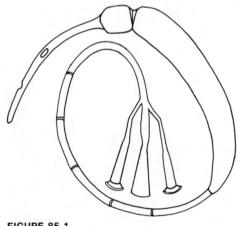

FIGURE 85.1

5. *Varices:* enlarged, twisted veins

C. Rationale for Actions

1. The intragastric tamponade attempts to collapse the venous channels in the cardia of the stomach, in an effort to stop the bleeding at its source.

2. The esophageal tamponade controls bleeding by compressing the varices and initiating firm clot formation.

II. NURSING PLAN

A. Objectives

1. To observe and report signs and symptoms of fluid and electrolyte imbalances

2. To maintain correct pressure of the esophageal and intragastric balloons to control bleeding

3. To provide a quiet environment

4. To allay apprehension and anxiety

5. To make the patient comfortable

6. To monitor vital signs to detect early warning of excessive bleeding

7. To begin discharge planning by teaching the patient and family about future nutritional needs

B. Patient Preparation

1. Elevate the head of the bed to prevent or alleviate nausea and gagging. This position also encourages stomach emptying.

2. Explain to the patient (if possible) and family the equipment and its purpose.

3. Tell the conscious patient that he will feel pressure in his nose and throat as the balloons and tube pass. There will also be a feeling of pressure and distension once the balloons are inflated in the stomach and esophagus. After the tube has been in place for a while, the discomfort will lessen. If medication is available to ease the pain, the patient may feel less apprehensive about the procedure. Stimulation of any kind should be avoided in a bleeding patient; this includes the stimulation brought on by fear and apprehension.

C. Equipment

1. Blakemore-Sengstaken tube

2. Glass Y connector

3. Disposable irrigation set

4. Suction machine

5. Three rubber-shod clamps

6. 75 cm (2½ feet) rubber tubing

7. Anesthetic nasal spray, as prescribed
8. Applicators
9. Water-soluble (K-Y) jelly
10. Blood pressure manometer
11. Adhesive tape, 1.3 cm (½ in) wide
12. Rubber band
13. Safety pin
14. Glass of water with straw
15. Emesis basin
16. Tissues

III. IMPLEMENTING NURSING INTERVENTION

A. Therapeutic Aspects

1. The balloons must be tested for air leaks before insertion. All air should then be evacuated and the rubber plugs reinserted. To facilitate passage by reducing friction, the tube and balloons should be lubricated with water-soluble jelly. The tube is passed by the physician to the 50 cm mark so that the numbers on the tubing will be along the right lateral aspect of the esophagus. If permitted, the patient may swallow water to facilitate passage.

2. With the numbers on the tube in the right lateral position, the cardia and fundus of the stomach will be engaged, thus putting pressure on the gastric veins (Fig. 85-2). The physician will inflate the retention balloon with 50 ml of air. The conical portion of this balloon is clamped 3 cm from the end. The physician will then inflate the stomach balloon with 300 to 400 ml of air; however, this degree of pressure can cause ulceration of the mucosa within a few hours.

3. To prevent undue pressure and irritation to the nostril, the tube may be padded. With a minimum of tension on the tube, a cuff of sponge rubber is placed around the tube next to the nostril and taped in place.

4. The esophageal opening is connected to the rubber tubing, the Y connector, and the blood pressure manometer. The physician will inflate the esophageal balloon to 25 to 30 mm Hg, to raise the pressure above the patient's portal venous pressure, thus applying pressure against esophageal varices.

5. All stomach contents are aspirated to clear the stomach of blood, since subsequent sampling will then be a true index of the effectiveness of hemorrhage control.

6. To prevent clotted blood from plugging the tube, the tube should be irrigated frequently with 50 ml of water.

7. Esophageal pressure should not exceed 45 mm Hg. When the balloon is in the proper position, the pressure will vary with respiratory

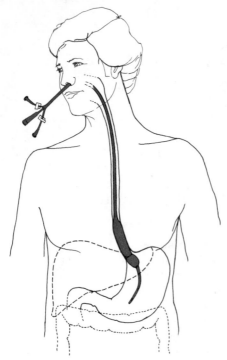

FIGURE 85.2

movement and esophageal contractions. The baseline pressure is the one of importance, however, not the transient peak pressure.

8. After the minimal effective pressure in the esophageal balloon has been determined by evidence of controlled bleeding, the tube leading to the esophageal opening is clamped to maintain a constant pressure against the esophageal varices.

9. After the stomach has been completely evacuated of blood, the stomach aspiration tube is connected to a suction machine.

10. The inflated esophageal balloon occludes the esophagus; thus, the patient cannot take anything by mouth or swallow his saliva. Tissues and an emesis basin should be provided. Gentle suction on the oral-nasal pharynx may be necessary for excessive secretions.

11. The nostrils should be kept clean, lubricated, and protected, so that tissues are not injured from pressure from the tube. Frequent oral hygiene is needed.

12. To ensure patency of the tube and constant gastric suction, the tube may be irrigated as prescribed. Regurgitation of the tube can occur if it becomes clogged and stomach contents accumulate.

13. Vomiting that occurs when an esophageal balloon tamponade is in use can lead to massive aspiration. Insertion of a nasogastric tube in the free nostril will provide drainage and prevent aspiration.

B. Communicative Aspects

1. *Observations*

   a. Check the manometer pressure every 15 to 30 min to guard against air leakage.

   b. Observe the patient for signs and symptoms of fluid imbalance. Evaluate, investigate, report, and treat them, as necessary, with appropriate nursing measures.

   c. Observe the patient for signs and symptoms of circulatory problems. Observation is of particular importance when the patient has a pathologic condition in which hemorrhage is a common complication.

   d. Observe the patient for signs and symptoms of respiratory problems, since asphyxiation can occur. If there is acute respiratory distress, cut the tubes to the balloons (to cause deflation) and remove the tubes if necessary.

   e. Observe the effect of treatment.

   f. Observe the reaction of the patient to the treatment.

   g. Note color, consistency, and amount of aspirated gastric content.

2. *Charting*

DATE	TREATMENT	TIME	OBSERVATIONS	SIGNATURE
6/1	Blake-more tube connected to suction	1320	Inserted by Dr. D. Patient had difficulty in swallowing. 200 ml bright red fluid obtained. Stomach irrigated with 400 ml ice water. No more red fluid obtained. Stomach balloon inflated with 300 ml air. Esophageal balloon inflated to 35 mm Hg pressure. BP 60/40, P 130, R 28. Demerol 50 mg IM given as prescribed. Placed in Fowler's position. Skin clammy, color ashen gray.	G. Ivers, R.N.
	Vaseline to lips and nostrils	1430	Rinsed mouth with mouthwash. Appears to be sleeping. BP 100/70. P 90, R 20.	C. Allen, L.V.N.

3. *Referrals*

   Not applicable

C. Teaching Aspects—Patient and Family

1. Explain to the family why visits should be short and pleasant (the patient needs rest and quiet).
2. Inform the family why the patient needs protection from infection.
3. Teach the family the patient's future nutritional needs.

IV. EVALUATION PROCESS

A. Did the nursing assessment include an evaluation of the emotional concerns of the patient and family?
B. Were measures taken to make the patient comfortable?
C. Is the patient in a quiet, safe environment?
D. Do the patient and family understand the importance of proper diet?
E. Was correct pressure maintained in the esophageal and intragastric balloons?
F. Were the desired effects of the treatment obtained?
G. Was adequate fluid and electrolyte balance maintained?

86

Cardiopulmonary Resuscitation (CPR), Closed Chest—Adult

I. ASSESSMENT OF SITUATION

A. Definition

The act of manually restoring the action of the heart and lungs

B. Terminology

1. *Anoxia:* deficiency of oxygen
2. *Arrhythmia:* abnormality of the heart beat

C. Rationale for Actions

1. To restore normal heart and lung function after an unexpected failure of these organs
2. To maintain adequate circulation until definitive treatment can be instituted

II. NURSING PLAN

A. Objectives

1. To prevent anoxia of the brain
2. To maintain adequate ventilation and circulation

B. Patient Preparation

Cardiac arrest is usually unexpected and calls for immediate nursing measures. The best preparation is to maintain a current stock of emergency drugs and of equipment in excellent working order.

C. Equipment

1. Airway
2. Cardiac arrest board
3. Self-inflating bag-and-mask device (AMBU bag)
4. Suctioning equipment, oral and gastric
5. Intravenous infusion equipment

III. IMPLEMENTING NURSING INTERVENTION

A. Therapeutic Aspects

1. Cardiac arrest is usually unexpected. The family should be notified as soon as possible, given a brief explanation, then kept informed of the continuing treatment.

2. When cardiac arrest occurs, the patient loses consciousness, has no obvious pulse or respiration, and has dilated pupils. With a patient suspected of being in arrest, the nurse should quickly check for respirations, carotid pulse (most easily palpable, Fig. 86-1) and dilated pupils. This should not take more than 15 sec. She should immediately call for help.

3. The heart may sometimes be reactivated within 5 to 15 sec after arrest by a sudden sharp blow on the lower third of the sternum. If pulse and respirations do not return, continue resuscitation.

4. An obstructed air passage prevents adequate ventilation of the lungs and hampers adequate gaseous exchange in the lungs. The air passage must be cleared by removal of any foreign material. The neck should be hyperextended, with the head tilted back. The jaw is pulled upward, and the patient's lungs should be quickly inflated two times, using the mouth-to-mouth or bag (if available) method. The AMBU bag is a commonly used device in resuscitation efforts (Fig. 86-2). It is an inflated bag attached to a mouthpiece. The mouthpiece either can cover the patient's mouth and nose, (in which case it must be pressed firmly against his face to prevent air leaks) or may be adapted to fit an endotracheal or tracheotomy tube (Fig. 86-3). Each time the bag is squeezed, it ejects air and forces it into the patient's lungs. The head may be tilted and the mask held in place with one

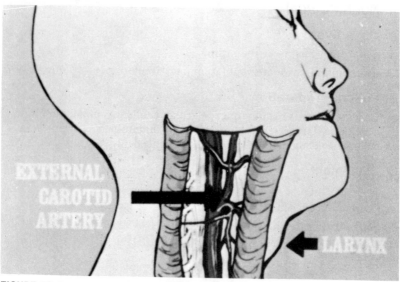

FIGURE 86.1

hand while the other hand is used to squeeze the AMBU bag. If two persons are available to operate the bag, one should use both hands to ensure an open airway and an airtight seal over the patient's nose and mouth while the other person compresses the bag.

5. External cardiac compression is effective only when the patient is on a firm surface, which allows for counterpressure. A cardiac arrest board should be placed beneath the patient's chest.

6. The heel of one hand is placed on the lower third of the sternum, over the heart. The other hand is placed over the first (Fig. 86-4). The sternum should be compressed 1 to 2 in (2.5 to 5 cm) directly downward. Care must be taken not to push too hard, because pressure on the xiphoid process may cause internal injury. Pressure on the ribs on either side of the sternum may cause rib fracture. A fractured rib may cause a punctured lung, leading to pneumothorax.

7. The normal heart rate is approximately 72 beats/min; respirations are normally 14 to 20/min. Adequate ventilation and circulation can be maintained by assisted respirations of 12/min and cardiac compressions of 60/min. When one person gives CPR, two inflations of the lungs should be interspaced with 15 consecutive compressions. When help arrives, the ratio should be one inflation to five compressions. The rhythm must be regular. The procedure must not be interrupted for over 5 sec for any reason.

8. The arrested heart may respond more quickly if a cardiotonic agent is administered by the intravenous (IV) route. An IV infusion should

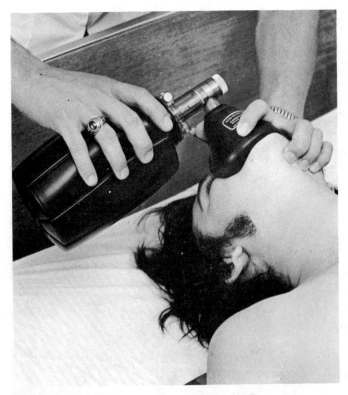

FIGURE 86.2

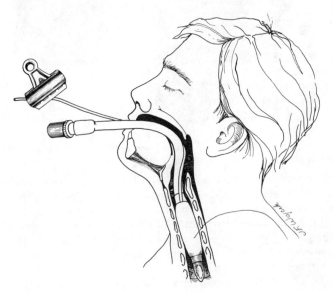

FIGURE 86.3

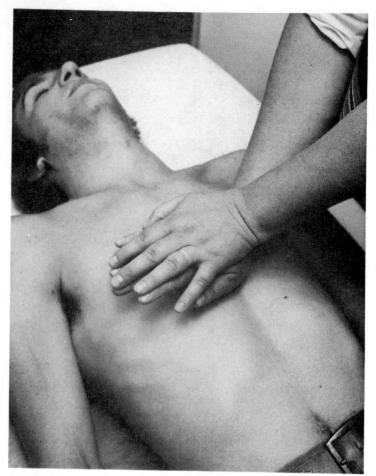

FIGURE 86.4

be started with an intravenous catheter to facilitate the administration of emergency drugs. Lactic acidosis occurs rapidly after cardiac arrest. The nurse should have sodium bicarbonate for IV administration on hand to lessen or prevent acidosis.

9. If closed chest massage produces no response, the physician may desire to mechanically defibrillate the heart. Many types of defibrillators are available; however, most work on the principle of passing an electrical current through the heart muscle in an effort to reestablish normal rhythm. Two paddles from the defibrillator should be placed on the patient's torso. Before placement, they must be well lubricated to prevent burning the patient (Fig. 86-5). Commercial electrode pastes are available. One paddle is placed on the upper left chest slightly toward the midline, and the other is placed somewhat below

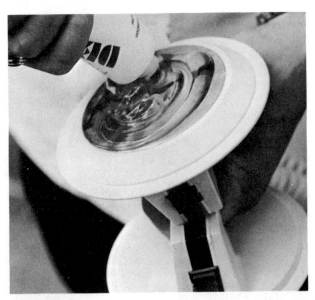

FIGURE 86.5

the left axilla. The exact location will vary with body size, but the desirable effect is to create a current in a straight line from paddle to paddle that will pass through the cardiac muscle. Since this current is highly transmissible, no member of the resuscitation team should be touching the patient at the time the current is released.

10. Successful cardiac output can be determined by return of the carotid pulse, by pupil movement (constriction), and possibly by spontaneous return of respirations.

11. To ensure a patent airway, a plastic oral airway device may be inserted. It serves to keep the tongue from falling against the roof of the mouth and to keep the teeth separated. Another means of maintaining an airway is by the insertion of an endotracheal tube into the trachea. This is accomplished by using a laryngoscope to visualize the trachea and by slipping the long tube through the scope, past the epiglottis, into the trachea. *This procedure should be performed only by specially trained personnel.* However, the nurse should be ready to care for the endotracheal tube once it is in place. Assisted breathing via the AMBU bag may be done through this tube. It should be tied or taped in place to lessen the possibility of its being aspirated.

12. During assisted or controlled respiration, the stomach may become dilated by air forced down the esophagus. Gaseous distension of the stomach can cause the gastric contents to be expelled through the mouth, leading to aspiration. Oral suctioning may be performed until a nasogastric tube can be inserted.

B. Communicative Aspects

1. *Observations*

   a. Circulation must be restored within 4 minutes of a cardiac arrest to prevent irreversible brain damage or death.

   b. A record must be kept that includes the following: the times resuscitation began, physician arrived, and resuscitation ended; drugs and techniques used; and the effectiveness of procedure.

2. *Charting*

DATE	TREATMENT	TIME	OBSERVATIONS	SIGNATURE
4/19	CPR begun	1015	Patient placed on cardiac arrest board. Resuscitation given by R.N. and L.V.N., at ratio of 5 compressions to 1 resp. "Code 99" called.	
		1020	Weak femoral pulse felt. Pupils constricted. Skin cool, moist and pale in color.	
		1025	Dr. D. here. Meds given as prescribed.	
		1045	Femoral pulse 72, good volume and regular rhythm.	
		1050	Spontaneous resp. 12/min. Radial pulse 76/min. Color good. Patient reacts to verbal stimuli. BP 92/60. Pupils equal and react.	
		1055	Physician explained emergency to family.	
		1130	Patient condition remains stable. Appears confused at this time. Clergy and family here with patient.	
		1200	V.S. stable. Patient asleep.	
		1300	V.S. stable. Patient asleep.	F. White, R.N.

3. *Referrals*

   Not applicable

C. Teaching Aspects—Patient and Family

1. Because time is a key factor during a cardiac arrest, all teaching of patient and family, other than notifying the family of the situation, is done *after* the emergency is resolved.

2. Instruct family to maintain a calm attitude when they are with the patient.

3. Instruct the patient to resume activity according to the physician's instructions.

4. Answer, as simply as possible, any questions the patient or family may have regarding the cardiac arrest.

IV. EVALUATION PROCESS

A. Have the fears and apprehensions of patient and family been eased?
B. Did the staff remain calm under emergency conditions?
C. Are physician's instructions written?
D. Are the patient's vital signs normal?
E. Is the patient mentally alert?
F. Was the resuscitation successful?

87

Cardioversion, Assisting With

I. ASSESSMENT OF SITUATION

A. Definition

A method of countershocking the heart at such a time in the cardiac cycle as to interrupt an abnormal rhythm and permit resumption of a normal rhythm

B. Terminology

1. *Arrhythmia:* abnormal heart action
2. *Atrial fibrillation:* disorganized and uncoordinated twitching of the atrial muscle
3. *Atrial flutter:* rapid, regular flutter of the atria, usually resulting in an atrial rate of 250 to 350 beats/min
4. *Cardiac cycle:* the electrical and mechanical activity involved from one point in a heartbeat to the same point in the next beat
5. *Hemoptysis:* blood tinged sputum
6. *Paroxysmal atrial tachycardia (PAT):* abnormally rapid heart rate (usually around 140 to 250 atrial beats/min)
7. *Sinoatrial node (SA node):* the area in the upper right atrium that initiates the electrical charge precipitating a heartbeat
8. *Ventricular tachycardia:* abnormally fast heart rate with decreased output manifested by ectopically caused erratic ventricular beats

C. Rationale for Actions

1. To convert the patient experiencing congestive heart failure and severe paroxysmal atrial tachycardia (PAT) back into normal sinus rhythm
2. To counteract the potential danger of atrial flutter or atrial fibrillation, attempting to reestablish normal rhythm
3. To reestablish normal sinus rhythm in the patient suffering from ventricular tachycardia that medications have failed to convert.

II. NURSING PLAN

A. Objectives

1. To return the patient to normal sinus rhythm
2. To eliminate a life-threatening arrhythmia
3. To assist the patient in cardiac rehabilitation, if appropriate
4. To monitor patients with potential cardiovascular problems carefully to ensure early and prompt treatment

B. Patient Preparation

1. The patient and family should understand why this procedure is necessary as well as what will take place. The patient should have at least a basic understanding of the cardiac irregularity necessitating cardioversion. A signed consent form signifying the patient's understanding of the procedure and his permission for it is usually required.
2. To ensure maximal effect and prevent the danger of drug-induced complications, diuretics and short acting digitalis preparations should be withheld for 24 to 36 hr. If possible, the patient should fast for 6 to 8 hours before cardioversion.
3. A 12-lead ECG should be done before cardioversion.

C. Equipment

1. Electrical defibrillator
2. Electrode paste
3. Suction machine
4. Endotracheal intubation setup
5. Emergency cardiac medications
6. Continuous cardiac monitoring equipment
7. 12-lead ECG machine

III. IMPLEMENTING NURSING INTERVENTION

A. Therapeutic Aspects

1. Cardioversion is extremely effective in the treatment of atrial flutter. It is also used for atrial fibrillation and ventricular fibrillation,

though sometimes not as effectively. Cardioversion can be extremely dangerous when the patient has been taking digitalis, since this externally caused stimulation of the heart muscle can precipitate ventricular fibrillation.

2. The goal in cardioversion is to avoid timing the shock to coincide with the T wave (see Technique 6, Electrocardiogram). To relieve the arrhythmia and restart the heart's beating in normal sinus rhythm, the physician initiates an electrical shock of relatively light intensity through the heart muscle. If the shock passes through the myocardium during the repolarization phase (T wave segment of the ECG), ventricular fribrillation may be induced. Therefore, the patient is attached to a cardiac monitoring device, and the pattern is watched carefully to assess the proper time to countershock.

3. A patent line for intravenous infusion is usually desirable in case of cardiac emergency. Emergency drugs and resuscitation equipment should be nearby.

4. The nurse should apply electrode paste liberally to the flat polished surface of the paddles. The physician places the paddles firmly against the chest wall in such a position as to direct the current through the heart muscle. The paddles are not to be placed near the electrodes since a spark could cause a burn on the skin. Employing the minimum effective electrical charge reduces the possibility of complications. Usually the starting level is 50 watt-sec or less. If this proves unsuccessful, the voltage may be changed to 100 watt-sec and increased by 100 watt-sec increments up to 400 watt sec. As a safety factor, all personnel should move away from the bed before shock is administered.

5. The patient will warrant careful monitoring for several hours after cardioversion has been completed. Visual cardiac monitoring, as well as frequent vital sign observation, is appropriate. The nurse should report any irregularities to the physician immediately. Emergency cardiac resuscitation equipment and drugs should be kept nearby until the patient's condition has stabilized.

B. Communicative Aspects

1. *Observations*

   a. The patient's monitor pattern should be carefully observed for conversion to normal sinus rhythm and to ensure that he does not lapse back into arrhythmia during the postconversion period.

   b. Since pulmonary embolism is a possible, though rare, complication of cardioversion, the patient must be observed for shortness of breath, cyanosis, chest pain, rapid respirations, and hemoptysis. The pain from pulmonary embolism may be discriminated from coronary pain in that it will be increased during respiration and decreased when the patient is holding his breath. Coronary pain is usually unrelenting and unaffected by respiration.

2. *Charting*

DATE	TREATMENT	TIME	OBSERVATIONS	SIGNATURE
5/4	Cardioversion from atrial flutter to normal sinus rhythm	1015	Rate before cardioversion, 140/min, 2-1 block. After cardioversion normal sinus rhythm of 86. ECG done. Cardiac monitor continuously. BP 136/88, R 18.	F. White, R.N.

3. *Referrals*

    a. The American Heart Association may be of assistance in helping the patient adjust to his cardiac rehabilitation program.

    b. Many cities have organized local groups of people who have suffered coronary problems. These groups may offer tremendous support and inspiration to coronary patients.

C. Teaching Aspects

1. The patient should be instructed to report any chest pain immediately.

2. Many coronary patients have difficulty accepting the dependent status necessary for recovery from cardiac problems. Even the simplest activities of everyday life, such as eating and elimination, are in the hands of other people. Acceptance of this dependent state can be facilitated by a matter-of-fact attitude on the part of the nurse, accompanied by careful explanations of the importance of rest and immobility to the recuperation process.

IV. EVALUATION PROCESS

A. Has the patient accepted his coronary problems and the ensuing limitations?

B. Was the patient informed about the cardioversion procedure; was he relaxed?

C. Is the patient's heart in normal sinus rhythm?

D. Has recurrence of the arrhythmia been decreased or eliminated?

88

Central Venous Pressure (CVP)

I. ASSESSMENT OF SITUATION

A. Definition

The measurement, in centimeters of water, of the pressure in the vena cava or right atrium, using a catheter threaded into the subclavian vein

B. Terminology

1. *CVP:* central venous pressure
2. *Hypervolemia:* increased volume of circulating blood
3. *Hypovolemia:* decreased volume of circulating blood
4. *Vena cava:* the major vein returning blood to the right atrium of the heart

C. Rationale for Actions

1. To determine blood volume
2. To evaluate the effectiveness of the pump mechanism of the heart
3. To evaluate vascular tone

II. NURSING PLAN

A. Objectives

1. To obtain an accurate reading
2. To allay the patient's fear
3. To prevent infection
4. To maintain fluid and electrolyte balances
5. To prevent air embolism

B. Patient Preparation

1. To allay anxiety and promote cooperation, the patient should be told he will not feel anything during the reading. He should understand why he must lie flat in bed with no pillow.
2. A central line connected to the right atrium or vena cava acts as an extension of the patient's vascular system. The venous pressure set, with a four-way stopcock, is connected to the subclavian intravenous (IV) line (Fig. 88-1). (See directions on the box of the venous pressure set.)

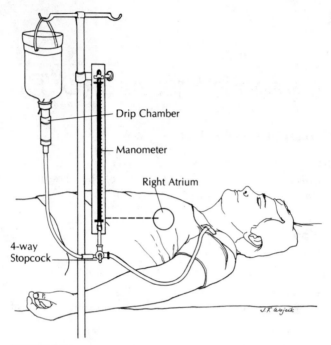

- Drip Chamber
- Manometer
- Right Atrium

4-way
Stopcock

FIGURE 88.1

3. An inaccurate zero point results in inaccurate CVP readings. The zero point on the centimeter scale tape must be at the level of the patient's right atrium. This is approximately midway between the anterior and posterior chest walls when the patient is in a recumbent position.

4. Circulatory dynamics are most stable while the individual is supine, since the arteries and veins are horizontally oriented at near-heart level. The patient must be flat in bed, with no pillows.

C. Equipment

1. Disposable venous pressure set, connected to IV infusion
2. Centimeter scale attached to IV standard
3. 18-ga airway needle

III. IMPLEMENTING NURSING INTERVENTION

A. Therapeutic Aspects

1. A vacuum within a bottle will not permit fluid to drip. If the vacuum is not released, the patient's blood will be drawn into the tubing and bottle. An 18-ga airway needle inserted into the stopper of the IV solution container will release the vacuum.

2. The venous pressure tubing should be filled with fluid to evacuate air because air in the line interferes with the pressure reading and could cause an air embolism. To fill, the stopcock is turned so that fluid does not fill manometer.

3. Introduction of pathogens can cause infection. All connections should be kept sterile while venous pressure tubing is being set up.

4. Respirators should be detached, if possible, during venous pressure readings. Artificial ventilators increase inspiratory pressure in the chest and will cause a higher CVP reading.

5. Occlusion of the patient's tubing by turning the stopcock allows fluid to enter the manometer. It is not necessary that fluid go all the way to the top of the manometer, but it should go far enough above the estimated CVP level so that one can see a free fall of fluid when the stopcock is opened toward the patient. In a disposable set, the fluid should not go all the way up the manometer tubing to wet the cotton air filter.

6. The stopcock is turned so that it is level with the IV tubing, allowing the solution from the manometer to communicate with the patient's venous tubing. The fluid in the manometer will drop until its hydrostatic pressure is equal to the patient's venous pressure. The solution in the manometer should fluctuate with each phase of respiration.

7. The scale on the manometer should be read at eye level; variations in reading will occur if the scale is viewed from different angles. Usual normal range is 5 to 12 cm H_2O. Reading should be taken at the point where fluid descent stops.

8. A continuous flow of solution will keep the tubing patent. The stopcock lever must be positioned to reestablish communication between the venous catheter and the IV solution. The fluid should drip at the rate prescibed by the physician.

B. Communicative Aspects

1. *Observations*

   a. If the fluid in the manometer drops rapidly (it normally fluctuates with the patient's respirations), check for a leak in the tubing or attachment points.

   b. If the fluid does not fall, drops sluggishly, or drops and stops intermittently, the catheter may have a clot in it, completely or partially occluding the flow of fluid.

   c. Check all tubing for kinking before each reading.

   d. A position change of the patient or equipment may produce a variance of more than 2 to 3 cm H_2O and result in an inaccurate reading.

   e. Check the dressing of the subclavian catheter insertion for bleeding or dampness. This may occur if the catheter becomes disconnected from the IV tubing.

f. Venous pressures are not usually taken with whole blood infusions, because blood may clot in the stopcock and cause mechanical difficulties.

g. Keep a record of each CVP, and notify the physician if a drastic increase or decrease in the CVP occurs. The upward or downward trend the CVP takes is much more important than the absolute value of one reading.

h. An elevated CVP may indicate hypervolemia, whereas a low CVP may indicate hypovolemia.

2. *Charting*

DATE	TREATMENT	TIME	OBSERVATIONS	SIGNATURE
5/31	CVP	0900	CVP is 4 to 5 cm; respirator removed during CVP reading.	
		0905	Patient turned to left side. IV running 33 drops/min.	G.Ivers, R.N.

3. *Referrals*

Not applicable

C. Teaching Aspects—Patient and Family

1. Instruct the patient and family about the hazards involved in their handling the equipment.

2. Explain the need for frequent readings of the CVP.

IV. EVALUATION PROCESS

A. Do the patient and family understand the reason for taking the CVP?

B. Is each reading properly recorded on the chart?

C. Was the patient left in a comfortable position after the reading was taken?

D. Was an accurate reading obtained?

E. Was the fluid flowing at the proper rate after the CVP was taken?

F. Does the intake and output record reflect fluid balance?

G. Is each reading properly recorded on the chart?

89

Chest Drainage (Closed)

I. ASSESSMENT OF SITUATION

A. Definition

1. The evacuation of air or fluid or both from the pleural cavity through a closed drainage system. Types are the following:
   a. Closed chest drainage without suction (by gravity)
   b. Closed chest drainage with suction (by pump)
   c. Closed drainage set up with one, two, or three bottles, depending on the physician's preference.

B. Terminology

1. *Atelectasis:* an airless state, causing collapse of lung tissue
2. *Bronchi:* tubes leading to the alveoli of the lungs
3. *Pleural cavity:* potential space between the two pleura covering the lungs
4. *Subatmospheric pressure:* pressure below that of the atmosphere

C. Rationale for Actions

To reestablish subatmospheric pressure in the pleural cavity, thereby permitting reexpansion of the lung

II. NURSING PLAN

A. Objectives

1. To maintain an airtight system preventing complications and infections
2. To relieve the patient's anxiety and discomfort
3. To teach the patient the importance of turning, deep breathing, and coughing
4. To prevent postural deformities and contractures
5. To record observations accurately
6. To promote adequate gaseous exchange

B. Patient Preparation

1. The patient and family should understand why the chest tube is being inserted and be informed of the measures taken to prevent com-

plications such as kinked tubing, leakage in the system, or elevation of the drainage bottle above the patient's chest.

2. Clamps should be placed in a convenient, conspicuous place for use after insertion, should the airtight system develop a leak.

C. Equipment

1. Sterile chest drainage set, containing:
   a. 2,000 ml glass bottle or plastic container
   b. Rubber stopper with holes and tubing
   c. Rubber tubing
   d. Plastic connector(s)
2. 1 liter sterile water
3. Adhesive tape and safety pins
4. Thoracic pump, if suction prescribed
5. Chest bottle protector (wooden box)
6. Clamps
7. Additional 2,000 ml bottles, rubber stoppers, and tubing if two- or three-bottle setup is needed

III. IMPLEMENTING NURSING INTERVENTION

A. Therapeutic Aspects

1. Pathogenic microorganisms may be present on the skin and equipment. Hands should be washed thoroughly. Equipment attached to the patient's chest catheters must be sterile.

2. Water-sealed drainage facilitates escape of air and fluid from the pleural cavity (Fig. 89-1). The water acts as a seal and keeps air from being drawn back into the chest. The drainage tube(s) from the patient's chest is attached to the tubing that leads to a long tube. This tube should be submerged at least 1 in under sterile water.

3. As drainage accumulates, pressure will build up that will eventually halt the process, unless there is some escape of air from the water-sealed drainage bottle. A short tube must be provided to allow escape of air from the chest bottle. This tube is located in the rubber stopper and is open to the atmosphere. The tube is approximately 10 cm (4 in) long and is not submerged in the water.

4. The amount of drainage may be indicative of the effectiveness of the drainage system. Knowledge of the quantity of drainage also assists the physician in evaluation and treatment. The original fluid level should be marked on the drainage bottle with adhesive tape.

5. Kinking of the tube may result in obstruction of drainage. Looping or pressure on the drainage tube can produce retrograde pressure, thus forcing drainage back into the pleural cavity. All tubes should be taped to the plastic connectors. The tubing should be fastened to the

From
Patient

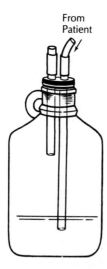

FIGURE 89.1

sheet with adhesive tape and a safety pin for optimal gravitational flow. The tubing should not loop or interfere with the movements of the patient.

6. The tubing may become obstructed with clots and fibrin. It should be "milked" every hour to prevent obstruction, by compressing the tubing manually in a progressive manner from patient to drainage receptacle.

7. Oscillation of the water level in the tube shows that there is effective patency between the pleural cavity and the drainage bottle. Oscillation will normally decrease as the lung reexpands. It may cease before reexpansion, because of clots and fibrin sealing off the tube.

8. *The drainage bottle must never be elevated above the level of the patient's chest, since the fluid may flow back into the patient's chest.*

9. If any part of the apparatus is damaged, the closed system will be destroyed. If a negative pressure is lost, atmospheric pressure in the pleural space will cause collapse of the lung. The drainage bottle must be stabilized in a protector on the floor. The bed should be in the high position. A hissing noise may indicate a leak. Visitors and personnel should be cautioned against handling equipment or displacing the bottle. Clamps should be kept nearby. Chest tubes should be clamped as near the patient's chest as possible, should damage to the apparatus occur.

10. Suction may be prescribed to hasten reexpansion of the lung or to compensate for a persistent air leak in the closed system. The physician will prescribe the amount of suction. A two-bottle setup may be used, with the second bottle attached to the first by rubber tubing to a short tube (Fig. 89-2). A long glass tube is submerged under water and opened to the atmosphere. This tube controls the amount of suc-

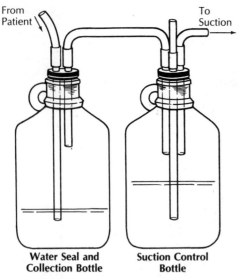

From Patient

To Suction

Water Seal and Collection Bottle

Suction Control Bottle

FIGURE 89.2

tion applied. The deeper it is submerged, the higher the vacuum. A third length of tube is connected to suction apparatus.

11. Direct observation of drainage aids in diagnosis and treatment. A three-bottle system is necessary for this (Fig. 89-3A, B). The first trap bottle permits visualization of fluid drainage. The second bottle, in combination with the first, can operate as a simple water seal. The third bottle controls the amount of suction by the depth of the tube submerged in water.

12. Coughing and deep breathing assist in raising the intrapleural pressure, clearing the bronchi, expanding the lung, and preventing atelectasis. The patient should be encouraged and assisted to breathe deeply and cough at hourly intervals.

13. Immobilization causes postural deformities and contractures. Proper body alignment should be encouraged.

14. Because of pain and discomfort, the patient may favor the arm and shoulder on the affected side. These body parts should be put through range-of-motion exercises several times daily.

15. The thoracic pump acts as a seal when it is not functioning. Therefore, the chest drainage bottle must be vented to the atmosphere when the pump is disconnected or malfunctioning.

B. Communicative Aspects

1. *Observations*

   a. Observe and immediately report symptoms of respiratory embarrassment, pressure in the chest, or hemorrhage.

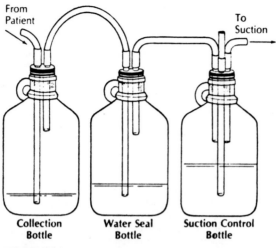

FIGURE 89.3A

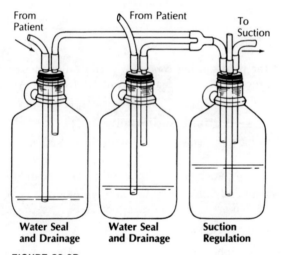

FIGURE 89.3B

b. Chart color, consistency, and approximate amount of drainage every 8 hr. (This can be estimated by marking a tape on the bottle.) The physician usually changes or empties the bottles when indicated. If the bottle is full or the physician gives an instruction to empty the bottle, be sure to clamp the tubes near the chest before disturbing the closed system.

c. Observe the apparatus frequently for proper functioning. *Be certain that the system is airtight and the tubes are open.*

d. Include the amount of drainage on the intake and output record of chart.

2. *Charting*

DATE	TREATMENT	TIME	OBSERVATIONS	SIGNATURE
5/22	Chest tubes attached to sterile under-water seal drainage system. 20 cm suction with electric pump.	0900	200 ml bright blood obtained initially. Fluid fluctuating in tube. BP 120/80, P 80, R 24; no cyanosis noted. R shallow. Patient encouraged to breathe deeply.	
		0905	Patient continues to have shallow resp. Turned to left side, P 88, R 26. IM med for discomfort given.	
		0920	R improved. Family with patient. Explanation given to patient and family regarding chest drainage.	F. White, R.N.
		1000	Tube remains patent. Approx 400 ml red fluid returned. Resting quietly.	B. Smith, L.V.N.

3. *Referrals*

Depending upon the predisposing condition necessitating chest tube insertion, some financial assistance may be available from the American Lung Association.

C. Teaching Aspects—Patient and Family

1. Explain the reason for and principles of the drainage system to patient and family.

2. Caution the family and patient not to handle the equipment.

3. Encourage the patient and family to report any symptoms of respiratory difficulty or discomfort to the nurse immediately.

IV. EVALUATION PROCESS

A. Is the patient as comfortable and relaxed as possible?

B. Do the patient and family understand the reason for and the expected results of the chest tube system?

C. Is the patient coughing, turning, and breathing deeply, properly, and regularly?

D. Are treatments and observations properly charted?

E. Is the system patent?

F. Is adequate gaseous exchange occurring, as evidenced by blood gas studies or patient's coloring?

G. Has the patient maintained proper body alignment?

H. Has clotting, kinking, or disassembly of the tubing been prevented?

90

CircOlectric Bed and Foster Frame

I. ASSESSMENT OF SITUATION

A. Definition

Devices for periodically changing a patient's position from prone to supine and vice versa, with little or no active participation on the part of the patient. (A Stryker frame is similar to but lighter than a Foster frame.)

B. Terminology

1. *Anterior frame:* frame on which the patient rests when in a prone position
2. *Posterior frame:* frame on which the patient rests when in a supine position
3. *Prone:* lying stomach-side down, with the face downward
4. *Supine:* lying on the back, with the face upward

C. Rationale for Actions

1. To secure a higher degree of immobilization
2. To maintain the desired body alignment while administering needed physical care
3. To maintain a position of hyperextension at adjustable points and heights
4. To maintain traction during the turning process, if desired
5. To change points of greatest pressure on body

II. NURSING PLAN

A. Objectives

1. To allay the fears and anxieties of the patient and family
2. To provide a safe and therapeutic environment
3. To prevent tissue breakdown due to pressure
4. To maintain a position of hyperextension
5. To observe the reaction of the patient while being turned
6. To plan and adhere to a turning schedule most compatible with patient and family needs

7. To record and report observations accurately

8. To ensure that hydration and elimination needs are being met

9. To provide some source of diversional therapy

B. Patient Preparation

1. Because of the helplessness caused by his condition, the patient will usually face the idea of turning with some degree of apprehension. The procedure must be thoroughly explained before the patient is turned the first time, if he is conscious. The nurse should emphasize the extra precautions taken to ensure that he does not slip or fall. Moreover, the patient should be reassured *each* time he is turned that he is safe and will not fall.

2. To facilitate the turning process, all equipment (*e.g.,* straps, pillows) should be available within easy reach.

3. When the patient is placed on the CircOlectric bed, he should be told that initial dizziness is to be expected.

C. Equipment

1. Foster frame

   a. Frames with canvas strips

   b. Pillows and foam pads

   c. Three restraining straps

   d. Footboard and armrests

   e. Tray table

   f. Bedpan holder

   g. Springs

   h. Linen

   i. Two security pins

2. CircOlectric bed

   a. Frames (basic and anterior)

   b. Foam mattress

   c. Special sheet

   d. Restraining straps

   e. Footboard and side rails

   f. Forehead and chin straps

III. IMPLEMENTING NURSING INTERVENTION

A. Therapeutic Aspects

1. Foster frame (Fig. 90-1)

   a. Patient safety is of primary importance in this procedure. Pillows and padding make the patient more secure in the frame, protect

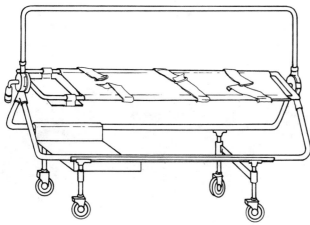

FIGURE 90.1

the female patient's breasts, and prevent limbs from slipping during the procedure (Fig. 90-2). Armboards should be lowered or removed. When the patient is being turned from supine to prone, pillows are placed over the chest and lower legs. When the patient is being turned from prone to supine, the padding should be over the back and lower legs, unless contraindicated. The arms should be placed at the sides, with a sheet tucked around the entire body to secure them.

b. Two frames enhance the immobilizing potential of the Foster orthopedic bed. The appropriate frame is placed over the entire length of the patient's body (Fig. 90-3). The security pins are inserted in the appropriate holes at the head and foot of the frames to lock them into place.

c. Use of headbands provides maximum support and comfort for the patient. The headbands on the anterior frame support the patient's chin and forehead.

d. Restraining straps add an extra margin of safety. The three straps go around both frames at the levels of shoulders, hands, and knees.

e. Two persons should turn the frame. Both anterior and posterior frames have been fitted on a standard with a pivoting device. The frame must be held securely while the lock at the head of the frame is released. The patient is turned in one smooth motion, neither too fast nor too slow.

f. While continuing to hold the frame securely, the nurse at the head secures the head lock in the turning mechanism. Once the frame is securely locked in place, the restraining straps, security pins, top frame, and padding are removed. The patient should be covered with a sheet.

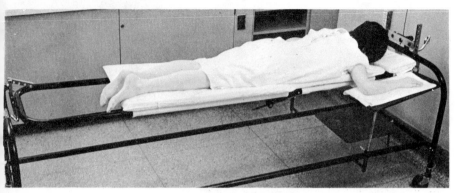

FIGURE 90.2

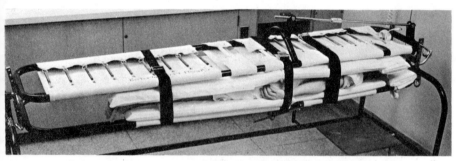

FIGURE 90.3

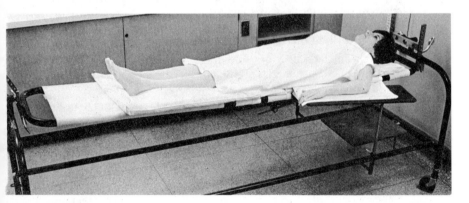

FIGURE 90.4

g. The armrests should be replaced and adjusted (Fig. 90-4). They prevent adduction contractures of the shoulders and flexion contractures of the elbows. The rests also provide a means of assuming a comfortable arm position. On the posterior frame, the armrests should be level with the frame. On the anterior frame, they should be below the level of the frame, in most cases.

h. The tendons of the calf muscles tend to shorten if the foot is allowed to rest in an unsupported position, whereas the muscles in the anterior portion of the leg become stretched. Therefore, when the patient is in the supine position, the feet should be planted firmly against a footboard in normal position. Having the feet hang over the end of the anterior frame prevents extreme plantar flexion of the feet with resultant foot drop and heel cord shortening and also prevents pressure on the dorsa of the feet. When the patient is in prone position, there must be adequate clearance for both feet to hang over anterior frame in normal position.

i. When the patient is in the prone position, the reading board is adjusted for his use and comfort in reading, eating, writing, and occupational therapy. Adequate lighting will prevent eyestrain.

j. The perineal section of the frame may be removed for using the bedpan while the patient is in the supine position. The bedpan is placed in a special rack. After its use, the perineal section should be replaced to prevent poor spinal alignment resulting from the buttocks being deprived of support for a long period.

k. The patient should be bathed daily. The patient's front is bathed as he lies on the posterior frame. The bath is completed when he is turned to the prone position. Sheets are changed in the same consecutive manner.

l. Traction may be attached to the frame. It is used to produce a state of equilibrium and must, therefore, be maintained continuously.

2. CircOlectric bed (Fig. 90-5)

a. In using the CircOlectric bed, many of the considerations involving safety, position, cleanliness, and traction are the same as for the Foster frame. Special considerations of the CircOlectric bed follow.

b. The usual purpose of the CircOlectric bed is maintenance of stable body alignment. Therefore, when a patient is transferred to this bed, his body must be kept in alignment. A minimum of three or four people is required.

c. After the patient is secured, as in the Foster frame procedure, the patient is slowly turned to the prone position by pressing the "face" position button. Gradual turning prevents vertigo and loss of consciousness.

d. To prevent falls, restraining straps are used when the patient is in the prone position, since the side rails cannot be used.

e. The circular metal plate and mattress section under the perineal area are removed to place the bedpan in the CircOlectric bed.

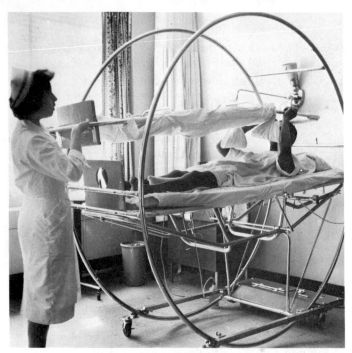

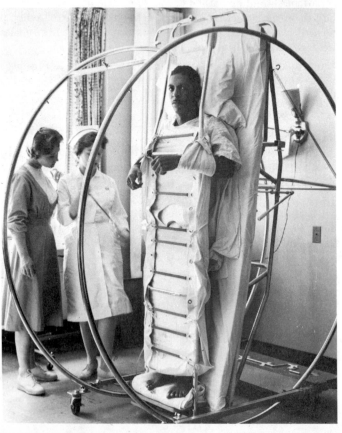

FIGURE 90.5

The bedpan is held in place by fasteners. To facilitate elimination, the bed may be tilted slightly, if permitted.

f. By manual adjustment, the bed may be placed in a sitting or semireclining position.

B. Communicative Aspects

1. *Observations*

   a. Observe and record the patient's reactions during turning.

   b. Note the appearance of the body, with particular reference to any pressure areas.

   c. Note any treatments the patient receives and his reactions to them.

   d. The frequency of turning and position should be noted. The patient should be turned at least every 2 hr.

   e. Check any tubings from body orifice (*e.g.*, Foley catheter, Levin tube), and secure these before turning.

2. *Charting*

DATE	TREATMENT	TIME	OBSERVATIONS	SIGNATURE
6/4	Turned to prone position	0900	Procedure explained to patient while preparing for turning. Patient seemed apprehensive about being turned but tolerated procedure well. No reddened areas on posterior area of body. Reading board adjusted.	F. White, R.N.
		1100	Patient writing letters. Tolerated turning very well; seems less apprehensive. Bedpan requested; voided 300 ml. Patient requested pan be kept in place so she wouldn't have to disturb nurse. Explanation given about why request could not be granted.	B. Smith, L.V.N.
		1200	Sleeping.	B. Smith, L.V.N.

3. *Referrals*

   If the patient has a debilitating injury that will cause immobilization for a prolonged period, early referral to a physical therapy program is essential.

C. Teaching Aspects—Patient and Family

1. Instruct the patient and family about the importance of frequent turning and good skin care.

2. Instruct the patient and family in the mechanism of the Foster frame or CircOlectric bed.

3. Encourage the family to help the patient occupy his time. Suggest activities such as new hobbies and watching television.

IV. EVALUATION PROCESS

A. Is the patient comfortable during and after turning?

B. Is the patient activity within the scope of his limitations?

C. Is the turning process being done frequently and safely?

D. Are observations being properly recorded?

E. Is the body in proper alignment?

F. Is the body free of pressure areas?

G. Has a proper elimination schedule been formulated and adhered to?

H. Has the patient maintained optimal mobility by a regular exercise schedule?

91

Heimlich Maneuver, Administration

I. ASSESSMENT OF SITUATION

A. Definition

A manual technique used on a person to dislodge foreign bodies or food from the airway, which was devised in 1974 by H. J. Heimlich, M.D.

B. Terminology

Residual air: Air remaining in the lungs after normal expiration

C. Rationale for Actions

1. To dislodge foreign bodies or food from airway

2. To establish and clear the airway

II. NURSING PLAN

A. Objectives

1. To ascertain, from the patient's signs and symptoms, whether the technique is needed

2. To perform the technique in a proper and efficient manner

3. To observe and record the patient's condition after the technique has been completed

B. Patient Preparation

Since this is an emergency maneuver, there is little time or necessity for patient preparation. The procedure can be done with the patient either standing upright or lying in a bed.

III. IMPLEMENTING NURSING INTERVENTION

A. Therapeutic Aspects

1. The main objective of the technique is to force the diaphragm up to cause the lungs' residual air to be forcefully exhaled, thereby dislodging the food or foreign body from the airway. To carry out this procedure, the nurse should act quickly once she observes that the individual is choking.

2. If the patient is lying in bed, the nurse should press the heel of her hand against the patient's abdomen in the midline just below the rib cage, providing quick upward thrusts against the diaphragm. If the patient vomits during or after the technique, his head should be turned to the side to prevent aspiration.

3. If the patient is standing, the nurse should stand behind him and wrap her arms around his waist—just above the belt line. The patient's head, arms, and upper torso are allowed to hang forward. The nurse makes a fist with one hand and grasps the fist with her other hand. She places the thumb side of her fist against the patient's abdomen slightly above the navel and below the rib cage. She then grasps her fist with the other hand and presses the fist into the patient's abdomen with a quick upward thrust. This movement will force the diaphragm up, thus increasing the pressure of the air in the tracheobronchial tree. A second person should be prepared to remove the foreign body from the patient's mouth if necessary.

4. The maneuver may have to be repeated several times.

B. Communicative Aspects

1. *Observations*

Watch the patient for signs of inadequate oxygenation as evidenced by dyspnea, restlessness, and cyanosis due to incomplete dislodgment of the obstruction.

2. *Charting*

a. If obstruction occurs in the hospital, the following information should be charted:

(1) Time technique was started

(2) Condition of patient before and after technique was administered

(3) Any evidence of foreign bodies expelled, such as food or bones

(4) Pulse and respiration following technique

DATE	TREATMENT	TIME	OBSERVATION	SIGNATURE
4/20	Heimlich maneuver	0330	Pt. found choking while lying in bed in room. Pressure applied with heel of hand against abdomen. Small bone dislodged. Pt. resting quietly. Color good. P 86, R 22.	J. Stokes, R.N.

3. *Referrals*

Not applicable

C. Teaching Aspects—Patient

Technique may be demonstrated to the patient after he has regained his normal health status, since this is an excellent technique for all the public to learn.

IV. EVALUATION PROCESS

A. Has the patient been made comfortable?

B. Have the vital signs of the patient returned to normal?

92
Neurologic Signs

I. ASSESSMENT OF SITUATION

A. Definition

The evaluation of the neurologic status of a patient by obtaining certain pertinent data

B. Terminology

1. *Hypoxia:* varying degrees of lack of oxygen

2. *Intracranial pressure:* pressure within the cranium

3. Levels of consciousness

   a. *Alert:* awake and oriented to time, place, surroundings, and so forth

b. *Comatose:* responsive only to painful stimuli; no spontaneous movement

c. *Confused:* awake but disoriented as to time, place, and so on

d. *Somnolent:* drowsy; sleeps when left alone; may be confused when awake

e. *Stuporous:* difficult to arouse; may be combative when aroused

f. *Semicomatose:* very little spontaneous motion unless aroused by vigorous stimuli

4. *Pulse pressure:* the difference between systolic and diastolic blood pressures

5. *Vital signs:* see Technique 83, Vital Signs

C. Rationale for Actions

1. To aid in the recognition of increased intracranial pressure

2. To aim for early prevention of increased intracranial pressure and its effects

3. To aid in determining the degree of paralysis

4. To aid in determining the level of consciousness

II. NURSING PLAN

A. Objectives

1. To protect the patient from further neurologic damage

2. To allay the fear and anxiety of the family and patient

3. To record and report observations accurately

4. To gain data on which to base further medication and treatment regimens

B. Patient Preparation

1. The patient, if he is conscious, should be told why the neurologic signs are being checked. Even if the patient is unconscious, the nurse should tell him when the light will be shined in his eyes, since the degree of perception, even when the patient is apparently unconscious, cannot be accurately determined.

2. The patient and his family should be told why neurologic signs are checked frequently. Before beginning, the nurse should have all of the equipment nearby, to avoid delays and patient discomfort.

C. Equipment

1. Flashlight

2. Stethoscope

3. Blood pressure cuff and gauge

4. Thermometer

III. IMPLEMENTING NURSING INTERVENTION

A. Therapeutic Aspects

1. Pressure on vital centers in the brain causes an increase in pulse, pulse pressure, and variable respirations. There is usually an associated hypoxia. Pressure on the hypothalamus may increase or decrease temperature. Before a neurologic exam, the vital signs should be checked: blood pressure, pulse, respirations, and temperature.

2. The center of consciousness is in the pons, a part of the brain stem. Any direct trauma or associated pressure on the pons will cause a change in the level of consciousness. The level of consciousness can be assessed by requesting the patient to speak. He may be directed to perform simple tasks, such as moving an extremity or gripping the nurse's hand, which will also demonstrate any hemispheric weakness. Response to painful stimuli should be noted when the patient is given an injection or is turned.

3. Edema of the pupillary muscle may result in an abnormal pupil size or a fixed pupil (Fig. 92-1A, B). The pupils are normally dilated or large when the eye is closed or the room dark. In the absence of trauma or abnormality, the pupil will quickly constrict (become very small) when a bright light is directed toward it. To check pupil size, the patient's eyes should be closed and the room darkened. One at a time, the eyes are gently opened by the nurse and a flashlight beam directed toward the pupils. Pupil size and configuration should be noted. Both pupils should react equally, with the same speed and to the same size. Dissimilarity may indicate neurologic damage.

4. Loss of motor function is an indication of increased intracranial pressure. As a patient's condition deteriorates, the extremities may become flaccid, with reflexes absent. To check and assess motor function, the nurse should direct the patient to move his extremities, one at a time, and to grip her hand with each of his hands, separately.

5. The nurse must remember that any neurologic trauma is a potentially critical situation. She must continually assess the patient's neurologic condition and report any sudden changes or abnormalities immediately. The family of this patient will need a great deal of explanation and realistic reassurance from the nurse.

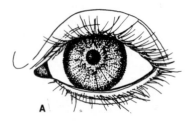
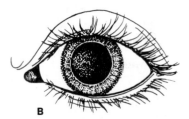

A   **B**

FIGURE 92.1

B. Communicative Aspects

1. *Observations*

   a. Report any change in pulse rate, pulse pressure, temperature, or respiratory rate.

   b. Report changes in size and reaction of pupils.

   c. Report changes in level of consciousness and motor functioning.

2. *Charting*

   Frequent notations of neurologic assessment should appear in nurse's notes (see Charting Sample on p. 538).

3. *Referrals*

   Not applicable

C. Teaching Aspects—Patient and Family

1. Explain to the family the reasons why the patient's neurologic signs are checked frequently.

2. Request the family to tell the nursing staff of any notable differences they observe about the patient, since they are more aware of patient's normal responses.

3. Encourage the family to ask questions regarding the patient's condition.

IV. EVALUATION PROCESS

A. Was the patient assessed for level of responsiveness and consciousness?

B. Has the patient been observed for changes in neurologic signs and vital signs?

C. Have pupillary changes been noted? Was the family advised regarding the checking of the neurologic signs?

D. Was an explanation of the neurologic sign procedure given to the patient regardless of his apparent level of comprehension?

CHARTING SAMPLE

DATE: ADMITTED TO ICU 5/26 AT 2258.
CONDITION: CRITICAL

DATE	HOUR	B.P.	P.	R.	TEMP.	STATE CONSCIOUSNESS	MOVEMENT EXTREMITIES	HAND GRIP	PUPILS: EQUALITY & REACTION	INTAKE	OUTPUT
5/26	2300	134/78	92	28		Stuporous	Moves with stimuli. Patient does not respond except to pin prick. Pulse of good quality; respirations regular. Head elevated 30°. Color good; no cyanosis noted.	none	Equal and react.		
5/27	2330	140/80	86	28		Stuporous	Moves with stimuli.	none	Equal and react.		
	2400	140/80	84	28		"	none	none	" "		
	0030	150/84	96	28		"	none	none	" "		
	0100	150/84	96	28		"	none	none	" "		
	0130	160/84	98	28		"	none	none	" "		
	0200	174/92	100	30	101ᴿ	Comatose	Patient's condition appears worse. Moderate amount of thick, white mucus suctioned. Dr. D. here. No bleeding from ear, nose, or mouth.	none	" "		
	0215						Oxygen 5 liter 1 mask. Visited by daughter. Explanation of patient's condition given to daughter by nurse. Patient's face appears to be more pale than on admission. No spontaneous moments observed.				
	0230	176/94	100	32		Comatose	none #16 Foley catheter inserted.	none	Equal and react.		

93

Pacemaker (Temporary), Assisting With Insertion

I. ASSESSMENT OF SITUATION

A. Definition

An electronic device to provide electrical stimulation of the heart muscle to ensure a satisfactory heart rate

B. Terminology

1. *Demand pacemaker:* an electrical impulse is emitted only after a predetermined interval has passed since the last spontaneous or induced ventricular impulse.
2. *Fixed-rate pacemaker:* impulses are generated at a predetermined rate set by the clinician.
3. *Synchronous pacemaker:* a sensing device in the atrium triggers an impulse to the ventricles after a predetermined appropriate interval.

C. Rationale for Actions

1. To initiate and maintain the heart rate when the natural pacemakers of the heart are unable to do so
2. To prevent circulatory failure resulting from inadequate cardiac output
3. To reduce the risks associated with long-term cardiac drug therapy
4. To suppress rapid arrhythmias that do not respond to drugs or cardioversion

II. NURSING PLAN

A. Objectives

1. To reestablish normal heart rhythm
2. To avoid cardiac override
3. To prevent infection and thrombophlebitis
4. To be constantly alert for failure of the heart to respond to the pacemaker stimulus
5. To have emergency equipment and drugs nearby in case of emergency

B. Patient Preparation

1. Once the physician decides that a temporary pacemaker is necessary, the patient should be informed about why and how it will be accomplished. Emphasis should be placed on the benefits derived from being able to control the heart rate in the prevention of serious complications.

2. An operative consent form should be signed.

3. The subclavian area (or area chosen by the physician for insertion) should be shaved and cleaned with an antiseptic solution.

4. The patient and family may have great reservations about the terms dealing with "electrical" stimulation. An explanation consistent with the patient's ability and desire to understand should be offered about the natural pacemaker and the electronic impulses found naturally in the body.

C. Equipment

1. Pacemaker

2. Transvenous catheters

3. Subclavian IV setup (see Technique 96, Subclavian Intra-Cath, Assisting with Insertion)

4. Image intensifier

5. Sterile gloves

6. Sterile knife blade

7. Suture

8. Defibrillator

III. IMPLEMENTING NURSING INTERVENTION

A. Therapeutic Aspects

1. The pacemaker will be inserted by the physician. All unnecessary furniture should be removed from the room, including the patient's bed. The patient should be placed on a surgical lift for easy mobilization and to facilitate accessibility by the physician and nurses. A defibrillator and image intensifier should be in the room. The image intensifier will enable the physician to ensure the proper location of the pacemaker catheter.

2. The patient will usually be sedated before catheter insertion. The physician inserts the pacemaker electrode into the vein and directs it to the desired area. Strict aseptic technique is observed. The free end of the catheter is then attached to an external pulse generating device for temporary pacing. For permanent pacing, the device is surgically implanted into the subcutaneous tissue. However, the temporary pacemaker is usually worn strapped around the patient's chest or waist.

3. Patients with newly inserted pacemakers should be carefully moni-

tored to ensure proper functioning of the pacemaker. Immediately after insertion, the tip of the catheter may float freely in the ventricle for a time. However, the catheter is soon coated with fibrin and eventually becomes embedded in the right ventricle. During the free-floating period, ECG tracings may show displays of varying intensity. However, this should be a short-lived phenomenon. Continuous monitoring will allow the nurse to be aware of pacemaker problems. The pacemaker artifact is usually represented as a thin, straight stroke on the cardiac monitor.

4. In the patient with a temporary pacemaker, a highly conductive direct route exists from the external catheter to the heart. The exposed electrodes where the catheter leaves the body can be insulated by placing the pacing unit in a rubber glove. Extreme caution must be utilized to ensure that all equipment in the room is properly grounded; only one machine connected to a wall outlet should be used at any time.

B. Communicative Aspects

1. *Observations*

   a. Absence of the pacemaker artifact may indicate faulty equipment or, more seriously, failure to pace because of malposition of the catheter, dislodging of the catheter, catheter breakage, or a rise of the pacing threshold due to tissue reaction to the catheter or to infection.

   b. To determine the efficiency of each pacing stimulus, the nurse takes the patient's pulse while simultaneously observing the cardiac monitor.

   c. The pacemaker insertion site should be observed for signs of localized phlebitis and cellulitis. The dressings should be watched for drainage.

   d. Hiccups may cause current leakage across the diaphragm or perforation of the ventricle by the catheter.

2. *Charting*

DATE	TREATMENT	TIME	OBSERVATIONS	SIGNATURE
4/9		0800	Permit for pacemaker signed by patient. States he understands necessity of procedure as well as what will occur.	F. White, R.N.
		0805	Sedative given as prescribed. BP 118/74, P 42, R 18	G. Albert, L.V.N.
	External transvenous pacemaker inserted	0830	Insertion under sterile conditions accomplished by Dr. S. via R subclavian vein. Catheter placement verified by image intensifier. Electrodes connected to demand pace-	

DATE	TREATMENT	TIME	OBSERVATIONS	SIGNATURE
			maker, set at 80. Monitor pattern shows pacemaker blip present. Patient tolerated procedure well. Resting quietly. P 84.	F. White, R.N.

3. *Referrals*

   a. The American Heart Association may be of assistance in helping the patient understand and accept his cardiac condition.

   b. Many cities have organized local groups of people who have coronary problems. These groups may offer tremendous support to the cardiac patient.

C. Teaching Aspects—Patient and Family

1. Place the pulse generator in a secure area; it should be immovable and there should be no tension on the wires. The patient should not be able to manipulate the controls. Stress to the patient and his family the importance of not tampering with this device.

2. Stress to the family the importance of grounding all electrical equipment so that no visitor brings ungrounded devices into the patient's room.

3. Explain to the patient the limitations on mobility as well as exercise progression, which will be determined by the physician.

4. The patient may view his dependence upon a "machine" with fear or rebellion. Allow him to express his feelings.

IV. EVALUATION PROCESS

A. Did the patient and his family understand why the pacemaker was needed?

B. Were fears and anxieties allayed by careful explanations and attentiveness by the nurse?

C. Did the patient comply with activity restrictions?

D. Has normal cardiac rhythm been established?

E. Is the pacemaker functioning properly?

F. Have complications been avoided?

G. Were emergency drugs and equipment readily available?

94

Pericardiocentesis

I. ASSESSMENT OF SITUATION

A. Definition

Aspiration from the pericardial sac of fluid that may accumulate because of pericarditis, effusion from malignant neoplasms or lymphoma, trauma, or acute rheumatic fever

B. Terminology

1. *Cardiac tamponade:* compression of the heart by blood, effusion, or a foreign body in the pericardial sac, with the effect of restricting normal heart activity
2. *Epicardium:* the innermost sac outlining the heart; separated from the pericardium by a space that normally contains a very small amount of fluid
3. *Paradoxical pulse:* lessening in pulse amplitude during inspiration followed by the prompt reappearance of the pulse upon expiration
4. *Pericardium:* the outermost sac surrounding the heart muscle
5. *Pulse pressure:* the difference between the systolic and diastolic pressure

C. Rationale for Actions

1. To relieve the pressure from pericardial effusion that results in cardiac tamponade
2. To prevent death caused by severely depressed cardiac output

II. NURSING PLAN

A. Objectives

1. To prevent complications
2. To monitor vital signs correctly during and after the procedure
3. To offer reassurance to the patient and enhance his cooperation during the procedure

B. Patient Preparation

1. The need for aspirating fluid from the heart sac should be carefully explained to the patient and his family. Since this is often an emergency, the stress level of the patient and family will probably already

be high. A calm and positive approach may relieve much of the tension.

2. Premedication is usually not required, though a sedative may be given.

3. The necessity for the patient to remain quiet and still during the procedure should be emphasized. If the nurse offers assurance that she will be with him, his anxiety may be lowered.

C. Equipment

1. 5- and 50-ml syringes
2. 14-, 18-, and 20-ga needles, 3 in long
3. Three-way sterile stopcock
4. Rubber connecting tubing
5. Sterile alligator clamp
6. Skin antiseptic
7. Local anesthetic
8. Sterile gloves
9. Cardiac monitor
10. Intubation equipment and AMBU-bag
11. Defibrillator

III. IMPLEMENTING NURSING INTERVENTION

A. Therapeutic Aspects

1. The patient should be placed in a comfortable position with the head of the bed or treatment table raised to a 60° angle. To provide a means of continuous monitoring, the ECG leads should be applied to the patient's limbs. In addition to the ECG, blood pressure and venous pressure should be monitored constantly during pericardiocentesis.

2. Because the release of pressure may cause dangerous arrhythmias, the defibrillator should be preset and ready for use, along with other emergency equipment.

3. Using sterile technique, the physician will administer local anesthesia. The V lead of the ECG may be connected to the shank of the aspirating needle after it has been connected to the syringe and stopcock. The ECG machine must be properly grounded. The needle will be advanced slowly with continuous gentle suction until fluid is found, usually at a depth of 3 to 4 cm.

4. A change in the ECG pattern will indicate contact with the epicardium. These changes may be marked ST-segment elevation, ventricular ectopic beats, or elevation of the PR segment with atrial ectopic beats. When these changes occur, the needle should be slightly withdrawn.

It will then be in the pericardial space and the fluid may be freely withdrawn.

5. After the fluid has been removed and the needle withdrawn, a small sterile dressing should be applied. The patient must be closely monitored for any indication of complications.

B. Communicative Aspects

1. *Observations*

   a. Notation should be made of the amount and appearance of fluid aspirated. Pericardial fluid usually does not clot.

   b. Careful monitoring should be employed to detect signs of a decline in venous pressure and a rise in systolic blood pressure.

   c. The area over the heart should be auscultated for clarity of heart rate and inappropriate sounds.

   d. Surgical intervention may be indicated if the following problems occur:

      (1) Repeated accumulation of pericardial fluid

      (2) Unsuccessful aspiration

      (3) Development of complications

   e. Possible complications include the following:

      (1) Inadvertent puncture of the heart chamber

      (2) Arrhythmias

      (3) Puncture of the lung, stomach, or liver

      (4) Laceration of a coronary artery or the myocardium

2. *Charting*

DATE	TREATMENT	TIME	OBSERVATION	SIGNATURE
7/12	Pericar-dio-centesis done by Dr.T	0845	30 ml. reddish fluid returned. ECG remained stable. CVP 11, BP 118/84; calm during procedure. Sterile dressing applied. Spec. to lab for analysis	F. White, R.N.

3. *Referrals*

   Not applicable

C. Teaching Aspects—Patient and Family

1. The patient and family should be given a basic understanding of cardiac anatomy. They should understand that there are several layers of lining around the heart and that actual penetration of the heart itself is not the goal of pericardiocentesis.

2. If the cardiac tamponade is due to a chronic problem, surgical intervention may be necessary at a later time.

IV. EVALUATION PROCESS

A. Did the patient and family understand the procedure and the need for it?

B. Did the patient remain still during the procedure?

C. Were complications prevented or handled efficiently?

D. Were vital signs, ECG, and central venous pressure (CVP) continuously monitored?

E. Was a significant amount of fluid returned?

95

Peritoneal Dialysis

I. ASSESSMENT OF SITUATION

A. Definition

The instillation of a solution and its subsequent removal from the peritoneal cavity with the purpose of removing harmful substances or correcting chemical imbalances

B. Terminology

1. *Dialysate:* the solution used to irrigate the peritoneal cavity
2. *Paracentesis:* withdrawal of fluid from the peritoneal cavity

C. Rationale for Actions

1. To remove harmful substances from the body
2. To correct electrolyte imbalances
3. To decrease edema

II. NURSING PLAN

A. Objectives

1. To keep an accurate record of the patient's weight and vital signs
2. To keep an accurate record of the patient's intake and output
3. To observe carefully for signs of complications, such as change in

level of consciousness, hallucinations, tachycardia, and severe abdominal pain

B. Patient Preparation

1. Baseline vital signs from which physiological changes can be measured must be taken before commencing the procedure. These include weight, temperature, pulse, respiration, and blood pressure.

2. Before the tube is inserted, the patient should fully understand what will take place. He should be told that there will be initial discomfort when the paracentesis is done; however, after this, he should be comfortable. There may be some pressure as the fluid is instilled, causing shortness of breath. This can usually be relieved by elevating the head of the bed.

C. Equipment

1. Incision tray, including blade, handle, suture with needle, Y connector, and gauze pads

2. Tubing and clamp

3. Two bottles of dialysate (usually 1 liter each)

4. Two bottles for drainage (usually 1 liter each)

5. Sterile sutures and dressings

III. IMPLEMENTING NURSING INTERVENTION

A. Therapeutic Aspects

1. To monitor the patient's reaction, an accurate record must be kept of his weight and intake and output. He should be weighed before the procedure is begun and daily on the same scale. Blood pressure, pulse, and respirations are also taken and recorded every 15 min during the first dialysis, then hourly. Output may exceed input; however, if the excess is more than 500 ml, the physician should be notified.

2. So that the nervous system is not shocked by a wide temperature variation, the dialysate should be at room temperature before being administered.

3. Diffusion can occur in both directions through the peritoneal membrane. For this reason, the nurse must ensure that each bottle of dialysate is hypertonic. Great care must be taken so that isotonic or hypotonic solutions, such as intravenous fluids, are not mistakenly used.

4. To perform the dialysis, the physician places a tube into the abdominal cavity by paracentesis and may suture it in place. Two bottles of dialysate are connected to a Y connector, which is attached to the tubing in the patient (Fig. 95-1). The solution is left in the patient for the time prescribed by the physician. At the end of this time, the drainage tube is unclamped and the fluid allowed to return by gravitational flow. Drainage may be facilitated by a position change or elevation of the head of the bed.

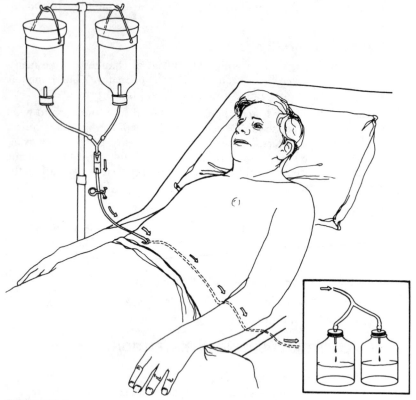

FIGURE 95.1

5. Some residual fluid may remain after the drainage tube is removed. A dressing should be applied. If it becomes saturated, a dry dressing should be applied.

B. Communicative Aspects

1. *Observations*

   a. During the procedure, the abdominal dressing should remain dry. If leakage occurs, the physician should be notified.

   b. The patient must be observed for bleeding, for dyspnea due to pressure on lungs, and for dehydration if too much fluid is removed from the body. Vital signs must be carefully monitored.

   c. Hourly urine excretion should be recorded and any change in output reported.

   d. If return drainage slows down greatly, the physician should be notified, unless the amount returned equals or exceeds the amount instilled.

e. Weight must be accurately taken before and after dialysis, then daily at the same time, on the same scale.

2. *Charting*

a. Peritoneal dialysis sheet

| | | | | OUTPUT | | | V/S | |
DATE	TIME	SOLUTION	WEIGHT	PERITONEAL	URINE	B/P	P	R
7/4	0800	1,000 ml	61 kg (136 lb)			126/60	82	12
	0805					130/70	88	18
	0810					128/68	88	16

b. Nurses' notes

DATE	TREATMENT	TIME	OBSERVATIONS	SIGNATURE
7/4	Peritoneal dialysis completed	1000	VS have remained stable; patient alert and awake. 1,000 ml instilled; 1,040 ml returned. Weight now 61 kg (135 lb). Urine output steady, 16 to 24 ml/hr. Sensorium intact. Skin turgor good. Tube removed, and sterile dressing applied.	G. Ivers, R.N.

3. *Referrals*

Not applicable

C. Teaching Aspects—Patient

1. The patient should be told to notify the nurse if he becomes short of breath or experiences abdominal pain once the procedure has begun.

2. The patient must be cautioned about avoiding excessive moving around in bed, which could cause the tubing to dislodge.

IV. EVALUATION PROCESS

A. Was adequate understanding of the procedure evidenced by the patient's willingness to remain quiet in bed with minimal movement?

B. Did the patient seem comfortable throughout the procedure?

C. Were weight and vital signs accurately measured and recorded? Are any great discrepancies or fluctuations noted?

D. Was the intake and output record kept accurately? Were discrepancies reported to the physician?

E. Did any side effects occur?

F. Did the amount returned equal or exceed the amount instilled?

96

Subclavian Intra-Cath, Assisting With Insertion

I. ASSESSMENT OF SITUATION

A. Definition

Introduction of a polyethylene catheter into the subclavian vein

B. Terminology

Pacemaker electrode: a medium intervening between a cardiac pacemaker and the heart

C. Rationale for Actions

1. To monitor central venous pressure (see Technique 88, Central Venous Pressure [CVP])
2. To rapidly administer fluids
3. To administer fluids when peripheral veins are collapsed
4. To provide a route for prolonged intravenous (IV) therapy
5. To provide a route for the insertion of a temporary pacemaker electrode
6. To provide a safe route for infusing irrigating solutions

II. NURSING PLAN

A. Objectives

1. To ensure continued patency of the subclavian catheter
2. To prevent the possibility of an air embolus
3. To allay the anxieties of the patient and family
4. To secure the tubing to prevent complications

B. Patient Preparation

1. The patient and family should receive a thorough explanation of what will occur during the procedure, if this is appropriate.
2. Fluids should be ready for administration and the IV tubing should be cleared of air before the subclavian puncture is made.

C. Equipment

1. Subclavian tray
   a. Large Intra-Cath

    b. Antiseptic solution

    c. 4-in tape

    d. 4 in x 4 in gauze pads

    e. 5 or 10 ml syringe, with plain tip

2. Fluids, as prescribed

3. Venous pressure set, if prescribed

4. Pacemaker electrode, if prescribed

III. IMPLEMENTING NURSING INTERVENTION

A. Therapeutic Aspects

1. Since pathogens may be transferred by needle puncture of the skin, aseptic technique should be used during the procedure. The area of venipuncture should be cleansed with the antiseptic requested by the physician.

2. The patient should be in the supine position so that the procedure site is accessible to the physician and the possibility of air embolus is reduced. Tension of the scalenus anterior muscle, engorgement of the subclavian vein, easy recognition of landmarks, and prevention of contamination are prerequisites to catheter insertion. The patient's face should be turned to the side opposite the puncture (Fig. 96-1A, B).

3. After insertion, movement of the polyethylene catheter may cause vessel irritation or inadvertent removal of the catheter from the vein. The catheter should be taped securely with large pieces of wide tape after a 4 in × 4 in gauze pad has been placed over the venipuncture site (Fig. 96-2A, B).

B. Communicative Aspects

1. *Observations*

    a. Bleeding at the site of the injection requires immediate attention.

    b. Dress the puncture carefully to prevent kinking the polyethylene catheter.

    c. Check the rate of infusion.

    d. Momentarily lower the infusion bottle below the level of the patient to check the free flow of fluid. You will see a return flow of blood in the catheter if it is in proper position and patent.

2. *Charting*

DATE	TREATMENT	TIME	OBSERVATIONS	SIGNATURE
5/15	Sub-clavian Intra-Cath	1100	Large Intra-Cath inserted into right subclavian vein by Dr. A. Infusion dripping well. No signs of bleeding.	G. Ivers, R.N.

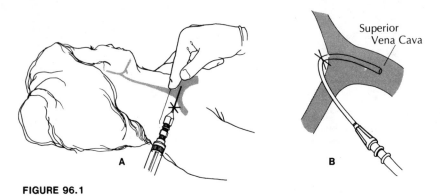

FIGURE 96.1

FIGURE 96.2

3. *Referrals*

Not applicable

C. Teaching Aspects—Patient and Family

1. Instruct the patient and family not to touch the dressing.
2. Instruct the patient in turning to prevent kinking the IV tubing.
3. Instruct the patient and family to call the nurse if the fluid ceases to drip.

IV. EVALUATION PROCESS

A. Is the patient comfortable?

B. Did the patient cooperate to the limit of his ability during insertion and during fluid administration?

C. Is the infusion proceeding at the prescribed rate?

D. Is the pacemaker attached to the patient and adjusted to the proper rate (if applicable)?

E. Is the Intra-Cath still positioned correctly in the subclavian vein?

97

Swan-Ganz Catheter, Removal of

I. ASSESSMENT OF SITUATION

A. Definition

A Swan-Ganz catheter is a balloon-tipped catheter that is inserted into a peripheral vein, usually the antecubital, and allowed to flow into the heart. Once it is in the superior vena cava, the balloon is inflated and flows through the heart until it reaches the pulmonary artery where it wedges because of the size of this artery. Pressure readings are then taken to measure the pumping force of the left ventricle.

B. Terminology

1. *Antecubital vein:* the vessel at the inner aspect of the bend of the arm
2. *Cardiogenic shock:* acute peripheral circulatory failure caused by failure of the left ventricle to pump sufficient oxygenated blood to meet the body's needs
3. *Pulmonary artery:* the vessel carrying unoxygenated blood from the right ventricle to the lungs
4. *Superior vena cava:* the principal vein draining the upper portion of the body

C. Rationale for Actions

1. To stabilize the condition of the patient who has suffered cardiogenic shock
2. To avoid complications associated with having the Swan-Ganz catheter in place for an extended period of time (thrombophlebitis, emboli, or sepsis)
3. To relieve the patient's anxiety caused by having a foreign body in his heart

II. NURSING PLAN

A. Objectives

1. To remove the catheter successfully without trauma to the heart or vessels
2. To monitor the patient's pulmonary artery pressure accurately

3. To ensure the patient's safety by having emergency equipment nearby if needed

4. To secure the patient's confidence and compliance through careful, understandable explanations

B. Patient Preparation

1. A clear and thorough explanation should precede removal of the Swan-Ganz catheter. The patient will be understandably apprehensive about his health status. If the nurse assumes a positive, self-assured attitude, this confidence will be imparted to the patient.

2. Skin preparation should be accomplished before removal of the catheter. A sterile gauze pad should be saturated with antiseptic, and the skin should be cleansed in a circular motion, working outward from the site of venipuncture. Three pads should be used to clean the area.

C. Equipment

1. Dressing tray with skin preparation solutions

2. Suture removal set

3. Paper sack for dressing disposal

4. ECG monitoring equipment

5. Emergency drugs and defibrillator

6. Sterile gloves

III. IMPLEMENTING NURSING INTERVENTION

A. Therapeutic Aspects

1. The Swan-Ganz catheter is inserted by the physician with the balloon deflated. After the catheter reaches the superior vena cava, the balloon is inflated and the catheter is allowed to flow freely through the right atrium and right ventricle, and out of the heart through the pulmonary artery. As it enters a branch of the pulmonary artery that has a diameter smaller than the inflated balloon, it becomes lodged. This is called the pulmonary wedge position, and the pressure is measured before the balloon is deflated to allow continuous blood flow to the lung. The deflated catheter will remain in the pulmonary wedge position. Pulmonary pressure can then be measured. Since the catheter is nearer the left ventricle, the reading is more accurate than a central venous pressure (CVP) reading. A maximum of 3 to 5 days is considered safe for leaving the Swan-Ganz catheter in place. It is sutured in place and covered with a sterile dressing. Removal of the catheter by the nurse is permissible provided she has adequate knowledge of the implications and procedures involved.

2. Before removal of the catheter, the suture must be removed. Direct visualization aids in accuracy. The knot of the first suture should be grasped with a sterile hemostat or forceps and elevated so that the portion below the knot is clearly visible. Using sterile scissors, the

nurse cuts one side of the suture below the knot next to the skin. This prevents drawing the exposed contaminated portion of the suture through the tissue.

3. The Swan-Ganz catheter with the balloon deflated is grasped firmly between the thumb and the index and middle fingers. Gentle pulling pressure should be applied and the catheter removed in one continuous motion. The cardiac rhythm and the pulmonary artery pressure reading must be monitored closely during this procedure.

4. Since pathogenic organisms may enter the bloodstream through any break in the skin, the insertion site should be cleansed with an alcohol sponge and covered with a sterile dressing.

B. Communicative Aspects

1. *Observations*

   a. Careful monitoring of the cardiac pattern should be maintained before, during, and after removal of a Swan-Ganz catheter.

   b. A tracing of the pulmonary artery pressure should be noted before and during the removal of the catheter. The normal pressure is 25/10 mm Hg. During pulmonary artery monitoring, a diastolic pressure over 12 mm Hg indicates left ventricle failure.

2. *Charting*

DATE	TREATMENT	TIME	OBSERVATIONS	SIGNATURE
5/9	Swan-Ganz catheter inserted by Dr. R	0815	Pressure in R ventricle is 20/0 mm Hg. PCWP* is 5 mm Hg. Balloon deflated and catheter sutured in place. PAP† is stable at 20/10. Patient tolerated procedure well. States he is not frightened and understands why the catheter is in place.	F. White, R.N.

* PCWP: Pulmonary capillary wedge pressure
† PAP: Pulmonary artery pressure

3. *Referrals*

   a. Referral to the American Heart Association may be appropriate after the initial coronary crisis has been overcome.

   b. Many cities have organized groups of people who have suffered coronary problems. These groups may offer tremendous support and inspiration to coronary patients.

C. Teaching Aspects—Patient

1. Instruct the patient to keep his fingers away from the wound.

2. Tell the patient to report any abnormality or pain in the venipuncture site.

3. Instruct the patient to report any chest pain, shortness of breath, increased anxiety, or other indications of cardiac problems.

IV. EVALUATION PROCESS

A. Was the patient informed about when and how the catheter removal would take place?

B. Did the patient seem relaxed and at ease about the procedure?

C. Was the proper aseptic technique maintained throughout the procedure?

D. Was the cardiac status carefully monitored during and after removal?

E. Was the catheter withdrawn with ease?

F. Did the pulmonary artery pressure monitoring result in clinical data enabling the physician to make an accurate diagnosis?

G. Was emergency equipment available and used if needed?

98

Tracheostomy Care

I. ASSESSMENT OF SITUATION

A. Definition

Aspiration of secretions from a tracheostomy wound by use of a sterile catheter connected to a suction machine and cleansing of the inner cannula of the tracheostomy tube and the anterior part of the neck

B. Terminology

1. *Cannula:* tube

2. *Hypoxia:* varying degrees of inadequacy of oxygen supply

3. *Patent:* open; unobstructed

4. *Tracheostomy:* the surgical creation of a vertical slit in the anterior portion of the neck (usually below the first or second tracheal cartilage) and the introduction of a single- or double-lumen cannula airway to facilitate adequate exchange of gases (Fig. 98-1). The outer cannula is held in place by ties around the neck. The inner cannula is locked into the outer cannula.

5. *Tracheostomy cuff:* a rubber balloon-type appliance placed around

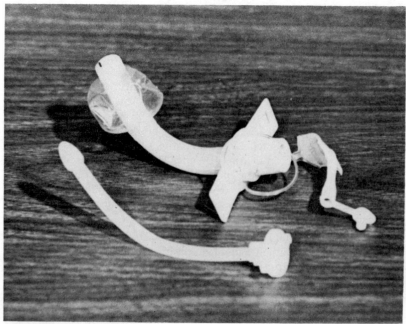

FIGURE 98.1

the lower two-thirds of the tracheostomy tube before insertion. After insertion, it can be inflated to prevent precipitous removal or air leaks if positive pressure inhalation devices are used.

C. Rationale for Actions

1. To facilitate adequate exchange of gases for maximum respiratory results
2. To limit the introduction of pathogens into the tracheobronchial tree

II. NURSING PLAN

A. Objectives

1. To maintain a patent airway to facilitate the therapeutic exchange of gases
2. To allay the fears and anxieties of the patient and family concerning the altered breathing route and loss of speaking ability
3. To prevent the transmission of pathogenic microorganisms
4. To prevent encrustation around the tracheostomy area
5. To provide adequate humidity

6. To provide adequate gaseous exchange

7. To provide optimal physical comfort

B. Patient Preparation

1. Diversion of the respiratory flow by means of a tracheostomy also directly alters the patient's ability to speak. Inability to speak or cry out adds to the emotional stress of the patient. Obstruction of the airway may cause a patient to panic. He should be closely observed at all times. A clear explanation of suctioning and other care will enhance his cooperation and security. Explanations should be given regardless of the apparent level of consciousness. The family, too, may exhibit increased anxiety over the inability to communicate with their loved one. Reassurance and clear explanations will help allay this anxiety. If the patient is able, he should be provided writing materials so that he can communicate with others.

2. Due to gravitational flow, secretions may collect in the tracheobronchial tree. The patient should be positioned on his side to facilitate drainage and aspiration of these secretions.

C. Equipment

1. Portable suction machine or gauge attached to a wall suction unit

2. Suction catheter, 12 to 10 French

3. Y connector

4. Container with sterile water

5. Sterile gloves

6. Hydrogen peroxide

7. Pipe cleaners

8. Sterile dressings

9. Umbilical tape

10. Cool or warm mist apparatus, as prescribed by the physician

III. IMPLEMENTING NURSING INTERVENTION

A. Therapeutic Aspects

1. Pathogenic organisms can grow and flourish in a warm, moist environment and are transmitted by direct contact. The nurse should use scrupulous handwashing techniques before and after this procedure. Sterile gloves should be worn.

2. Moistening the catheter tip with water will reduce friction and facilitate insertion.

3. The catheter is guided by the anatomic structure of the bronchi. It is inserted through the tracheostomy tube with the suction off. It may be directed to the right or left bronchus by having the patient turn his head to the opposite side (Fig. 98-2).

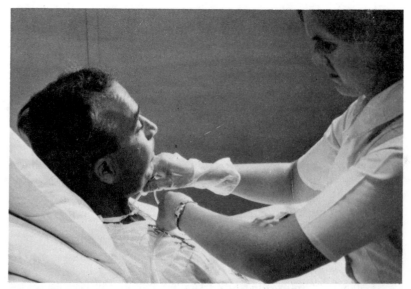

FIGURE 98.2

4. Changes in pressure inside a tube will cause secretions to move from areas of greater pressure to areas of lower pressure. A finger is placed over the opening of the Y connector to create suction, and the tube is withdrawn slowly, in a rotating motion, to prevent creation of excessive vacuum with resulting tissue damage.

5. The patient's airway is obstructed during suctioning, and hypoxia is intensified if suction is maintained too long. The maximum time for continuous suctioning is 15 sec, with a 3-min rest period between insertions, if the patient's condition permits.

6. The tubing should not be pinched, since this creates excessive negative pressure, with resulting danger of injury to mucous membranes.

7. Pressure on the walls of the trachea can cause decreased circulation, with resulting tissue damage. If a tracheostomy cuff is used, it should be deflated once each shift or as prescribed, to prevent damage to the trachea.

8. The patient should be left with a feeling of comfort and security. He should be positioned to facilitate optimal ventilation. The suction apparatus should be changed and left ready for immediate use in case of an emergency. All equipment should be changed or cleaned every 8 hr, to prevent the growth and spread of pathogens.

9. Moist air keeps the delicate mucous membranes of the respiratory tract from drying out and may keep secretions from becoming thick and viscous. A mist collar may be ordered for this purpose. It should be checked frequently for proper positioning, and excess moisture

should be drained off. Keeping the doors and windows closed will help maintain a high-humidity atmosphere.

10. The inner cannula becomes coated with mucus-containing proteins. It should be removed at least every 8 hr, washed with hydrogen peroxide and pipe cleaners, inside and outside, and rinsed thoroughly with water. It should then be gently reinserted into the outer cannula and locked in place.

11. The tracheostomy tube may accidentally become displaced by forceful coughing, confusion, or excessive movement. Except in emergencies, the outer cannula should be replaced by a physician. A sterile tracheostomy setup must be obtained. Forceps or some other dilating instrument in the trachea opening will prevent suffocation until a new cannula can be inserted.

12. Keeping the area around the tracheostomy clean and dry will discourage pathogenic processes and facilitate comfort. The neck area should be washed, rinsed well, and dried thoroughly with a soft towel. The area around the outer cannula may be cleansed with hydrogen peroxide to remove encrustations. A sterile dressing around the outer cannula will reduce irritation and absorb secretions.

B. Communicative Aspects

1. *Observations*

    a. Record the amount, consistency, color, and odor of secretions.

    b. Note the approximate length of time of suctioning.

    c. Note the area of skin around tracheostomy site for edema or redness.

    d. Record the reactions of the patient during the suctioning, cleaning of cannula, and care of neck.

    e. Care must be taken to use separate catheters and setups for tracheostomy and oral/nasal suctioning.

2. *Charting*

DATE	TREATMENT	TIME	OBSERVATIONS	SIGNATURE
5/23	Tracheostomy suctioned and cleaned	0900	Patient positioned on left side. Large amt white mucus aspirated. Patient positioned on right side. Large amt of thick, white, blood-tinged mucus obtained. Patient appears frightened; reassured that staff is available. Inner cannula cleaned and reinserted. Clean tapes applied to outer cannula. Trach. dressing applied.	B. Smith, L.V.N.

3. *Referrals*

If the tracheostomy is permanent, the patient may be referred to a speech therapist for training in communication skills.

C. Teaching Aspects—Patient and Family

1. If the patient has a temporary tracheostomy, he can be taught to speak by placing his covered finger over the opening of the inner cannula. Depending on the patient's condition, the cannula may be plugged for short periods of time, if prescribed.

2. The patient and family need instruction about the purpose of a tracheostomy.

3. If the tracheostomy is to be permanent, the patient should be taught to suction and clean it when he is physically and psychologically able. The family should be included in this teaching.

IV. EVALUATION PROCESS

A. Has the patient exhibited feelings of comfort and security?

B. Has a means of communication been established?

C. Have the fear and anxiety levels of the patient and family been reduced?

D. Is the airway patent?

E. Is the environment free of infectious hazards?

F. Are the cannula and tracheostomy wound free of secretions?

G. Has an adequate degree of humidity been maintained?

H. Does the patient's intake and output record indicate adequate fluid balance?

4

Techniques for Obstetric Patients

99

Admission to Labor Room

I. ASSESSMENT OF SITUATION

A. Definition

Labor is a process that results after 40 wk of gestation. The exact time may vary. The process consists of three stages:

  a. The time of the onset of labor through dilatation of the cervix

  b. The period from complete dilatation of the cervix through the birth of the child

  c. The period from the birth of the child through the expulsion of the placenta and membranes

B. Terminology

  1. *Amniocentesis:* the introduction of a needle into the uterus through the abdominal wall to puncture the amniotic sac and withdraw a fluid specimen

  2. *Antepartal care:* refers to care given the pregnant mother from conception to the onset of labor

  3. *Cesarean section:* the removal of a fetus through an incision into the uterus and the abdominal wall

  4. *Dorsal (supine) position:* a position in which the patient is on her back, with the knees flexed and separated

  5. *External fetal monitor:* an audible record of the heartbeat of infant in the uterus; used to keep a constant record of the regularity of the fetal heart during labor

  6. *False labor:* contractions known as Braxton Hicks contractions; an irregular tightening and relaxing of the uterine muscle, with no accompanying dilation of the cervix

  7. *Internal fetal monitoring:* a system that detects and displays the fetal heartbeat or maternal contractions or both, through the use of an electrode and intrauterine catheter

  8. *Lithotomy position:* a position in which the patient is on her back, with the knees separated and flexed on the abdomen or supported in stirrups

  9. *Perineum:* in the female, the area between the vagina and rectum

  10. *Significant others:* a term applied to other members of the family or associates (*e.g.,* husband, relatives, friends)

11. *Stillborn:* any product of conception born dead that is 5 mo or more gestational age, 26 cm or more in length, or more than 500 g in weight or a combination of the latter two

12. *Toxemia of pregnancy:* a condition resulting from poisonous products being distributed throughout the body from disordered metabolic or hormonal states

13. *Vulva:* the external genital organs in the female, including the lower pubis to the perineum

C. Rationale for Actions

1. To gather data regarding pregnancy as a basis for present planning
2. To totally assess the present status of the mother and fetus
3. Total assessment provides for individualization of care for the mother and her spouse or significant others
4. To prepare the patient and her spouse for the delivery process
5. To monitor the progress of labor
6. To provide an aseptic environment

II. NURSING PLAN

A. Objectives

The objectives for the labor and delivery process can be best accomplished through the combined efforts of the physician, the nurse and staff, the expectant parents, and significant others.

1. To make the total labor process a meaningful and learning experience
2. To create an environment of trust and support
3. To allay the fear and anxieties of patient and her spouse by keeping them informed of the progress of labor and by offering reassurance
4. To make a psychosocial assessment as early as possible, encouraging the patient to express fears and concerns and reducing anxiety as much as possible
5. To employ all appropriate available methods to alleviate discomfort and fear
6. To keep an accurate record of the observations of maternal and fetal status
7. To keep the physician informed of the progress
8. To obtain complete obstetric history (time permitting)

B. Equipment

1. Physician prescriptions and instructions
2. Labor record form
3. Labor and delivery form

4. Medication and graphic sheet

5. Patient teaching guide

6. Patient identification cards (overhead and room door holder)

7. Thermometer, sphygmomanometer, and stethoscope

8. Sterile glove (for vaginal or rectal exam)

9. Fetoscope

10. Amniotome

11. Clock with second hand

12. Razor and shaving cream, preparation tray

13. Enema setup

14. Rectal and vaginal gloves, clearly labeled

15. Povidone iodine (Betadine) solution

16. Paper towels

17. Lubricant

18. Gown, clothing tags.

III. IMPLEMENTING NURSING INTERVENTION

The assessment of the antepartal care record by each patient will provide the basis for the individual patient care plan. Upon admission to the labor room, antepartal care in the broadest sense provides for the physical, emotional, and social needs of the expectant mother and her family. The degree to which these needs have been met must be determined by the nurse. It is the responsibility of the nurse to assess effectively the total situation and to plan accordingly.

A. Psychosocial Aspects

Psychosocial aspects of care are the extension of care beyond the physical-therapeutic realm of care. As a basis for meeting the patient's psychosocial needs, the nurse will need a thorough knowledge of human development. Available references should be reviewed and used.

1. Nursing deals with helping the patient through the total delivery process. This period of care is often very short; therefore the nurse must be very knowledgeable and well organized.

2. To provide humanized care, the nurse must understand cultural variations that influence attitudes and behavior.

3. The nurse recognizes that all behavior is meaningful and utilizes her background to understand the specific needs of all ethnic groups.

4. Nurses assess the cultural norms relating to the father's role during the birth process. Fathers need to be involved in making contributions to the process.

5. The nurse considers the meaning of children in different cultural

groups. Parental behaviors toward the child should not be considered good or bad. The cultural significance should be considered.

6. Parental responses to pregnancy, labor, and delivery are reflective of the life-style of each family.

7. Cultural assessment provides the basis for understanding the behavior of the patient and her family.

8. A woman's concept of the "mother role" will be based on the ethnic group, social class, and the culture of which she is a part and the socialization that has occurred in her life.

B. Therapeutic Aspects

1. Admission to the labor suite will elicit a variety of responses from the patient: relief that her time of waiting is nearly finished; fear of what lies ahead; excitement at the prospect of having her baby; and anxiety over her own helplessness in the situation. Her initial contact with labor room personnel will have a profound and lasting effect on her. She should be greeted with cordiality, friendliness, and reassurance.

2. A complete medical and antepartal history is invaluable in assessing each individual patient's needs and anticipating complications. Some patients may have had no preparation at all; others may have attended prenatal classes, which vary in content and approach. If birth is imminent, the minimum essentials should be obtained: vital signs, fetal heart tones, maternal allergies, time labor started, frequency of contractions, status of membranes, previous pregnancies, physician contacts, and if the mother is unmarried, if she will keep the baby.

3. The nurse is primarily interested in maternal and fetal health and well-being. Initially, she ascertains the status of the mother and baby. She listens to fetal heart tones with a fetoscope (see Technique 106, Fetal Heart Tones), notifies the physician of the progress of labor, and informs the family.

4. To promote a feeling of trust, the nurse will do the following:
   a. Introduce herself and never appear rushed or hurried
   b. Look for signs of anxiety and stress
   c. Engage in therapeutic listening according to good communication techniques
   d. Provide eye-to-eye contact while listening and provide feedback
   e. Use "touch" in a soothing and appropriate manner, which is very important in establishing confidence and trust
   f. Consider each patient's level of pain tolerance and special needs
   g. Include the father and the family in the labor and delivery process as much as possible, depending on their wishes

5. Admission procedure includes the following:
   a. Assist the patient to the room.

b. Explain the policies, procedures, and routines to husband and family.

c. Direct the husband to the admitting office if this has not been taken care of.

d. Assist the patient in undressing.

e. Perform the initial check of the fetal heart tones, contractions, and vital signs. This assessment needs to be made as soon as possible.

f. Do an examination unless the patient is bleeding or in premature labor.

g. Give valuables to the father or send them to the safe. Keep clothing together and labeled. Also give prostheses, such as contact lenses and partial plates to the father or place them with the mother's belongings. The chart should reflect these items and their disposition.

h. Notify the physician of the patient's present status.

i. Place Ident-a-card or other identification on the patient and explain the purpose.

j. Review the patient's prenatal record, if available.

C. Communicative Aspects

1. *Orientation to the labor room*

   a. If the antepartal care has been adequate, the mother will know what to expect; if it is not adequate, explain the preliminary procedures in more detail.

   b. Orientation should include all aspects of the process of labor and the physical environment.

   c. The preparation for delivery will vary in different hospitals; however, the basic principles are the same.

2. *Observations*

   a. Observe for signs of maternal distress
      (1) Sudden change in blood pressure
      (2) Elevated temperature and pulse
      (3) Continued sustained contraction with no relaxation phase
      (4) Extreme continued abdominal pain unrelated to contractions
      (5) Extreme emotional distress.

   b. Watch for signs of fetal distress
      (1) Change in fetal heart rate
      (2) Passage of meconium (unless it is a breech presentation)
      (3) Prolapsed cord
      (4) Bright red, frank bleeding

(5) Hyperactive fetus

c. Observe the progress of labor by assessing the contractions, vital signs, and maternal responses.

d. Crowning is an indication birth is imminent; have the patient taken to delivery room at once.

3. *Charting*

DATE	TREATMENT	TIME	OBSERVATIONS	SIGNATURE
5/1	Admitted to labor room 4	1345	24-year-old female, para ī grav īī admitted in active labor. Membranes have ruptured. Dilated 6 cm, effacement complete. Prep has been done. Dr. B. here. Rings and contacts to husband. Contractions q 3 min, approx. 45-60 sec duration. Nurse with patient.	G. Ivers, R.N.

D. Teaching Aspects—Patient and Family

1. Teach patient who has not had prenatal classes and instructions about when to breathe evenly and regularly (during the first stage of labor) and when to bear down (during second stage of labor). She will also need added explanations and reassurance.

2. Use visual aids to explain the physiology of labor.

3. Teach the father how to help: to coach the mother about breathing, to rub her back, to hold her hand, and so on. If he is not available, have some other person provide the support.

IV. EVALUATION PROCESS

A. Did the patient progress through each stage of labor satisfactorily and within normal limits?

B. Did the patient seem calm and confident?

C. Was the progress of labor adequately monitored and reported?

D. Is the obstetric history complete?

E. Were any abnormalities detected early?

F. Did the patient have a normal, uncomplicated delivery?

G. Was the father included in the total process?

H. Was the instruction plan understood and was it adequate?

100
Amniocentesis

I. ASSESSMENT OF SITUATION

A. Definition
A procedure in which a needle is inserted through the abdominal and uterine walls into the amniotic fluid for the withdrawal of a fluid specimen or for the injection of a fluid substitute

B. Terminology
1. *Amnion:* of the two fetal membranes, the inner membrane that forms a sac and contains the fetus and the fluid
2. *Amniotic fluid:* the liquid surrounding the fetus in the inner membrane (amnion)
3. *Amnionitis:* infected amniotic fluid

C. Rationale for Actions
1. To allow early prenatal detection, clinical diagnosis, and evaluation of genetic or acquired disorders and abnormalities that may afford the option of intrauterine treatment or a therapeutic abortion
2. To assess fetal maturity
3. To relieve hydramnios
4. To follow up isoimmune disease patients
5. To inject substances into the uterus

II. NURSING PLAN

A. Objectives
1. To inform the patient of the purpose of the examination and the procedure to be followed
2. To provide emotional support before and during the procedure
3. To serve as a caring, knowledgeable, and resourceful person
4. To assist in the procedure

B. Patient Preparation
1. Explain the procedure and reassure the patient and family.
2. Obtain the necessary legal permits.
3. Check vital signs before the procedure.

4. Catheterize the patient, as prescribed, before the procedure.
5. Place the patient in a comfortable position.
6. Perform surgical preparation of the abdomen.
7. The procedure may be performed in the radiology department so that ultrasound identification can be made of fetal parts before the aspiration.

C. Equipment

1. Amniocentesis tray
2. Local anesthetic of physician's choice, syringe, and needles
3. Sterile vaginal examination tray
4. 2% tincture of iodine (not iodine soaps or other solutions), alcohol sponges
5. Sterile gloves
6. Band-Aid
7. Small brown paper bag or other light-excluding container if bilirubin is to be measured
8. Label for tubes
9. Dye for fetal identification in multiple pregnancy
10. For amniocentesis done for hydramnios, the additional equipment:
    a. Ten extra 20 ml glass syringes
    b. Sterile saline
    c. Pan set
    d. Measuring pitcher

III. IMPLEMENTING NURSING INTERVENTION

A. Therapeutic Aspects

1. Amniotic fluid studies are usually performed between the 14th and 16th weeks of gestation.
2. The procedure is usually done under local anesthetic at the suprapubic site, after localization and manual elevation of the fetus (Fig. 100-1).
3. Put the specimen in the appropriate containers. If bilirubin studies are requested, place the specimen containers in a brown paper sack or wrap them in foil *immediately;* do not expose to light. Label tubes correctly and send to lab immediately.
4. Amniocentesis is indicated if the following conditions exist:
    a. Family history of genetic disorders
    b. A pregnant woman over 40 yr of age, because of the higher incidence of fetal chromosomal aberrations
    c. Couples who have at least one child with genetic disorders

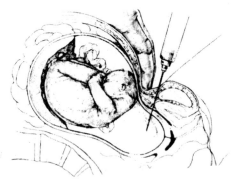

FIGURE 100.1

B. Communicative Aspects

1. *Observations*

    a. Monitor the general condition of the patient very closely.

    b. Check vital signs and fetal heart tone every 30 min.

    c. Watch for vaginal show or bleeding.

    d. Observe for the loss of amniotic fluid or signs of labor.

    e. Instruct the patient to remain on complete bed rest unless notified otherwise.

    f. Follow the same procedure for the injection of an abortifacient.

2. *Charting*

DATE	TREATMENT	TIME	OBSERVATIONS	SIGNATURE
4/7	With-drawal of 30ml amniotic fluid. Specimen to lab for studies.	0910	BP 120/60. P 80, R. 20, FHT 130. No evidence of vag. bleeding or loss of amniotic fluid.	J. Jones, R.N.

3. *Referrals*

Not applicable

C. Teaching Aspects—Patient and Family

1. Instruct the patient and husband and family about the purpose of the examination and the information that can be obtained.

2. If indicated, provide additional information in genetic counseling and other abnormal conditions existing in childbearing.

3. Instruct the patient and husband, if appropriate, concerning further pregnancies and alternate considerations.

IV. EVALUATION PROCESS

A. Did the patient and family understand the purpose of the examination?

B. Was there acceptance of the possible results?

C. Was there an open, frank discussion of the possibilities?

D. Was the procedure carried out without any difficulty?

E. Were proper precautions taken in handling the specimen?

F. Did the patient experience any ill effects?

101

Amniotomy

I. ASSESSMENT OF SITUATION

A. Definition

A procedure to release the amniotic fluid and initiate a shortened labor

B. Terminology

1. *Amnion:* inner membrane

2. *Amniotic fluid:* fluid surrounding the fetus in the amnion. The term fetus is immersed in about 1 liter of this clear liquid.

3. *Chorion:* outer membrane

4. *Complete rupture of membranes:* amnion and chorion completely ruptured

5. *Sepsis:* the presence of pathogenic microorganisms or their toxins in the blood or other tissues

C. Rationale for Actions

1. To assess the condition of the patient and the fetus and the progress of labor

2. To assess carefully the basis for selection and alternatives in the modes of care

3. To monitor progress in normal labor, which can be predicted as a constant entity; deviations or interventions are necessary in some situations.

II. NURSING PLAN

A. Objectives

1. To alleviate the delay in the spontaneous rupture of the membranes
2. To provide supportive measures to the patient and family
3. To ensure sterile technique and all necessary precautions to avoid infections
4. To provide technical assistance with the procedure

B. Patient Preparation

1. Explain the procedure and what will be accomplished.
2. Reassure the patient and family.
3. Take the fetal heart tone (FHT) immediately before and after the membrane ruptures and after the first contraction.
4. Caution the patient to remain in bed after the membrane ruptures.
5. Prepare the patient for a vaginal examination.
6. Explain to the patient that she must not get out of bed or sit up in bed but that she may turn from side to side or lie on her back.

C. Equipment

1. Cleansing solution
2. Amniotome
3. Sterile vaginal glove
4. Lubricant
5. Fetoscope

III. IMPLEMENTING NURSING INTERVENTION

A. Therapeutic Aspects

1. In a high percentage of cases, labor is initiated by the spontaneous rupture of the membranes.
2. Labor usually begins within 12 hr after the membranes have ruptured.
3. During amniotomy, the nurse should remain with the patient and assist the physician. She should provide emotional support to the patient and family. The patient is in the lithotomy position and draped. The nurse should provide an antiseptic preparation of the vulva. After the procedure is done, the nurse should note the color and odor of the fluid; check the FHT immediately and after the first contraction; and observe closely for cord prolapse or any sign of fetal distress. The nurse should give perineal care, change the hip pad, and keep the patient in bed unless the fetal head is well engaged in the pelvis and dilatation is less than 5 cm. After contractions start, the nurse should

check the FHT every 15 to 30 min. The time, the condition of the fluid, and FHT should be charted.

4. After the membranes have ruptured, the chances of infection increase in proportion to the length of time between the rupture and the completion of labor.

5. After the membranes have ruptured the temperature should be checked every 2 hr.

6. After the membranes have ruptured spontaneously or by amniotomy, the induction of labor is indicated. If this is not successful, a cesarean section may be necessary.

7. Amniotic fluid serves several functions important to the development of the fetus:

   a. It allows freedom of movement.

   b. It facilitates the development of the fetus.

   c. It plays a major factor in maintaining constant body temperature in the fetus.

   d. It is a source of oral liquid.

   e. It protects the fetus from direct trauma.

   f. It equalizes the pressure on the cervix during uterine contractions.

B. Communicative Aspects

1. *Observations*

   a. Have the patient void.

   b. Membranes should remain intact as long as possible unless the vertex is presenting and engaged.

   c. Almost constant monitoring of the fetus will be necessary.

   d. Observe vaginal bleeding and fluid discharge.

   e. Check FHT before the procedure, immediately following it, and after each contraction.

   f. Check the frequency and duration of contractions every 30 min.

   g. Measure the vital signs every 3 to 4 hr and blood pressure every hour.

   h. Perform rectal examinations at periodic intervals to determine the stage of labor.

   i. Report any changes to the physician immediately. Be prepared for emergency measures.

2. *Charting*

   Chart the procedure, the mother's vital signs, the FHT and the condition of the amniotic fluid.

3. *Referrals*

   Not applicable

C. Teaching Aspects—Patient and Family

1. Explain in detail the necessity of doing an amniotomy.
2. Make the patient aware of the progress that should occur following the amniotomy.

IV. EVALUATION PROCESS

A. Was the procedure accomplished with minimal stress to the patient?
B. Were techniques sterile and properly carried out?
C. Was the patient relaxed and cooperative?
D. Did the vital signs and FHT remain stable?

102

Antepartal Care

I. ASSESSMENT OF SITUATION

A. Definition

The antepartal period extends from conception to the onset of labor.

B. Terminology

1. *Amenorrhea:* absence of menstruation
2. *Amniocentesis:* a procedure in which a needle is inserted through the abdominal and uterine walls into the amniotic fluid
3. *Antenatal:* before birth; refers to fetal care
4. *Antepartal:* before delivery; refers to maternal care
5. *Auscultation:* listening for sounds produced within the body
6. *Cervix:* lowest and narrow end of the uterus, extending into vagina
7. *Conception:* the process of becoming pregnant, involving fertilization of the ovum and implantation
8. *Embryo:* early development of the unborn human from second week until the 7th or 8th wk of gestation when the skeleton begins to form
9. *Family:* a unit of individuals engaged in intimate interactions in daily living patterns, for example, two parents and children
10. *Fetus:* the unborn human from the 7th wk of gestation until birth
11. *First trimester:* period between the last menstrual period until the

14th wk of gestation, during which the fetus begins to develop and, in the mother, physical and psychological changes are observable

12. *Gestation:* period of development from conception through birth
13. *Multigravida:* a woman who has had two or more pregnancies
14. *Nulligravida:* a woman who has never been pregnant
15. *Para:* parturition, delivery of a viable fetus
16. *Primigravida:* a woman who is pregnant for the first time
17. *Second trimester:* the 15th to the 28th wk after last menstrual period, during which the uterus extends to above the umbilicus and fetal movements are evident
18. *Third trimester:* the end of the 28th wk of gestation until delivery, during which fetal growth is rapid

C. Rationale for Actions

1. People who wish to bear children should have adequate health services and resources available.
2. Proper antepartal and antenatal care is necessary to ensure and maintain the health of the expectant mother and infant.
3. High-risk situations can be identified early and dealt with effectively in most situations.
4. The infant mortality rate can be reduced significantly by improved maternity care.
5. The patient's bill of rights ensures each individual the right to the best health care available.

II. NURSING PLAN

A. Objectives

1. To direct the course of a normal pregnancy by providing the essential services
2. To teach parenting skills
3. To provide early detection and treatment of maternal diseases that may affect the course of the pregnancy
4. To reassure the patient and family members, if appropriate
5. To identify abnormalities or other problems that may prevent the normal process of a pregnancy
6. To establish a therapeutic relationship with the patient and her family

III. IMPLEMENTING NURSING INTERVENTION

A. Therapeutic Aspects

1. Recognize the common symptoms and signs of early pregnancy: amenorrhea, nausea and vomiting, urinary frequency, breast sensi-

tivity, listlessness, fatigue, quickening, leukorrhea, abdominal enlargement, skin changes, and changes in internal genitals.

2. Positive signs of pregnancy are the following:

   a. Laboratory tests showing the presence of human chorionic gonadatropin (HCG) in urine

   b. Fetal heartbeat heard with the use of a clinical stethoscope or electronic means such as fetal electrocardiography

   c. Palpation of fetal outline around 24th wk

3. Most obstetricians and clinics establish a general plan, such as a monthly visit until 8th mo, then a visit every 2 wk or weekly.

4. Routine care generally includes the following procedures:

   a. Obtain initial data, health history, and social data.

   b. Note the initial weight and weight gain. Develop an overall plan for weight gain.

   c. Do a urinalysis, the specimen from first morning voiding. Check for protein and glucose.

   d. Measure blood pressure.

   e. Do a complete nutritional analysis.

   f. Collect data as to the patient's well-being, problems, complications, and concerns.

   g. Develop a teaching plan.

   h. Acquaint the patient with community resources, such as prenatal classes, hospital services, and LaMaze classes.

   i. Instruct the patient in the common discomforts generally associated with pregnancy

      (1) Backaches: demonstrate the techniques for rest and relaxation, and better posture (pelvis tilted forward).

      (2) Headaches: discuss methods to lessen physical and emotional stress. Identify causes.

      (3) Constipation: determine causes, encourage fluid intake, diet, and exercise.

      (4) Leg cramps: usually caused by pressure on the nerve to the lower extremities. Check calcium and phosphorus intake, clothing worn, and personal habits.

      (5) Nausea and vomiting: causes may vary, including anxiety, emotional stress, poor eating habits, altered hormone levels, and metabolic changes. Tell the patient that relief may be obtained by eating small amounts of dry or bland foods during the day.

      (6) Urinary frequency: this is usually due to the growth of the uterus resulting in pressure on the bladder. Check for infections or abnormal conditions.

(7) Varicose veins: recommend elastic support stockings.

(8) Ankle swelling: check for hypertension or proteinurea. Encourage elevation of the legs and hips several times during the day, the use of support hose, and fluid intake.

5. Health counseling involves the following points:

a. Drugs

(1) No drug should be taken unless prescribed by a physician.

(2) All drugs, including aspirin and some of the more common self-treatment drugs, can be dangerous, especially during the first trimester.

(3) A careful record of all drugs taken should be maintained.

b. Alcohol

(1) The excessive use of alcohol during pregnancy could result in premature delivery, other complications, or abnormal pregnancies.

(2) The occasional use of alcohol beverages is presently being questioned and is generally not considered safe.

c. Smoking

Studies have shown that heavy cigarette smoking may cause fetal growth retardation and result in perinatal and infant mortality.

d. Clothing

(1) Loose clothing is advised; constricting garments such as girdles, stretch pants, tight waisted clothing, garters, and high heels should be avoided.

(2) Maternity girdles that can be easily adjusted may be indicated in some situations.

e. Exercise and physical activity

(1) Simple exercises are encouraged.

(2) A program of physical activity should be outlined according to the mother's prior activity regimen and her present state of health.

f. Personal care

(1) Bathing: tub bathing is permitted until the membranes rupture.

(2) Figure: positive efforts should be directed toward maintaining the figure, including exercise, breast support, good nutrition, personal cleanliness, and good hygiene.

(3) Dental care: good dental care is essential to prevent infections or dental caries.

(4) Immunizations: some immunizations are advisable, others are not. The killed-virus immunizations for influenza and the Salk poliomyelitis vaccine are indicated because of the wom-

an's increased susceptibility. The "live" or attenuated virus immunizations are not indicated, including those for measles, German measles, and mumps.

6. Common nursing techniques in the antepartal period include the following:

   a. Initial interview-intake process

     (1) Personal data: obtain birthdate, place, marital status, husband's occupation and age, occupation, education, children in family, living habits, church affiliation, and ethnic and cultural background.

     (2) Family history: note siblings, health status of family, history of serious illnesses, chronic diseases, hereditary diseases, deformities, mental illness, epilepsy, and multiple pregnancies.

     (3) Medical history: ask about childhood diseases, operations, menstrual history, conditions relating to body systems (endocrine, gastrointestinal, cardiovascular, muscular, urinary, respiratory, sensory), menstrual history, obstetric history (para, gravida, abortions, premature deliveries, type of deliveries, outcomes), and medications, smoking, alcohol use.

     (4) Attitudes toward childbearing: inquire about the background of knowledge, past problems, plans for infant (type of feeding, babysitters), plans for self (school, stay at home), review purposes of available classes on cooperative childbirth, provide brochures.

   b. Physical assessment

     (1) Assist patient in undressing and drape for complete examination.

     (2) Check vital signs: temperature, pulse, respirations, blood pressure, weight, height.

     (3) Obtain specimen for urinalysis for glucose and albumin, if indicated, culture, and sensitivity.

     (4) Physical examination is completed by the physician, including eye, ear, nose, and throat, vital organs (heart, lungs), abdomen, thyroid, breasts, abdominal palpation, and external observations.

     (5) Laboratory tests, as prescribed by the physician, include microscopic urinalysis, wet mount for bacteria, cervical smear for cancer, and gram stain and anaerobic culture for gonorrhea. Blood work involves testing for complete blood count, blood type, Rh factor, syphilis, rubella antibodies, and sickle cell anemia.

     (6) Pelvic examination is performed to check the vagina for growths or weaknesses in the posterior and anterior walls; examine the uterus for consistency and size and adnexa; check

the cervix for color, consistency, erosion; check the pelvis for adequacy for vaginal delivery; examine the external genitalia, the anal sphincter, the perineal body, and the urethral meatus.

    (a) Assemble equipment

        (1) Vaginal speculum

        (2) Sterile gloves for vaginal examination

        (3) Clean gloves for rectal examination

        (4) Forceps

        (5) Uterine swabs

        (6) Sterile lubricant

        (7) Sponges

        (8) Applicators

        (9) Vaginal pipette with rubber bulb

     (10) Slides

     (11) Spatula for pap (Papanicolaou) smear, fixative

     (12) Saline solution, KDH, dropper

     (13) Media for cultures

    (b) Explain the entire procedure to the patient.

    (c) Have the patient void.

    (d) Position the patient in the lithotomy position.

    (e) Warm the speculum in a pan of water.

    (f) Instruct the patient in pant-breathing.

    (g) Assist the physician as indicated. He will use sterile gloves. Lubricate speculum (unless contraindicated) and gently insert it (Fig. 102-1).

    (h) Provide wipes following exam.

(7) The pap smear is done to detect abnormalities of cell growth in the cervix.

    (a) Instruct the patient not to use vaginal medications for the 10 to 12 hrs before the test.

    (b) Help the patient assume the lithotomy position.

    (c) Fill out the appropriate laboratory form to accompany the specimen.

(8) There are generally three indications for douching: cleansing, application of heat, treatment with local medication.

    (a) Equipment needed includes vaginal tablets, suppositories, or tampons.

(9)   For the urine specimen, give the patient the following instructions:

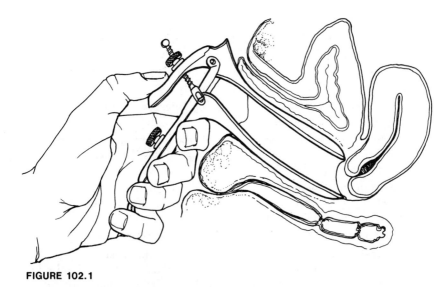

FIGURE 102.1

 (a) Use a clean container with lid.

 (b) Obtain the first voiding in the morning, if possible.

 (c) Clean the vulval and rectal areas with a damp cloth, always wiping from front to back.

 (d) Void a small amount first, then obtain specimen; usually 60 ml (2 oz) are adequate.

B. Psychosocial Aspects

1. During the initial intake process, a social history is obtained. This provides the data base for meeting the patient's needs psychologically and emotionally.

2. It is very important for the staff to understand a person's cultural background and the customs that are characteristic to certain ethnic groups. A good reference source in this area should be made available to all staff.

3. When possible, husbands or significant others should participate in an instructional conference.

4. Establishing a good relationship with the patient is very important and greatly enhances the patient's trust and openness with the staff.

5. Psychological and social changes evolve during pregnancy; the patient's self-image may undergo considerable change, and mood changes are common. Emotional support during this time is a major component of care. It is important for the staff to have a good knowledge and background in psychosocial nursing. Most recent maternity textbooks include this content and should be used by the staff.

C. Communicative Aspects

1. A written plan of care during the antepartal period should be developed and shared with the patient and family.

2. The patient must understand her role and responsibilities in the total plan. The objectives are developed jointly.

3. The physician's instructions must be interpreted and the patient helped to understand them.

4. A schedule of routine visits will enable the patient and staff to review together the progress being made and to discuss problems, changes, and concepts.

5. The staff must be very observant each visit, noting weight changes, blood pressure trends, edema, uterine enlargement, laboratory reports, and emotional changes.

6. The nurse must record all findings in the appropriate record.

7. Referrals include community activities, expectant parents classes (International Childbirth Education Association literature), La Leche League and literature, March of Dimes educational programs, genetic counseling, other medical consultation, if indicated, and psychosocial counseling, if indicated.

D. Teaching Aspects—Patient and Family

1. A systematic plan for patient and family teaching is a vital component of antepartal care.

2. The plan should include written materials, visual aides, and library resources list.

3. The patient care plan for the period of gestation should be reviewed with the patient.

4. The content of the instruction program should cover the process of pregnancy and the postnatal period.

    a. Developmental changes in the mother

    b. Development of the embryo/fetus

    c. Essential maternity care

    d. Personal hygiene

    e. Diet

    f. Dental care

    g. Rest and relaxation

    h. Dealing with common problems related to pregnancy

    i. Changes to be noted and reported to physician or nurse immediately

    j. Plans for hospitalization

    k. Process of labor, what to expect

    l. Postnatal period, what to expect

m. Care of the newborn infant

n. Breast care

o. Breast-feeding

p. Other methods of infant feeding

q. Child growth and development

r. Psychosocial changes

IV. EVALUATION PROCESS

A. This is an ongoing process throughout the pregnancy period. During each visit an assessment should be done.

1. Is the pregnancy progressing normally, and according to the plan?

2. Is the patient fulfilling her responsibilities: adhering to regular visits, weight control, dietary habits, personal hygiene, dental care; reporting changes and symptoms; following the physician's instructions?

3. Has the educational process been successful? What about feedback from the patient?

4. Does the patient demonstrate good or poor psychosocial adjustment?

5. Does the patient demonstrate good physical adjustment to the pregnancy?

6. Are members of the family involved in the planning?

B. The final assessment should be done at the time of delivery and the postpartum period.

1. Did the total gestation period progress according to goals and the plan?

2. What were the complications? How could these have been avoided?

3. What is the general condition of the mother, physically and emotionally?

4. Was the husband and family involvement satisfactory?

5. Were preparations for the infant adequate?

103

Breast Care

I. ASSESSMENT OF SITUATION

A. Definition

Care given to a recent postpartum patient who is not breast feeding. (For care of the breasts of nursing mothers, see Technique 104, Breast-feeding.)

B. Terminology

None

C. Rationale for Actions

1. To maintain proper support and cleanliness
2. To prevent trauma to the nipples and infection
3. To correct existing conditions such as inverted nipples

II. NURSING PLAN

A. Objectives

1. To teach the patient breast care
2. To teach the patient the changes she can expect to occur in the breasts due to pregnancy
3. To prevent infection in the baby's mouth and mother's breast
4. To teach routine self-check of the breast

B. Patient Preparation

1. Special care of the breasts during the antepartal period is essential in preparing to breast-feed the infant. Care during this period includes the following:

   a. The breast and nipples must be cared for daily. Early in pregnancy the breasts secrete colostrum, a milky, sometimes yellowish orange fluid. Unless this secretion is cleaned off regularly, infection may occur, or the drying may result in crusts that irritate the skin.

   b. Breasts become heavier and fuller, as a result of pregnancy hormones. Therefore, a good support brassiere is needed.

   c. The nipples can be toughened for nursing by rubbing with a rough towel during the last trimester.

d. The physician may advise the use of a nipple cream.

e. The three types of nipples are normal, flat, and inverted (Fig. 103-1). The inverted type of nipple is given special attention. Care to correct this should begin in the 5th mo of pregnancy. The general procedure consists of the following (Fig. 103-2):

(1) The thumbs are placed close to the inverted nipple, pressed

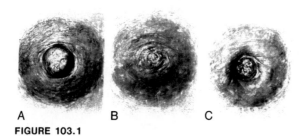

A   B   C

FIGURE 103.1

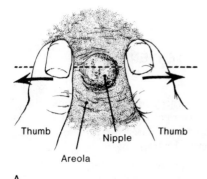

Thumb   Nipple   Thumb

Areola

A

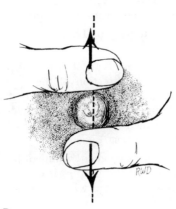

B

FIGURE 103.2

firmly into the breast tissue, and gradually pushed away from the areola.

(2) This should be done several times daily.

f. Manual expression of colostrum starting the 8th mo of pregnancy is recommended by some physicians. This technique keeps the milk ducts open. The procedure is simple to follow:

(1) Hands are washed.

(2) The breast is cupped in the hand; the thumb is placed above the nipple and forefinger below the breast at the edge of dark area.

(3) The thumb and finger are squeezed.

(4) The hand is moved back and forward in order to stimulate all milk ducts.

C. Equipment

1. Mild soap and warm water
2. Clean washcloth and towel
3. Well-fitting support brassiere
4. Nipple cream, if prescribed

III. IMPLEMENTING NURSING INTERVENTION

A. Therapeutic Aspects

1. If the mother will not be breast-feeding her infant, she may be given medication within the first few hours after delivery to suppress lactation. This may save much discomfort later, because once lactation has begun, drugs are not effective in stopping it.

2. Pathogens on the skin and hands may cause infection in the breast tissue. The patient should always wash her hands thoroughly before handling the breasts. The breast is washed with warm water and soap on a washcloth, using circular motions from the nipple out.

3. A dry environment discourages bacterial growth. The breasts should be dried well but gently.

4. All postpartum patients should wear some type of breast support that lifts the breasts upward and in the direction of the opposite shoulder. This serves to relieve discomfort, especially if breast engorgement occurs. The support will also encourage the breasts to return to normal muscle tone. A well-fitting brassiere (Fig. 103-3) or a breast binder will provide the needed support.

5. A damp and soiled environment provides a good environment for the growth of infection-producing bacteria. If the nipples leak, nursing pads should be used for protection and changed when they become soiled.

6. Tender, painful, cracked nipples should be exposed to the air to promote healing. Medication may be prescribed.

7. For several weeks after delivery the nipples should be washed and dried thoroughly after each feeding.

8. If the breasts become engorged, priority must be given to relieving the engorgement and making the mother comfortable. A tight-fitting binder is indicated (see Technique 30, Binders, application of). It usually goes beneath the axillae and around the back and laps over the front. In placing the binder, the breast tissue should be equally distributed so that the nipples are in the center. It may be secured by a series of safety pins. Ice packs to the breast may also bring relief. Pain medications may be prescribed.

9. If the nipples become eroded and cracked, a heat lamp is used after each feeding, suckling time is limited, or a nipple shield used.

B. Communicative Aspects

1. *Observations*

   a. Watch closely for signs of infection, such as redness and heat.

   b. Check daily for cracks and fissures.

2. *Charting*

DATE	TREATMENT	TIME	OBSERVATIONS	SIGNATURE
9/1	Breast care	0800	No discomfort or signs of infection or engorgement.	F. White, R.N.

3. *Referrals*

   Not applicable

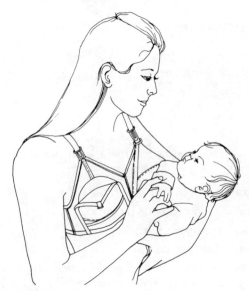

FIGURE 103.3

C. Teaching Aspects—Patient

1. Teach the mother the inspection and palpation of the breast to be done routinely.

2. Instruct the woman in routine care procedures.

3. Inform the mother of the cause of engorgement and assure her that congestion usually subsides in 1 to 2 days without treatment if the baby does not suck and if the milk is not expressed.

4. Inform the patient that hormone drugs given to dry up the breasts may cause vaginal bleeding after cessation of therapy.

IV. EVALUATION PROCESS

A. Does the mother understand and practice good breast care?

B. Has infection been prevented?

C. Are the breasts properly supported?

D. Has the patient been properly instructed regarding regular examination of the breasts?

104

Breast-Feeding

I. ASSESSMENT OF SITUATION

A. Definition

Feeding the infant from lactating breasts

B. Terminology

1. *Areola:* a ring of darker color around the nipple

2. *Lactation:* secretion of milk

3. *Nipple:* protuberance on each breast, from which lactiferous ducts discharge

C. Rationale for Actions

1. To provide the most suitable food for the infant

2. To facilitate involution of the uterus

3. To foster a closer mother-child relationship

4. To help the woman feed her infant with the method that is the most convenient and that, for most women, provides greater emotional satisfaction than bottle-feeding

II. NURSING PLAN

A. Objectives

1. To help the mother to meet the infant's nutritional needs
2. To assist the mother in becoming skillful in suckling her infant
3. To maintain the comfort of the mother and infant during feeding
4. To teach proper breast care

B. Patient Preparation

1. Evaluate each baby's condition. A small baby tires very easily.
2. Determine the baby's readiness for feeding. Note behaviors such as swallowing reflexes, alertness, mouth activity, and sucking.
3. Give the baby a few sips of sterile water after birth to initiate the sucking process. Later dextrose can be added.
4. Vital signs should be stable before feeding is attempted.
5. Have the mother hold the child in a semireclining position.
6. Tell the mother to feed the baby slowly and burp frequently.
7. Tell the mother not to overfeed; the stomach capacity at birth is approximately 60 ml (2 oz). If the capacity is exceeded, vomiting and diarrhea result.
8. Provide rest periods during feeding.
9. After feeding, position infant on his abdomen. This prevents aspiration if regurgitation or vomiting should occur.

C. Equipment

1. Pillow
2. Footstool
3. Nursing pads
4. Supporting brassiere
5. Sterile water and cotton balls

III. IMPLEMENTING NURSING INTERVENTION

A. Therapeutic Aspects

1. Encouragement can help allay anxiety in a new experience. The nursing mother needs teaching and encouragement, especially if this is her first attempt at nursing.
2. The nurse should instruct the mother about adequate diet during lactation.
3. Comfort greatly enhances breast-feeding effectiveness. The mother should sit with her feet on a footstool and a pillow in her lap to support the infant (Fig. 104-1). Or she may lie down, well supported by pillows, to nurse the infant.

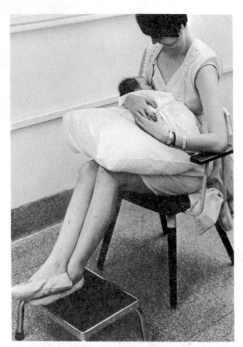

FIGURE 104.1

4. Proper care of the nipples is extremely important for the nursing mother. Pathogenic microorganisms may be transferred by direct contact. The nipples should be washed with a fresh, clean cloth every morning before the shower or bath. They should also be rinsed with plain water before each feeding. Handwashing by the mother is essential before each feeding.

5. Physiological changes in the breasts may cause pain and difficulty in suckling the infant. If the nipples are flattened because of engorgement, they may be pulled out with a breast pump. Tender nipples may be helped with a nipple shield. If the nipples become cracked or bleed, nursing should be stopped until they have time to heal. Breast-feeding may cause an increase in after pains, but this will soon cease.

6. Nipples may become sore after the first feeding. Breast-feeding time should be very brief at first, 1 to 2 min at each breast, then gradually increasing to 15 to 20 min. Initially, both breasts should be nursed at each feeding.

7. To remove the infant from the breast, the mother should first depress the areola area and release suction.

8. The natural reflexes possessed by the baby at birth will aid the learning experience. Brushing the baby's cheek with the nipple or a fingertip will cause him to turn in the direction of the stimulus and

grasp the nipple. The mother must take care that her breast does not obstruct the infant's breathing.

9. Breasts will generally fill by the 3rd day postpartum (sometimes later following cesarean section).

B. Communicative Aspects

1. *Observations*

   a. Observe nursing techniques, and offer support and encouragement.

   b. Observe the nipples for redness, cracking, and bleeding, which may indicate the necessity for alternate feeding measures.

   c. Observe the breasts for engorgement, adequate emptying, and proper support.

2. *Charting*

DATE	TREATMENT	TIME	OBSERVATIONS	SIGNATURE
1/5	Infant to breast	0800	First attempt to nurse; nipples cleansed. Nursed 2 min each breast. Sucking reflex on infant good. No distress or discomfort noted. In chair with feet elevated. Appears comfortable.	F. White, R.N.

3. *Referrals*

   Not applicable

C. Teaching Aspects—Patient

1. Instruct the mother about breast care and the techniques of infant feeding.

2. Explain that an occasional bottle of expressed milk or formula will allow the mother to have some time to herself.

3. Emphasize the need for a properly fitting and supporting bra.

4. Review the usual diet and suggest modifications to include additional calories and fluids if necessary.

5. Instruct the mother to report any breast tenderness, masses, or fever.

IV. EVALUATION PROCESS

A. Can the mother properly nourish her infant by breast-feeding?

B. Is the mother comfortable and the infant supported during feeding?

C. Does the mother understand and practice proper breast care?

D. Is the infant gaining weight?

E. Are the mother's breasts engorged?

105

Cesarean Section

I. ASSESSMENT OF SITUATION

A. Definition

An operative procedure to deliver a fetus by an incision through the abdominal wall and the uterus

B. Terminology

1. *Abruptio placentae:* partial or complete separation of the placenta before the delivery of the infant
2. *Breech presentation:* in labor the presentation of the buttocks or feet (or both) of the fetus; occurs in approximately 3% of deliveries
3. *Dystocia:* difficult delivery; prolonged because of the size of the fetus or the pelvis of the mother, or inadequate uterine muscular contractions
4. *Eclampsia:* severe complications of pregnancy characterized by albuminuria, high blood pressure, edema, convulsions, and coma
5. *Hypoxia:* insufficient available oxygen to the tissues
6. *Placenta previa:* a placenta that is abnormally planted in the uterus, partially or completely occluding the internal cervical os
7. *Transabdominal:* through the abdomen
8. *Vaginal:* vaginal cesarean section

C. Rationale for Actions

1. To protect the lives of the mother and the fetus
2. To enhance the chances of health for mother and fetus

II. NURSING PLAN

A. Objectives

1. To assess the anxiety level of the patient and family
2. To prepare the patient mentally and physically for the procedure
3. To maintain close contact with the family, assisting them through the process
4. To provide preoperative preparation
5. To determine if the mother plans to breast-feed the baby; if she does intend to breast-feed, explain that nursing her baby will help the uterus to contract and reduce bleeding.

B. Patient Preparation

1. Explain the reasons for the surgical procedure to the patient and family, and answer questions.

2. Give the patient the opportunity to express her feelings and fears.

3. Assist the family in understanding the various tests and procedures that are done.

4. The surgeon and consultant should discuss the reasons for this type of delivery with the patient and spouse so that *informed* consent may be obtained. The nurse supports the patient by reinforcing patient and fetal needs and clarifying statements when requested.

5. Preoperative preparation may include the following:

   a. Surgical preparation and obstetric preparation, if indicated

   b. Enema

   c. Insertion of a retention catheter. (Trauma to the uretha must be avoided. If the patient has been in labor and the presenting part is posterior to the symphysis pubis, the urethra will be compressed and elongated.)

   d. Appropriate laboratory reports recorded on the chart

   e. Blood, typing and crossmatching usually done

   f. Intravenous infusion, as prescribed

   g. Administration of preoperative medications, when prescribed

   h. Record checked for consultation reports

   i. Clean gown, personal attention

   j. Routine care such as removal of contact lenses, rings, dentures, fingernail polish

6. The surgical procedure may be performed in the operating room or in the obstetric unit, depending on the hospital. The role of the maternity nurse will vary, depending on hospital policy and procedures. The maternity nurse may accompany the patient to the operating room suite to assist the pediatrician with the infant.

7. Proper identification of both mother and infant is the primary responsibility of the nurse.

C. Equipment

1. Enema tray

2. Retention catheter setup

3. Surgical preparation tray

4. Intravenous infusion tray and fluid

5. Preoperative medication

6. Gown

7. Equipment needed for infant

   a. Transport with oxygen

   b. Infant resuscitation setup

   c. Fetoscope and stethoscope

   d. Umbilical cord clamp

   e. Infant linen pack

   f. Delivery room notes for report to nursery staff

   g. Infant warmer

III. IMPLEMENTING NURSING INTERVENTION

A. Therapeutic Aspects

1. Cesarean section deliveries have a higher maternal and fetal mortality rate than normal deliveries.

2. Indications for a cesarean section are fetopelvic disproportion, dystocia, fetal distress, placenta previa, abruptio placentae, positive stress test, preeclampsia, herpes II virus, previous cesarean delivery, previous surgery involving reproductive organs, pelvic tumors, recent pelvic fracture, and any maternal illness in which labor would be hazardous.

3. A postmortem cesarean section performed a few minutes after the mother's death should result in living baby. Hypoxia is the major concern.

4. For patients having elective cesarean sections (usually repeat cesarean section), there is ample time for teaching, psychological preparation, and support. The apprehension felt by the mother is generally the same as for any surgical procedure.

5. Patients who face an emergency cesarean delivery may find it very traumatic. This reaction should be anticipated and efforts should be directed toward preventing an emotional crisis.

6. Postoperatively, time should be spent reviewing the events to ensure the patient's understanding and acceptance. The patient should be informed that future deliveries will be elective cesarean section.

B. Communicative Aspects

1. *Observations*

   a. Be aware of the psychological effects of a cesarean section.

     (1) The patient may exhibit a sense of failure or defeat because she could not complete the normal process.

     (2) The grieving process may be evident and generally relates to being unable to perform.

     (3) The anxiety level may be extremely high.

     (4) The mother may express feelings of fear, concern for the welfare of the baby, and death fears.

     (5) Some patients believe cesarean delivery is easier than labor; they may welcome it as a relief from pain.

b. Maintain a deep appreciation for the fears and concerns of the patient undergoing cesarean section.

(1) As early as possible, assess how the patient and family are reacting.

(2) Provide adequate information, allow for the expression of feelings, and answer questions.

(3) Provide as much opportunity as possible for the husband and family to be with the patient; prevent isolation and loneliness, if possible.

(4) Constantly provide reassurance in the form of verbal and nonverbal support. The presence of the nurse by the patient's bedside may be advisable.

(5) Do not sacrifice interpersonal nursing activities for technical functions unless it is a crisis situation.

(6) Promote a constant environment of caring and support.

c. Continuously observe the following:

(1) Fetal heart tones

(2) Fetal positioning

(3) Contractions, interval and duration

(4) Vital signs

(5) Vaginal discharge

(6) General condition of patient

d. For the patient with a preexisting disorder, maintain the medical regimen, as prescribed.

e. Postoperative observations include the following:

(1) Complications

(2) Paralytic ileus

(3) Hemorrhage

(4) Infection, especially if membranes ruptured early

(5) Inflammation and drainage of the incision

(6) Thrombophlebitis

(7) Pulmonary embolus

2. *Charting*

Report all pertinent data in the patient's chart

3. *Referrals*

a. Chaplain

b. Medical consultant for maternal or infant condition

C. Teaching Aspects—Patient

1. When a cesarean section is indicated, it may be an emergency situation or the patient may be exhibiting a high level of anxiety and

stress. In both situations, refrain from adding to the stressful situation by presenting too much information. The patient's ability to assimilate information at this time is probably very limited.

2. Present information in a clear, concise manner; the key role is to be present, to listen, and to clarify.

3. Sometimes time is limited for a woman to prepare for the reality of a cesarean section. Therefore, combine the time needed for technical procedures and psychological support.

IV. EVALUATION PROCESS

A. Did the patient exhibit a feeling of confidence?

B. Was the physical and emotional support system adequate?

C. Were the purposes (objectives) for doing the cesarean section met?

D. Were the technical measures performed safely and effectively?

E. What could have been done differently?

F. Was there a follow-up conference with the patient and family to determine effectiveness of the plan?

106

Fetal Heart Tones (FHT)

I. ASSESSMENT OF SITUATION

A. Definition

Periodic auscultation of the fetal heart. Heart beat of the fetus is normally 120 to 160 beats/min and is generally heard at 20 wk.

B. Terminology

1. *Auscultation:* the act of listening for sounds within the body

2. *Funic souffle:* murmur or whizzing sound caused by blood rushing through the umbilical cord; sometimes mistaken for FHT because it is synchronous with it

3. *Uterine souffle:* murmur or rushing sound caused by blood rushing through the large vessels of the uterus; should be synchronous with maternal heart rate

C. Rationale for Actions

1. To evaluate the condition of the fetus and detect any fetal distress
2. To diagnose a multiple pregnancy
3. To ascertain fetal position

II. NURSING PLAN

A. Objectives

1. To provide for the safety and welfare of the infant
2. To count and record FHT every hour in the latent phase of labor, or more often if indicated
3. To count and record FHT every 30 min in the active phase of labor, or more often if indicated
4. To count and record FHT every 5 min during the second stage of labor; it may be necessary to monitor constantly

B. Patient Preparation

1. Explain the purpose of evaluating the FHT to the patient.
2. Explain the equipment being used and what is expected of the patient.
3. If unable to hear the FHT, briefly explain the immediate plan of care to the patient; avoid showing concern or anxiety.

C. Equipment

1. *Bell fetoscope:* a weighted stethoscope useful under sterile drapes to check FHT
2. *Head fetoscope:* a stethoscope with a fitted headpiece, allowing for conduction of sound through the frontal bones as well as through the eardrum of the listener
3. *Doppler probe:* an instrument capable of detecting fetal cardiac activity by low energy ultrasound; applied externally for heart monitoring when necessary in pregnancy and labor; very useful in detecting hard-to-hear FHT and in localizing the placenta
4. *Fetal phonocardiography:* a method of obtaining FHT by placing a microphone to the maternal abdomen; also amplifies other sounds

III. IMPLEMENTING NURSING INTERVENTION

A. Therapeutic Aspects

1. The fetal heart rate is an indicator of fetal status. It should be checked on admission, every 30 min during the relaxation phase of labor, every 15 min during the transition phase, and every 5 min during the beginning of the second stage. It is heard by placing the bell of the head fetoscope or the weighted bell fetoscope firmly on the skin of the maternal abdomen (Fig. 106-1). Before auscultation, ma-

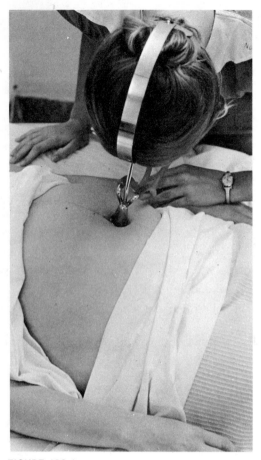

FIGURE 106.1

ternal abdomen is palpated to assess the fetal presentation, position, and lie.

2. FHT is best heard through the fetus's back, so the optimal location to place the fetoscope will vary according to fetal position. If the fetus is in the usual vertex presentation (head first), the sound will usually be best heard in the lower right or left quadrant of the maternal abdomen. However, if the infant is breech (feet or buttocks first) or in transverse lie (lying crosswise in the uterus), it will be more difficult to locate the actual FHT, and extra care must be taken not to confuse it with the uterine souffle.

3. In order to avoid mistaking the uterine souffle for the fetal heartbeat, the nurse first counts the mother's radial pulse and then listens to the FHT.

4. Rupture of the uterine membranes is serious for the fetus. The gush of water that ensues may cause cord prolapse. Therefore, the FHT must be checked immediately after the membranes rupture.

5. During contraction, there is interference with the audibility of the FHT. It is advisable to wait at least 30 sec following contractions before attempting to listen, in order to get a baseline reading. During the progressive activity of normal labor, the FHT must be listened for during the entire period of the contraction and ensuing relaxation to assess the quality of the FHT. Fetal heart rate is measured for 1 full min.

B. Communicative Aspects

1. *Observations*

    a. Checking the fetal heart beat is an important responsibility of the nurse. Abnormalities must be recognized for the safety of the mother and infant.

    b. The normal fetal heart rate is 120 to 160 beats/min. The FHT should be checked for rate, regularity, and strength, and any deviations must be reported immediately.

2. *Charting*

    The FHT should be charted when taken, along with the location on the abdomen where the FHT was obtained.

DATE	TREATMENT	TIME	OBSERVATIONS	SIGNATURE
6/15	FHT	0910	FHT taken. 142 beats/min heard in right lower quadrant.	F. White, R.N.

3. *Referrals*

    Not applicable

C. Teaching Aspects—Patient and Family

Emphasize the importance of monitoring the FHT to both the father and mother early in labor, to prevent undue concern over the frequency of taking it. It also serves as a reminder to the parents that the mother and fetus are being watched closely.

IV. EVALUATION PROCESS

A. Was FHT monitored throughout pregnancy and labor?

B. Were any deviations noted in FHT? If so, were they reported to the physician?

C. Did the patient understand the need for monitoring and observation?

107

Fundus, Checking (Postpartum)

I. ASSESSMENT OF SITUATION

A. Definition

The assessment of uterine involution; observation and intervention that prevents or alleviates complications resulting from a "relaxed" fundus after delivery

B. Terminology

1. *Fingerbreadth:* the width of the examiner's finger
2. *Fundus:* the upper portion of the uterus, between the points of insertion of the fallopian tubes
3. *Hemorrhage:* loss of 500 ml of blood or more
4. *Involution:* the retrogression of the female reproductive organs to the normal, nonpregnant state

C. Rationale for Actions

1. To check progress of involution
2. To prevent hemorrhage from the placenta site
3. To ensure a contracted uterus

II. NURSING PLAN

A. Objectives

1. To prevent the fundus from becoming boggy and soft
2. To evaluate the involutional process
3. To prevent shock and hemorrhage

B. Patient Preparation

1. If the patient is awake or reacting, explain what is being done and the importance of ensuring that the fundus is firm.
2. Communication with the patient will depend on her level of consciousness and general condition.

C. Equipment

None

III. IMPLEMENTING NURSING INTERVENTION

A. Therapeutic Aspects

1. The time of greatest danger of hemorrhage is immediately after delivery. The fundus should then lie at or below the level of the umbilicus and be contracted and firm. At times, the uterine muscles may relax, and excessive bleeding may occur. Holding the uterus by grasping the lower portion directly above the symphysis pubis with one hand and holding the top of the fundus with the other hand should quickly aid its contractile power (Fig. 107-1). The uterus should be checked and massaged, if needed, every 15 min during the first 90 min after delivery.

2. Overmassage will cause the mother considerable pain. It also stimulates premature uterine contractions, thereby causing undue muscle fatigue which results in uterine atony.

3. After delivery, there are large open vessels at the placenta site. With the muscle fibers contracted, the bleeding is controlled. If the uterus becomes tonic, blood and clots may collect in the cavity. They may be manually expelled by firm but gentle force in the direction of the outlet. This is done only after the fundus has been massaged. If done before massage, it could result in uterine inversion, an exceedingly serious complication.

4. As involution progresses, the uterus recedes in size. The height of the fundus is checked daily in relation to the umbilicus. It is measured in fingerbreadths and expressed as follows (Fig. 107-2):

    1/U: uterus 1 fingerbreadth above the umbilicus
    U/U: uterus level with the umbilicus

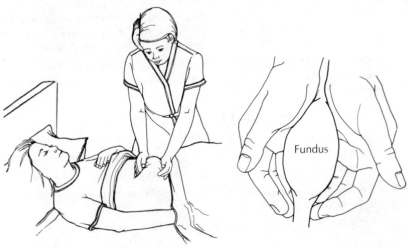

Fundus

FIGURE 107.1

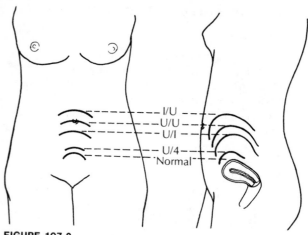

FIGURE 107.2

U/1: uterus 1 fingerbreadth below the umbilicus
U/4: uterus 4 fingerbreadths below the umbilicus
Receded: uterus not palpable

5. Immediately after delivery, the fundus is below the level of the umbilicus and symphysis pubis. As it changes its shape after completion of oxytocic stimulation, it will rise to the umbilicus (the grandmultipara has a larger, more fibrous uterus than the primipara). Day by day, it decreases in size at a rate of approximately 1 fingerbreadth a day. By the 10th day, it should no longer be palpable.

6. A full bladder inhibits contraction of the uterus by elevating it high in the pelvis, displacing it from the midline, and preventing normal contraction. Mothers who have had a caudal or saddle block often do not experience the urge to urinate during the first hours postpartum. The mother should thus be checked for a full, distended bladder.

7. "After pains" or cramps are experienced by multiparas. These contractions are usually severe enough to warrant the use of analgesics, especially at bedtime.

B. Communicative Aspects

1. *Observations*

   a. Check the consistency of the fundus (*e.g.*, boggy, firm).

   b. Check the height of the uterus (measured in fingerbreadths).

   c. Observe vital signs; even a slight deviation may indicate internal hemorrhage.

   d. Observe the mother's behavior; restlessness and anxiety are other signs of shock.

   e. Notify the physician of any marked delay of involution, so immediate care can be given.

2. *Charting*

DATE	TREATMENT	TIME	OBSERVATIONS	SIGNATURE
9/14	Fundus massaged; U/U	0800	Fundus at umbilical level, boggy. Massaged for 30 sec until firm. Large amount clots expelled. Physician notified.	F. White, R.N.

3. *Referrals*

Not applicable

C. Teaching Aspects—Patient and Family

Give explanation to the mother and family on the necessity of checking and massaging the fundus, in order to relieve their fears and anxiety.

IV. EVALUATION PROCESS

A. Was the correct method used?

B. Was the fundus kept contracted?

C. Were hemorrhage and shock prevented?

D. Is the mother comfortable?

E. Has the uterus regained its normal, nonpregnant state?

108

Labor and Delivery, Nursing Care During

I. ASSESSMENT OF SITUATION

A. Definition

1. *Normal labor:* Progressive dilatation and effacement of the cervix until the expulsion of the products of conception. Normal labor has four stages:

   a. *First stage:* the onset of labor until the cervix is completely dilated

   b. *Second stage:* complete dilatation of the cervix until the infant is delivered

    c. *Third stage:* from the birth of the infant until the placenta and membranes are delivered

    d. *Fourth stage:* the immediate postpartum period; duration usually 1 to 2 hr

B. Terminology

1. *Dilatation of cervix:* enlargement of cervical os from a few millimeters in size to an opening large enough to permit passage of the fetus

2. *Effacement:* shortening of the cervical canal from 1 to 2 cm in length to practically no canal. The inner cervix is pulled up into the lower segment of the uterus as the outer cervix dilates, resulting in thinning and eventual disappearance of all but the circular margins of the cervix. A nulliparous patient may have complete effacement ("paperthin cervix") before dilatation becomes progressive. A multiparous patient has concurrent dilatation and effacement of the cervix.

3. *Fetus:* child *in utero* from approximately 8 wk gestation to birth

4. *Infant:* child under 1 yr of age

5. *Uterine contractions of labor:* rhythmic, progressive muscular activity of the body of the uterus, resulting in shortening and thickening of the upper uterine segment and dilatation and thinning of the lower (passive) segment

    a. *Acme:* the height of the contraction

    b. *Decrement:* the release and decrease in intensity of the contraction

    c. *Duration of a contraction:* in active labor, generally ranges from 45 to 60 sec

    d. *Increment:* the increase in intensity of the contraction

C. Rationale for Actions

1. To provide an environment that will contribute to the best outcome for the mother and fetus

2. To provide the planned support system that is needed to provide optimal care to the mother during this difficult period

3. The nurse assumes most of the responsibility for the laboring process, making the initial assessment of the patient's status and the ongoing assessment of progress during labor; immediately observing deviations from the norms; and keeping the physician and family informed of the progress.

II. NURSING PLAN

A. Objectives

1. To review pregnancy history. If not previously recorded, obtain and record the necessary data, including the patient's preparation for childbirth and her plans for the infant.

2. To assess the pregnancy status, progress of labor, and fetal condition

3. To develop a relationship of trust and confidence with the patient, husband, and family

4. To provide direct, individualized care during the entire birthing process, encouraging the patient and her husband to verbalize feelings, and providing support for the manner of birthing they have chosen

5. To keep the patient and family informed of the progress

6. To provide information according to their levels of comprehension

7. To relieve discomfort as much as possible

8. To monitor fetal condition during the first and second stages of labor

9. To report the significant changes in the progress of labor, maternal or fetal health, and fetal presentation and position, as they occur

10. To prepare and maintain a safe and suitable delivery room

11. To assist in the delivery of the fetus

12. To provide immediate care for the newborn

13. To promote the prompt, safe delivery of the placenta

14. To observe the mother closely during the fourth stage of labor until her signs and symptoms indicate recovery from the delivery

B. Patient Preparation

1. Welcome the patient to the labor room. Demonstrate an interest and concern during the orientation procedures.

2. Outline the individualized plan of care, as indicated by the physician.

3. Explain the need for the initial assessment.

4. Briefly explain the routine to be followed: present the information slowly, giving the patient time to adjust to the new surroundings. Allow ample time when circumstances permit and encourage questions.

5. Ensure that the patient understands the physician's instructions to her.

6. Encourage the patient to express minor discomforts and fears.

7. Provide continuous support to the patient during the emotional changes that usually occur during labor and delivery.

C. Equipment

1. Physician's prescriptions

2. Medical records (including a copy of the physician's record of antepartal care; labor record form, labor and delivery form, medication and graphic sheet)

3. Patient care plan and teaching guide

4. Patient identification cards (overhead and room door holder)

5. Clothing wrapper and luggage tags

6. Thermometer, sphygmomanometer, stethoscope, and fetoscope

7. Sterile gloves for vaginal examination, nonsterile gloves for rectal examination

8. Gown, hip pads, and washcloths

9. Clock with second hand

10. Amniotome

11. Tray for vulval skin preparation, cleansing solutions, as prescribed

12. Lubricant

13. Enema setup

III. IMPLEMENTING NURSING INTERVENTION

A. Therapeutic Aspects

1. To provide skilled and therapeutic care the nurse must be knowledgeable about the stages of labor and skilled in the application of the nursing techniques pertinent to patient care during each stage.

2. The process of labor is complex and is subject to unforeseen difficulties and emergencies. The nurse must be capable of assessing, planning, interviewing, reassessing, and evaluating the mother as she progresses through labor.

3. The emphasis in this section is on the nurse's therapeutic role and her constant interaction with the patient. To assist the nurse in her therapeutic role, an aid for visualization of cervical dilatation has been included (Fig. 108-1).

   a. First stage of labor

   (1) *Latent phase:* onset of labor; 2 to 5 cm dilatation. Duration of first stage is usually 8 to 10 hr, which may include a latent period of several hours.

   (2) *Active phase:* from 3 to 8 cm dilatation to 8 to 9 cm (complete) dilatation.

   (3) *Transition phase:* 8 to 10 cm dilatation. This is the most painful and difficult time for the mother. There is an increase in the amount of bleeding (show). The first phase is characterized by dilatation and effacement of the cervix, which is due to uterine contractions.

   (4) The nurse's role in the first stage is the following:

      (a) Make a nursing assessment before reporting to the physician about the patient's admission.

      (b) Compile physical assessment data: data regarding the pregnancy; physical assessment form completed as required by the hospital; required lab work prescribed by physician.

      (c) Make immediate observations:

         (i) Fetal heart rate, rhythm, stability

         (ii) Membranes: intact or ruptured, time of rupture

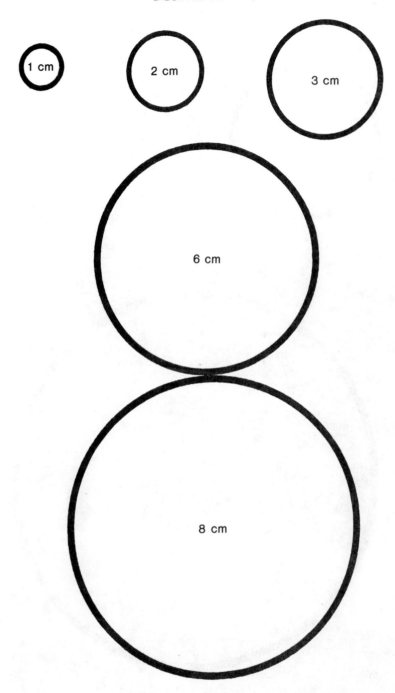

FIGURE 108.1   Aid for Visualization of Cervical Dilatation

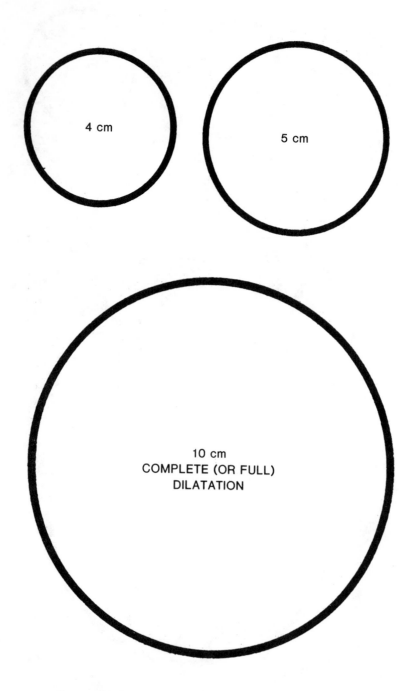

FIGURE 108.1   Aid for Visualization of Cervical Dilatation (cont'd)

    (iii) Vaginal discharge ("show" or bleeding)

    (iv) Vital signs

    (v) Stage and phase of labor

    (vi) Behavior and needs of the patient

    (vii) If the patient is not known to the physician, additional data about the age, parity, and gravidity of the patient and other pertinent information

(d) Obtain psychosocial data: knowledge the patient has about the delivery process; attendance at prenatal classes; completeness of her education and information from the attending physician or prenatal clinic; instruction in relaxation techniques. These techniques can be explained if the patient is admitted in early labor.

(e) Obtain personal data: person available to assist the patient. Provide a brief orientation and instructions to the patient's companion.

(f) Make periodic assessments to determine the progress of labor. These include at least the following:

    (i) Contractions: frequency, duration, quality

    (ii) Vital signs

    (iii) Fetal observations: FHT, activity, position, presentation, condition of the fetal membranes

    (iv) Membranes: time of rupture, color, odor

    (v) Vaginal examinations: condition of the cervix and presenting part. The examinations include determining the station and palpating the sagittal suture; identifying the posterior fontanelle; and identifying the anterior fontanelle (Fig. 108-2, A, B, C). (These examinations should be limited and should not be substituted for nursing attention to the maternal indices of the progress of labor.)

    (vi) Maternal position and activity: most patients should be able to walk and socialize until the cervix is dilated 5 cm. Thereafter, lateral positions should be assumed to relieve uterine pressure on the abdominal vessels supplying the fetus.

    (vii) Hydration and nourishment of the patient: to prevent dehydration, fever, circulatory problems, hypoglycemia, and other physiologic changes and physical discomforts.

    (viii) Elimination: urinary output, color, frequency; loss of body fluids through diarrhea, vomiting, excessive and prolonged perspiration.

    (ix) Vaginal discharges: the pink, scanty "show" of early

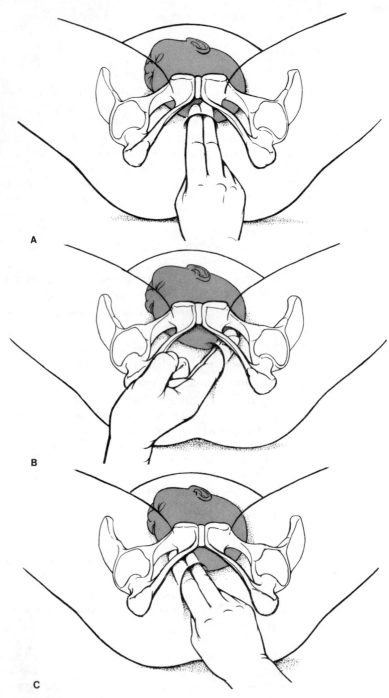

FIGURE 108.2

dilatation is usually absent during the period of 2 to 5 cm dilatation. When the cervix has dilated to about 6 cm, there will be a dark, red, heavy discharge.

(x) Examination of the vulva when the patient exhibits the desire to bear down

(xi) Observation of the abdomen for outline of bladder above symphysis pubis, when the cervix is dilated 6 to 10 cm. Bladder must be emptied; a full bladder retards labor and causes increased discomfort.

(xii) IV fluids if the patient has had nothing to eat for several hours

(xiii) 8 to 9 cm rim of cervix remains. Deceleration of labor is normal. Patient should be encouraged to rest. She will awaken for contractions.

(xiv) Patients who have chronic diseases: constant observation and additions to the nursing care plan as indicated by the physician for possible immediate termination of the pregnancy. Monitoring of the fetal condition is especially emphasized.

(g) Provide information as an ongoing process. See that the patient and husband are interacting, and encourage questions and participation.

(h) An immediate goal is to establish a feeling of trust and confidence. This can be accomplished by degrees.

(i) Make every effort to encourage the patient to verbalize fears.

(j) Establish an environment conducive to the total welfare of the patient. Make the patient feel that she is your only concern.

(k) Provide comfort measures, such as a back rub, positioning, wet washcloth, bathe face and hands. Remain with the patient and provide continuous emotional support during the active phase and later.

(l) Use doptone or fetoscope to determine FHT every 15 min in the latent phase and every 5 min in the active phase.

(m) A fetal monitor may be needed to more accurately observe for decelerations.

(n) Report any changes or stress signals immediately.

(5) The nurse's approach through the first stage of labor is to work with and for the mother and to include the father or significant others as a vital source of support.

b. Second stage of labor

(1) The second stage occurs when there is full dilatation of the cervix and the fetus is ready to descend through the vaginal

canal. The duration of the second stage for a nullipara is usually 40 to 50 min; for a multipara it is up to 30 min.

(2) This stage can be identified by a vaginal examination (sterile) revealing complete dilatation, or by observation of the patient (*e.g.*, bulging perineum). The head or presenting part should be engaged and descending.

(3) The transition from the first to second stage is marked by more frequent contractions and greater severity of pain.

(4) The patient may show some signs of frustration, fear, loss of control, total preoccupation with contractions, irritability, and signs of exhaustion.

(5) Physical problems may include nausea and vomiting, profuse perspiration, feeling of the need to defecate caused by rectal pressure, amnesia, pallor, and headache.

(6) Patient may have difficulty following instructions, be vague in communicating and fearful of losing control; may need reinforcement of directions. It is important to give simple, clear directions.

(7) A major role of the nurse during this stage will be to encourage and assist the patient in effective pushing and breathing.
   (a) Instruct the patient to take a deep, cleansing breath, then one short one, in and out; then to take another breath, hold it, and push for 6 sec, repeating the process until contraction ceases.
   (b) Place the patient in semi-Fowler's position, legs abducted, hands grasping legs behind knees, chin on chest. If the upper part of the body is elevated about 30° the patient can bear down more effectively. Drape properly and always protect patient's privacy.

(8) At all times, maintain aseptic technique to prevent contamination and infections.

(9) Keep the husband informed of all progress and changes.

(10) Observe closely for crowning.

(11) Move the patient to the delivery room at the appropriate time. This is usually determined by the duration of the early and midphases of current labor, the history of previous labors, and the pattern of labor. For the multipara, this should be when the cervix is dilated. For the nullipara, it usually is when the caput is visible.

(12) Nurse-patient contact in the delivery room is important. This can be done by touching and speaking softly if patient is conscious.

(13) During the second stage, the internal rotation of the fetus is

completed. In a vertex presentation, there is crowning, delivery of the head, external rotation, then delivery of the shoulders, anterior then posterior, with the entire body following (Fig. 108-3).

(14) If the father is to attend the delivery, give him instructions.

(15) Provide immediate attention to the newborn: position the infant on side, see that the airway is open, use suction bulb to clear mucus, dry the infant, record Apgar score, cover the infant, and place him in a warm crib. Some physicians order vitamin K, 1 mg IM, to prevent neonatal hemorrhage.

(16) Inform parents of health status and sex of baby.

(17) Permit mother to see and hold infant as soon as she is awake. The mother may exhibit various reaction patterns: happy, pleased, disappointed, angry, rejecting, unconcerned, ambivalent.

(18) Notify the father as soon as possible if he is not in the delivery room. Father can hold infant if the infant's condition is satisfactory and there are no complications.

c. Third stage of labor

(1) The third stage of labor consists of two phases:

(a) During the first phase, there is separation of the placenta. Following the delivery the uterus shrinks to a firm globular mass positioned just below the umbilicus. The uterus is somewhat relaxed; the uterus rests for several minutes before contractions continue, and during the contractions the placenta is separated from the uterine wall. There is an upward rise in the uterus. The lengthening of the cord as the placenta moves from its attachment on the uterine wall should be watched for.

(b) During the second phase, placenta is expelled (Fig. 108-4). There will usually be a sudden rush of blood accompanying the expulsion. The mother will need to bear down during the expulsion stage; if she is unable to do this because of anesthesia, then gentle pressure on the uterine fundus will assist. The uterus should be firm before manual pressure is applied to avoid inversion of the uterus.

(2) Uterine contractions following delivery will also prevent hemorrhage. Direct effort to decreasing the amount of bleeding during labor as much as possible.

(3) If the first and second stages have been completed within normal limits, the third phase is usually uneventful.

(4) Examine the placenta closely (Fig. 108-5) to ascertain that fragments are not remaining in the uterine cavity.

(5) Before the repair of the episiotomy, if one has been necessary,

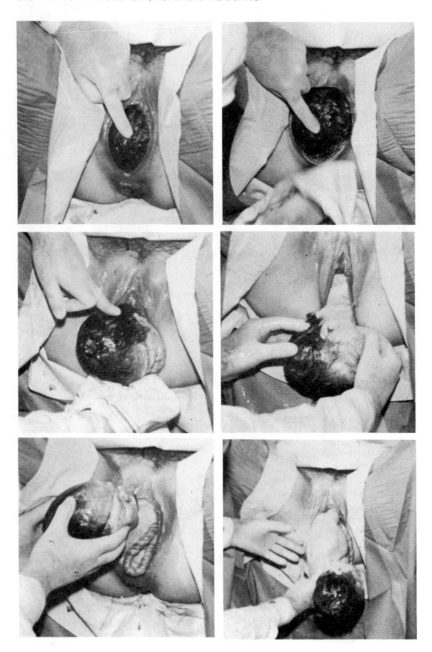

FIGURE 108.3

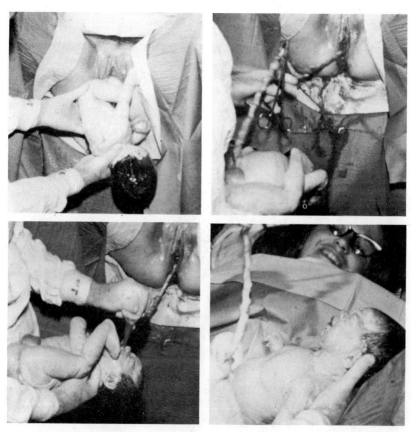

FIGURE 108.3 (cont'd)

a thorough examination is made by the physician. Strict aseptic technique is important: Clean sterile gloves are rinsed in
sterile water; vulva and perineum are cleansed. The vagina,
cervix, and perineum are examined closely for hematomas,
placental fragments, and lacerations.

(6) If the mother has decided to bottle feed, an antilactogenic hormone is usually administered prior to transfer from the delivery room.

(7) During the third stage, reinforce emotional support and encourage the interaction of the husband and wife.

(8) The mother should leave the delivery room clean, warm, and
relaxed. Assistance will be needed and the position will depend on the type of anesthetic administered.

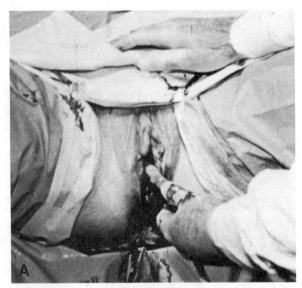

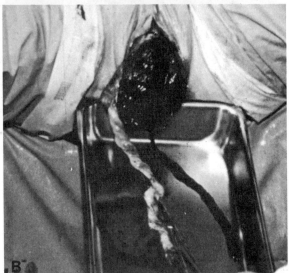

FIGURE 108.4

d. Fourth stage of labor

    (1) This stage of care is considered critical for the mother, and lasts from 1 to 2 hr.

    (2) The recovery room nurse should perform the following functions:

        (a) Provide an environment conducive to rest and relaxation.

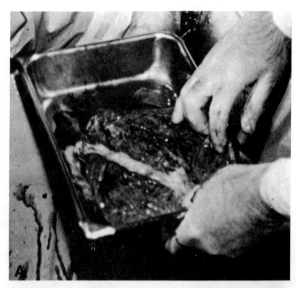

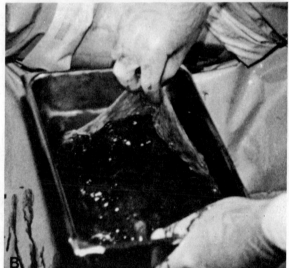

FIGURE 108.5

(b) Promote the patient's comfort by a quiet room; keep linen clean; change pads as needed; and provide fluid and food as tolerated.

(c) Perform routine checking for hemorrhage and changes in blood pressure, temperature, pulse, and respiratory rate.

(d) Palpate the fundus at intervals, noting position and consistency. Check the amount of vaginal flow.

    (e) Observe for bladder distension.

    (f) Apply an ice pack to the episiotomy if needed, to minimize edema and relieve the pain.

    (g) Administer analgesics, as needed, to multiparas for "after-pains."

    (h) Observe the patient's emotional state, noting any deviations. Encourage the mother to verbalize any anger or disappointment.

    (i) Reassure the mother about the health of the infant. Assess her ability to relate to the infant.

(3) At the end of the second hour, perform a thorough examination to determine if the physical condition has stabilized, then transfer the patient to the postpartum unit. A completed labor record will be taken to the unit and an oral report given to ensure continuity of care.

B. Communicative Aspects

1. *Observations*

  a. Determine the level of anxiety the patient is expressing. Identify major fears: death, body changes, isolation. Anxiety may hinder her ability to cope.

  b. The degree of discomfort expressed by the patient is not necessarily proportional to the force of labor or complication of labor.

  c. Immediately identify deviations from the normal, such as unusual abdominal shape, unusual presenting part, arrest of dilatation, or arrest of descent of presenting part. Meconium-stained amniotic fluid may indicate fetal distress, except with breech presentation. Communicate to the physician bright red bleeding that does not clot. Fetal distress is evident when fetal heart rate is below 100 beats/min or above 160 beats/min.

  d. Check the blood pressure every 4 hr if it is in the normal range; if not, check it every hour, or more often if indicated. Report elevations over 140/90 to the physician. Examine the patient for swelling of hands, feet, and face. A urine test for albumin should be done.

  e. Check temperature, pulse, and respirations every 4 hr until membrane ruptures; then check them every hour.

  f. Give immediate attention to an elevated temperature. Assess fluid intake, observe signs of dehydration, note time of rupture of membranes (a critical time for infections to develop), and the amount of vaginal discharge. Physician will generally order IV fluids.

  g. Check contractions every 30 min until the active phase, then assess them every 15 min.

h. Determine the progress of cervical dilatation every hour by rectal examination.

i. Observe the amount and type of vaginal discharge; record the time of observation and the color and odor of the discharge.

j. When the membranes rupture, note the time of rupture and the color, amount, and odor of the fluid.

k. Note the exact time of birth.

2. *Charting*

Recordings on the labor record are done as interviews and changes occur during the four stages.

DATE	TREATMENT	TIME	OBSERVATIONS	SIGNATURE
4/12	Vaginal exam performed	0815	Small amount of pink discharge. Cervical dil. approx. 2 cm, effacement 75%. Pt. relaxed and ambulating.	J. Brown, R.N.

3. *Referrals*

Not applicable

C. Teaching Aspects—Patient

1. Before and during the first phase of labor (latent phase) use every opportunity to provide information and to teach the patient. This must be done according to her level of understanding and comprehension.

2. The amount of information to be provided will depend on the patient's background, cultural orientation, number of deliveries, and participation in prenatal classes. Assess the level of knowledge and proceed accordingly.

IV. EVALUATION PROCESS

A. Did the patient respond to information and instructions provided by the nurse and the physician?

B. Was the psychosocial assessment successful in identifying the emotional needs and concerns of the patient?

C. Did the patient and family show signs of trust and confidence?

D. Did the patient use her energy constructively in relaxing and "working" with contractions?

E. Did the patient appear relatively free of anxiety and stress?

F. Did the husband or other member of the family provide the necessary support?

G. Was the mother's response to the infant positive?

H. Was the physical assessment complete and accurate?

I. Did the stages of labor proceed according to standard norms and without complications?

J. Were the complications identified immediately and corrective action taken?

K. Was the observation and monitoring of both mother and baby done efficiently and effectively?

109

Labor, Induction of

I. ASSESSMENT OF SITUATION

A. Definition

1. The process of starting labor by artificial means. In some situations, induction is used to intensify a labor that is progressing too slowly. Reasons for an induction may be medical or elective.

    a. Medical indications are primary uterine inertia, severe pre-eclampsia, prolonged pregnancy (43 wks), prolonged rupture of membranes, a mother with diabetes or severe isoimmunization, or a fetus with a hemolytic disease.

    b. Elective indications include convenience for the mother, multi-gravidas who have a past history of precipitate labor, and patients who must travel a long distance to the hospital.

    c. Another reason for inducing labor is the presence of any condition of the mother or fetus indicating the need for termination of the pregnancy by a method deemed to be safe if all the criteria for safety are met.

B. Terminology

1. *Fetal heart rate pattern*

    a. Normal: 120 to 160 beats/min

    b. Mild bradycardia: 100 to 119 beats/min

    c. Marked bradycardia: 99 or fewer beats/min

    d. Mild tachycardia: 161 to 180 beats/min

    e. Marked tachycardia: 181 or more beats/min

2. *Fetal heart rate variability:* the fluctuations that may occur, which may range from 5 to 10 beats/min

3. *Oxytocic agent:* drug that stimulates uterine contractions

C. Rationale for Actions

1. To safeguard the mother and fetus during a potentially hazardous procedure
2. To provide an individual choice by the mother or family for personal reasons

II. NURSING PLAN

A. Objectives

1. To support the patient through the procedure
2. To provide technical assistance throughout the induction process
3. To provide constant monitoring of the fetal heart rate
4. To maintain close contact with family members

B. Patient Preparation

1. Explain the procedure to the patient and her husband. Provide enough information so that they will understand the procedure.
2. Provide an ongoing support system and reassure the patient as needed.
3. Make the patient as comfortable as possible taking into account position, cleanliness, and the room environment.
4. Have the patient empty her bladder before the procedure begins.

C. Equipment

1. Stethoscope
2. Fetoscope
3. Fetal monitor, if available
4. Intravenous tray
5. Angiocath or Medicut intravenous catheter
6. Solution as prescribed by the physician
7. Volume infusion pump
8. Watch with second hand
9. Sterile gloves for vaginal examination
10. Sterile sharp instrument

III. IMPLEMENTING NURSING INTERVENTION

A. Therapeutic Aspects

1. A written report should be made by the physician and placed in the record documenting the following:
   a. Reason for doing an induction
   b. Position, presentation, and status of the fetus

    c. Dilatation and consistency of cervix before induction

    d. The estimated gestational age and size of the fetus and expected date of confinement

    e. Adequacy of the patient's pelvis

2. Criteria for stimulation of labor include the following:

    a. Engagement of presenting part

    b. 50% or more cervical effacement

    c. 2 to 3 cm cervical dilatation

    d. Adequate pelvis

3. Consultation with a second physician is required in many hospitals if conditions are present that would contraindicate induction, such as multiple pregnancy, abnormal presentation or position, abruptio placentae, placenta previa, previous cesarean section, or previous uterine surgery.

4. Common methods of induction are the following:

    a. Artificial rupture of membranes (amniotomy) by using a sharp instrument (long hook) or Allis clamp. Cervix should be soft, partially effaced, slightly dilated. Once the membrane is penetrated, the amniotic fluid will drain. Membranes serve as a barrier against infection; therefore, asepsis must be maintained and the delivery accomplished as soon as possible.

    b. IV administration of an oxytocic agent. The physician will order the exact drug, dosage, and method of administration. The nurse should start a main intravenous (IV) line solution as prescribed by the physician. This will hydrate the patient; it will be continued if the oxytocin has to be discontinued. The second IV containing the oxytocin solution is piggybacked to the main IV (Fig. 109-1). A pump for steady flow is desirable and may be obtained by an IV regulating device. The usual rate is 5 adult drops/min, increasing or decreasing the dose, depending on contractions. This is considered an efficient and safe method of induction. Oxytocin causes a marked contraction of the uterus and an antidiuretic side effect. Any deviations in the fetal heart tone (FHT) or contractions lasting up to 90 sec are danger signals, and the solution should be temporarily disconnected. A setup of 500 ml distilled water, 5% dextrose should be in use in order to maintain an open vein.

       The nurse should explain the procedure to the patient and family and assemble equipment. She should assist the physician in starting the IV. It is essential to provide emotional support to the mother and to reassure the patient as contractions increase in frequency and duration. Continuous and competent assessment is necessary; any deviations should be reported to the physician immediately. The flow of the oxytocin solution should be checked at regular and frequent intervals. Close monitoring of the intensity

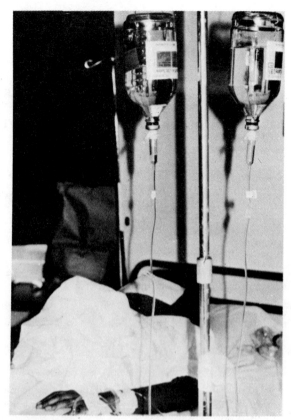

FIGURE 109.1

and duration of contractions, blood pressure, and pulse is necessary. FHT should be checked every 15 min. The nurse should monitor for tenderness of the abdomen, abruptio placentae, and vaginal bleeding.

Danger signs are an increase or decrease in blood pressure with increase or decrease in pulse, fetal hyperactivity, FHT or other sign of fetal distress, meconium stained amniotic fluid, contractions occurring more frequently than 90 sec or lasting more than 60 sec.

5. Other methods of induction that can be used with extreme caution are the following;

    a. Stripping of the membrane: the physician inserts a finger through the cervix around the internal os and strips the membranes off the internal cervix. Dangers of this method are sepsis, profuse bleeding, and prolapse of the cord. The procedure can cause amniotic fluid embolism.

b. Intraamniotic injection of hypertonic sodium chloride solution: nursing intervention here is extremely important. This method should not be used unless there is firm evidence that the fetus is dead, since the effect would be lethal for the fetus.

c. Intramuscular oxytocin: this method is dangerous because it is very difficult to control the effect of the drug. The result could be severe, prolonged uterine contractions.

6. The induction of labor is a traumatic experience for the patient. The nurse plays a vital role in providing the major support system.

7. The success and safety of the induction procedure will depend on the nurse's observation skills and ability to act in emergency situations.

8. Excessive uterine stimulation resulting in frequent contractions and intense labor may lead to fetal hypoxia.

B. Communicative Aspects

1. *Observations*

   a. Observe constantly during the IV infusion.

   b. Monitor contractions for duration and intensity.

   c. Count and record FHT at regular intervals. The FHT should return to the normal rate in approximately 13 sec after a contraction.

   d. Report frequently to the physician.

2. *Charting*

   The procedure used for induction, cervical dilatation, effacement, station of the presenting part, presentation, and the position of the fetus should be recorded on the patient's record.

DATE	TREATMENT	TIME	OBSERVATIONS	SIGNATURE
4/10	Induction of labor started. 1 liter 5% dextrose in H$_2$O. Oxytocin 10# IU added to fluid. Regulated at 5 drops/ min.	0900	Patient relaxed. BP 120/ 60.Temp 98.6, P 80. R 20. FHT 120 LLQ. No contractions at present time.	J. Brown, R.N.

3. *Referrals*

   Consultation with another physician may be advisable when situations are present that would contraindicate the use of an induction method.

C. Teaching Aspects—Patient

1. Explain the procedure and equipment used for induction.
2. Explain the necessity for proper positioning (being on right side, preferably).

IV. EVALUATION PROCESS

A. Was the patient able to accept the intervention without undue stress?

B. Did the husband and family understand the need for induction and cooperate during the induction period?

C. Did the patient exhibit a feeling of trust and confidence?

D. Did the team (physician, nurse, and others) work in harmony and in the best interests of the patient?

E. Did the mother respond satisfactorily as the contractions intensified?

F. Was there undue anxiety and concern about the fetus?

G. Was the mother kept apprised of the condition of her fetus?

110

Lochia, Observation of (Postpartum)

I. ASSESSMENT OF SITUATION

A. Definition

The discharge from the birth canal occurring after childbirth

B. Terminology

1. *Lochia alba:* slowing discharge occurring toward 10th day, which is thinner, greatly decreased in amount, and almost colorless
2. *Lochia rubra:* discharge occurring 1 to 3 days after birth, which is a reddish color and consists of blood with a small amount of mucus, particles of decidua, and cellular debris that escape from the placental site

3. *Lochia serosa:* discharge occurring 6 to 7 days after birth, which is reddish brown because of the exudate from healing surfaces and the breakdown of remaining debris

C. Rationale for Actions

1. To check the progress of postpartum healing and involutionary process of the uterus
2. To identify complications early

II. NURSING PLAN

A. Objectives

1. To teach the patient selfcare of the perineum, episiotomy, rectum, and vagina
2. To teach the technique of and the need for frequent changing of the perineal pad
3. To notice any signs of postpartum complications early and report them to the physician

B. Patient Preparation

1. Explain the purpose of regular checking.
2. Solicit cooperation and information from the patient.

C. Equipment

1. Perineal pad
2. Washcloth

III. IMPLEMENTING NURSING INTERVENTION

A. Therapeutic Aspects

1. The appearance of bloody vaginal discharge after birth is expected, both with vaginal delivery and cesarean section. Lochia is a mixture of the waste products left after birth. It is red at first, because of the bleeding of vessels in the placental attachment site. It slowly becomes pale and scant, and usually stops in 3 to 4 wk. A perineal pad, held in place with a belt, is used to absorb the discharge just as for menstrual flow. The patient must be warned not to use a tampon, because of the possible trauma of sensitive tissue and the possibility of uterine infection. The nurse should check the appearance of the lochia often during the first 24 hr, then daily.
2. Microorganisms are on the skin. To inhibit the transfer of bacteria from the rectum to the birth canal, the patient must be instructed to clean the vulva from front to back. Proper handwashing must be done before and after applying the pad, to prevent contamination of the perineum by the hands.
3. The characteristic odor of lochia is fresh and fleshy. A foul odor indi-

cates that some debris, placental or membrane tissue, has been retained and is necrotic. This may lead to serious infection unless expelled.

4. Bacteria tend to grow more readily on a moist surface. The pad should be changed every 4 hr, and the perineum cleaned and dried thoroughly.

B. Communicative Aspects

1. *Observations*

   a. Lochia should be checked frequently during the early postpartum period.

   b. Lochia should progress from reddish brown to pink to colorless. Bright red bleeding, clots, and tissue in the lochia are abnormal and warrant immediate attention.

2. *Charting*

DATE	TREATMENT	TIME	OBSERVATIONS	SIGNATURE
4/9	Lochia serosa	1800	Pad changed. Small amount of brown discharge.	L. Davis, N.T.

3. *Referrals*

   Not applicable

C. Teaching Aspects—Patient

1. Instruct the patient in the importance of maintaining cleanliness.

2. Emphasize the necessity of putting on the pad from front to back.

3. Forewarn the patient of changes in color and amount of discharge.

IV. EVALUATION PROCESS

A. Does the patient understand the procedure for perineal care?

B. Does the patient know what changes to expect in the lochia?

C. Has the patient been advised to report any abnormalities to her physician?

111

Perineal Light

I. ASSESSMENT OF SITUATION

A. Definition

The application of warmth to the perineal area with a heat lamp

B. Terminology

None

C. Rationale for Actions

1. To provide perineal heat for the comfort of the patient
2. To aid in the healing of the episiotomy or laceration by keeping the sutures dry

II. NURSING PLAN

A. Objectives

1. To facilitate healing by the optimal use of light and heat
2. To avoid burning the patient by prolonged exposure or too-close proximity to the light
3. To prevent cross-contamination by thorough cleaning of lights between patient use

B. Patient Preparation

1. Explain the purpose and the procedure.
2. Ask the patient to cooperate and to signal if the heat is too hot or uncomfortable.

C. Equipment

1. Perineal light
2. Padding for stirrups
3. Screen
4. Sterile perineal pad
5. Bag for disposal of used perineal pad
6. Medicated spray, if prescribed

III. IMPLEMENTING NURSING INTERVENTION

A. Therapeutic Aspects

1. After delivery, the perineum needs special care because it has been stretched, bruised, and often torn or cut during delivery. Exposure to dry heat several times a day seems to promote healing and relieve pain. This is accomplished with a heat lamp which must be placed far enough from the perineum to avoid burning the tender skin. Approximately 12 in is considered safe (Fig. 111-1).

2. A distended bladder may cause discomfort during the procedure. The patient should empty her bladder before the procedure.

3. A position of comfort and optimal exposure is desirable. The patient should be flat on her back in bed. If the perineal light has stirrups, they should be padded for comfort.

4. Plastic and rubber absorb and conduct heat. If an indwelling catheter is in place, a clean washcloth should be placed between it and the thigh, to protect the patient from being burned by the heated tubing.

5. Concentrated heat may cause burning. The bulb should be checked each time the lamp is used. A bulb over 60 W must never be used. The lamp should not be left on for longer than 20 min.

6. The equipment should be washed with a germicide in a utility room.

B. Communicative Aspects

1. *Observations*

    a. The patient should remain awake during the treatment and have a bedside signal available.

    b. The perineal area must be checked frequently during the proce-

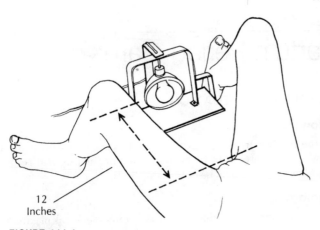

12
Inches

FIGURE 111.1

dure for redness, which would indicate the light was too hot or the time span was too long.

c. Sutures should be observed for proper healing and signs of infection, bleeding, or any other problems.

d. The patient's reaction must be observed to see that she does not become cramped or overtired from this procedure.

2. *Charting*

DATE	TREATMENT	TIME	OBSERVATIONS	SIGNATURE
4/1	Peri light for 20 min	0900	Tolerated well, without signs of fatigue. No redness noted. Suture line intact and clean.	G. Ivers, R.N.

3. *Referrals*

Not applicable

C. Teaching Aspects—Patient

1. Demonstrate how equipment works.
2. Be sure the patient understands the importance of proper perineal care.

IV. EVALUATION PROCESS

A. Did the patient rest better after the procedure?

B. Did the warmth seem to help the patient relax?

112

Postpartum Period Care

I. ASSESSMENT OF SITUATION

A. Definition

Care of the mother from the termination of pregnancy until the reproductive system returns to its normal state, or the physical recovery of the mother. This period lasts for 6 to 8 wk.

B. Terminology

1. *Involution:* the retrograde changes in the female genital organs that result in a return to normal size after delivery

2. *Mothering:* warm, tender behavior toward child; the ability to love unconditionally

3. *Puerperium:* synonymous with postpartum, "to bring forth"

C. Rationale for Actions

1. Recovery from parturition is not complete for 6 to 8 wk. Care and support are needed during this time.

2. The mother undergoes physiological changes in a very short period of time.

3. Psychosocial stress may be significant as the mother adjusts to herself, the baby, her husband, other children, and significant others.

II. NURSING PLAN

A. Objectives

1. To teach genital hygiene

2. To support and assist in the patient's full recovery from the delivery process

3. To promote mother-infant bonding

4. To assist the patient in establishing priorities and continued health goals

5. To help the patient understand the need for continued health care

6. To provide information and instruction on available methods of contraception

7. To promote the understanding of infant growth and development

8. To explain the physiological and psychological changes that are relevant to recovery

B. Patient Preparation

1. Review data from the antepartal, delivery, recovery, and immediate postpartum periods.

2. Evaluate the home environment and ongoing support system.

3. Assess the patient's emotional status and ability for self-care and infant care.

4. Encourage early ambulation to promote the recovery of strength and to reduce the incidence of thrombosis.

5. Urge the mother to express feelings of depression, generally known as "postpartum blues."

C. Equipment

Review the equipment needed at home to continue care of the mother and infant.

III. IMPLEMENTING NURSING INTERVENTION

A. Therapeutic Aspects

1. Many parents are poorly prepared to assume the responsibilities of parenthood. A major role of the nurse is to ascertain each situation and plan for continuing care on an individualized basis.

2. It is better to provide an environment of problem solving than to disseminate information that the mother may not fully understand.

3. Mothering may be a new and complex experience; the cultural background will play an important part in the role the mother assumes.

4. Some authorities believe that depression in the postpartum period is related to repression and preconscious maternal identification. To avoid the depressed state, an effort should be directed to seeing that the new mother has adequate rest, good nutrition, and a relaxing quiet environment, and that she avoids sensory overload.

5. Social relaxation for both the mother and father should be encouraged and planned during the postpartum period.

6. Most postpartum care occurs during the first 3 to 4 days, while the mother is in the hospital. Professional assistance should be available for at least 6 wk to assist the patient in making the major adjustments after leaving the hospital.

7. Home instruction should include the following:

    a. Avoidance of fatigue is very important; gradual increase in activities should be planned.

    b. Light housework may be done after several weeks; full activity should be delayed until the postpartum examination at 4 wk.

    c. An exercise plan should be developed to strengthen the pubococcygeal muscles and help the mother in trimming her figure back to normal. This should be done on a progressive basis.

    d. Food intake for lactating mothers should be around 3,000 calories/day, and for nonlactating mothers, about 2,300 calories/day.

    e. Patients should understand the process of the return of the reproductive organs to their normal state following a pregnancy:

        (1) The vagina will not lubricate normally because of steroid depletion; the response to sexual stimulus may be limited. A contraceptive cream or water-soluble gel can be used.

        (2) Psychological reactions to sexual relations may be reduced in intensity and level of response.

        (3) The vaginal walls are thin and red, comparable to atrophic vaginitis, resulting from the decline in hormones. The extended vagina usually returns to the prepartal condition in about 3 wk. The uterus rapidly involutes after delivery. Progesterone is not produced until the first ovulating period.

(4) The initial vaginal discharge following delivery is red for approximately 3 days; then the flow becomes pinkish brown. Odor is a very important sign of complications, as is temperature over 37.8°C (100°F). Usually within 10 days the flow will be yellowish white. If the lochia continues, this may indicate retained placental fragments, endometritis, or infection.

(5) Sexual intercourse can be resumed by the 4th wk if the episiotomy has healed satisfactorily and bleeding has ceased.

(6) Menses will resume in 6 to 8 wk, unless the mother is breast-feeding. Then menses will not resume for 4 mo or more, but the mother should be made aware that she still can become pregnant.

8. Postpartum care should be based on involutionary changes that generally occur on a continuing basis during the 5- to 6-wk period:

  a. During the first 2 wk the following changes occur:

    (1) Body weight immediately reduces 5 to 7 kg (10 to 15 lb).

    (2) Blood pressure is generally maintained at normal levels.

    (3) The involution of the uterus progresses normally, usually 1 cm/day until 10th day. Its size and position are regained by 5 to 6 wk, but it will be somewhat larger than before.

    (4) The vagina remains relaxed for a period of weeks.

    (5) The abdominal wall is weak and flabby. The recti muscles may have separated.

    (6) Temperature may be elevated because of low fluid intake. Elevated temperature and pulse may also indicate infection, hemorrhage, or hematoma. In infection, the pulse rate is elevated before the temperature rises.

    (7) Elimination patterns are quickly reestablished.

      (a) Urination is usually spontaneous by 6 to 8 hr unless the patient was allowed to become dehydrated; it is frequent for several days as retained interstitial fluid is eliminated.

      (b) Bowel habits usually return to normal.

    (8) Breasts immediately secrete colostrum. By the 3rd day they become engorged and tender. Pain and swelling subside in several days.

    (9) Depression reactions are common emotional responses. Responses may vacillate from happiness to sadness, fatigue, and frustration.

  b. During the 3rd to 6th wk, the physician's and nurse's responsibilities include the following:

    (1) Observe closely for any complications of the puerperium.

    (2) Make sure that the mother understands the need for continued health care: repeat examinations at 6-mo intervals.

(3) The 6-wk examination consists of the following:

    (a) Vulval and perineal examination.

    (b) Checking for condition and healing of episiotomy

    (c) Examination of the pelvic floor for uterine prolapse, cysto-cele, or rectocele

    (d) Checking the size of the uterus

    (e) Assessment of the condition of the cervix

    (f) Pap smear to check for normal estrogen pattern

    (g) Assessment of urinary tract functioning to detect problems of dysuria, frequency, or burning

    (h) Assessment of bowel functioning

    (i) Checking the condition of the breasts

    (j) Blood count to determine if hemoglobin is at normal level

    (k) Urinalysis (should reveal normal findings)

    (l) Measurement of vital signs (should be normal)

    (m) Measurement of blood pressure (should be stabilized at prepregnancy level)

    (n) Assessment of psychological, emotional functioning and wellbeing

B. Communicative Aspects

1. *Observations*

    a. The physical and psychological changes during the postnatal period should be observed closely as outlined under "Therapeutic Aspects."

    b. The patient's well-being can be greatly enhanced by nursing intervention in all phases of the recovery process: individualized planning, providing information, involvement of the mother and father in the planning, and planned follow-up care.

2. *Charting*

    a. Parents should be instructed about the data they should maintain at home on the mother:

        (1) Temperature recorded for several weeks

        (2) When lochia ceases

        (3) Vaginal discharges

        (4) Weight changes

        (5) Breast changes and amount of lactation

        (6) Bladder and bowel patterns

    b. Parents should be told to note the following information on the infant:

      (1) Weight

      (2) Eating habits

      (3) Sleeping habits

      (4) Development

3. *Referrals*

    a. Visiting home services

    b. Family planning clinics

    c. La Leche League

    d. Food assistance programs

    e. Social services

    f. Pediatrician

    g. Child development clinics

C. Teaching Aspects—Patient and Family

1. A major role of the nurse in the postpartum period is to inform and teach the new parents. Informed parents provide a much more favorable environment for the infant to develop in.

2. Content of instruction should cover the following:

    a. Physiological changes in mother and infant

    b. Psychological changes in mother and infant

    c. Total care of the mother through the 6-wk period and meeting her maturational needs

    d. Meeting the needs of the father and significant others

    e. The care of the newborn infant

    f. Preparation of other children, to minimize opportunities for sibling rivalry

IV. EVALUATION PROCESS

A. Was the support system planned for the mother following delivery? Was it adequate?

B. Did the mother and father participate in planning for the recovery period?

C. Was the planning done on a problem solving basis?

D. Was there continuity in the recovery following delivery—in the recovery room, postpartum unit, home, and follow-up clinic?

E. Was the plan for family planning implemented and effective?

F. Was there evidence of parent-infant bonding?

113

Postpartum Recovery Care

I. ASSESSMENT OF SITUATION

A. Definition
The recovery period following delivery of the baby, usually a 1-hr period, referred to as the third and fourth stages of labor

B. Terminology
1. *Cotyledons:* subdivisions of the uterine surface of a discoidal placenta
2. *Postnatal:* occurring after birth, refers to infant
3. *Postpartum:* after delivery or childbirth; refers to mother
4. *Puerperium:* synonymous with postpartum; time from giving birth until physical and psychological recovery; 6 to 8 wk

C. Rationale for Actions
1. To assist the mother, father, and the family to progress through fourth stage without complications
2. To assist in alleviating the psychosocial stress common after delivery
3. To provide support for the early mother-child relationship through early parental contact and interactions with the newborn

II. NURSING PLAN

A. Objectives
1. To assess the physical and psychosocial needs of the mother, and initiate immediate action to meet these needs during the third and fourth stages of labor
2. To provide safe, immediate care of the newborn
3. To manage the third and fourth stages of labor so that complications will not develop
4. To decrease environmental stimuli as much as possible, promoting rest and relaxation
5. To allow the parents to become acquainted with newborn; support parent-infant bonding in every possible way

B. Patient Preparation
1. Placenta expulsion—the third stage of labor
   a. If the mother is not heavily anesthetized, instruct her in bearing down to expel the placenta.

b. Gentle pressure on the uterine fundus may help; this should not be done unless the uterus is hard.

c. The contraction of the uterus produces placental separation and controls uterine hemorrhage.

d. Oxytocic drugs may be indicated. Have these readily available for use after the placenta has separated.

e. There is usually a gush of blood before the expulsion of the placenta. The fundus of the uterus rises in the abdomen when the placenta is in the vagina, and the cord lengthens. When this happens instruct the patient to push it out. Gently guide the placenta out by firm manual pressure on the fundus.

f. The placenta should be expelled within 5 to 30 min of delivery.

g. If a continuous intravenous (IV) infusion is running, oxytocin may be added to it, or a preexisting oxytocin "piggyback" may be reopened. Following placental delivery, adjust the flow to prevent exhaustion of uterine muscles, which may result in postpartum hemorrhage.

h. Episiotomy will need to be sutured before or following placental delivery.

i. Examine the placenta and membranes thoroughly to make sure that the cotyledons of the placenta fit together and the membranes are complete. Fragments left in the uterus will cause bleeding and infection. Record any unusual characteristics of the placenta and umbilical cord. A laboratory examination of the placenta may be prescribed

j. After the placenta is delivered and the episiotomy repaired, the physician checks the following:

　(1) Perineum, vagina, and cervix for lacerations or hematomas

　(2) Uterine cavity for retained placental fragments

　(3) Cervical lacerations, which will need repair

k. The uterus should be a firm, hard mass following delivery. It is easily movable during this time and can be manually moved upward into position for evaluation and massage, if necessary.

2. Immediate recovery care—the fourth stage of labor

a. Cleanse the vulva gently with warm sterile water; apply sterile perineal pad.

b. Cleanse upper portion of body as needed, dress in clean gown, remove drapes, and cover with a warm blanket.

c. Reposition the delivery table; and gently lower both of the patient's legs from the stirrups simultaneously

d. If spinal anesthesia has been used, the patient will need to remain in a supine position for 8 to 12 hr. This is to prevent headache. Assist the patient with foot exercises. Record functional use of lower extremities.

e. Before moving patient onto stretcher, check the following:

  (1) Any hemorrhage

  (2) Changes in blood pressure

  (3) Fundus tone and location

  (4) Bladder for distension

  (5) Color (should be pink)

  (6) Respirations (should be normal)

f. Routine care in the recovery room includes the following:

  (1) Put side rails up.

  (2) Check the fundus and lochia every 15 min. If the fundus is situated to the right of the midline, the bladder may need emptying. If it is soft, gently massage it until it contracts. Avoid unnecessary massage of fundus. Monitor parenteral fluids containing oxytocic agents, if prescribed. Clots are usually expelled. Immediately report heavy flow. Estimate blood loss and record on chart. If number of clots is excessive, place them in a measure and assume additional fluid loss. Some hospitals weigh all perineal pads as soon as they are changed, thereby measuring the entire clots, particles, and fluid component of the discharge (the weight of pads is known; subtract to find the difference). When the patient first arises, the lochia that has accumulated in the now relaxed vagina will flow freely. The uterus will contract and align in midpelvis when the patient gets up to void. Following her return to bed, palpate the uterus again and chart its position. If there is residual urine in the bladder, the uterus will remain elevated in the abdomen. Chart this finding and verbally report it, because a displaced uterus will not contract without stimulation.

  (3) Blood loss during delivery may result in a rising pulse and respiratory rate and a lowered blood pressure. Check the blood pressure every 15 min (blood pressure should return to normal within 1 hr); then every 30 min for 2 hr; then four times a day. Check pulse and respiration every 15 min for 1 hour.

  (4) Apply ice pack to perineum, as prescribed.

  (5) Chilling is a frequent reaction to loss of body mass, muscular effort of labor, perspiration, and exposure. Cover the mother with blankets as needed.

  (6) Measure intake and output and record on flow sheet.

  (7) It is important for the mother to see her husband in the delivery room, if she is awake, or in the recovery room. Both parents should see the baby together as soon as possible (Fig. 113-1).

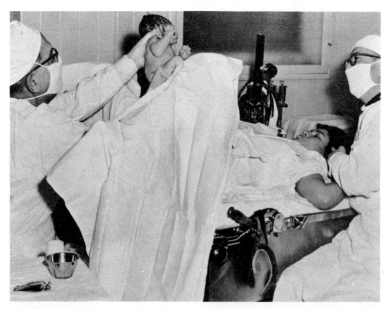

FIGURE 113.1

(8) Allow the patient to sit on the side of the bed for a while when arising, to recover from the effects of postural hypotension, and accompany her to the bathroom for the first few visits, since fainting can occur.

(9) Watch for vaginal or pelvic hematoma. Symptoms are severe pain (or no pain), rectal discomfort, and heat and bulging of the perineum or vulva.

(10) The mother is usually thirsty following delivery. Unless nausea is present, fluids are permitted.

(11) Do not remove the patient to the postpartum unit until vaginal bleeding is normal, the fundus is firm, and vital signs are stable.

(12) Clean and inspect the perineum. Report the number of pads used each hour; record the amount of clots (in milliliters).

C. Equipment

1. The recovery room
   a. Blood pressure cuff and sphygmomanometer
   b. Suction bottle, tip, and catheter
   c. IV equipment and supplies
   d. Tongue blade and airway
   e. Perineal pads

    f. Emesis basin

    g. Oxygen

    h. Recovery cart with side rails

III. IMPLEMENTING NURSING INTERVENTION

A. Therapeutic Aspects

1. The third and fourth stages of labor occur immediately following delivery. This is a critical period in the total labor process. Some major changes may evolve including the following:

    a. The mother begins to adjust to a nonpregnant state.

    b. Physiological instability occurs.

    c. Dangers, such as aspiration, hemorrhage, hematoma, urinary retention, and hypotension, may develop.

    d. Psychic states range from euphoria, a feeling of well-being, to listlessness and lack of awareness.

2. The immediate reaction of the mother to the birth process may indicate physical and nervous exhaustion.

B. Communicative Aspects

1. *Observations*

    a. Observe the patient constantly until stabilization has occurred.

    b. Note the color of the patient's skin, vital signs, position of fundus, amount of lochia, and mental alertness. Identify and report any abnormal symptoms immediately.

    c. Note the mother's reaction to the infant. This may be evident by rejoicing, excitement, laughing, or by anger, rejection, crying, withdrawal, ambivalence, or passivity.

    d. Observe for signs of hostility the mother may show toward the father.

    e. Observe for signs of physical exhaustion.

2. *Charting*

DATE	TREATMENT	TIME	OBSERVATIONS	SIGNATURE
7/12	Admission to recovery room	0910	Color of skin flushed. BP 120/70. P 80; R 20. Fundus firm. Midline at umbilicus. Lochia flow: pads clean. Awake.	S. White R.N.

3. *Referrals*

    Not applicable

C. Teaching Aspects—Patient

The opportunity for teaching will be limited during the recovery period. The patient should be allowed to know that she did well and is now going to rest; however, she may be too excited to do so.

IV. EVALUATION PROCESS

A. Did recovery proceed according to established norms?

B. Was mother's response positive and accepting?

C. Was father assisted as a part of the support system?

D. Was the parents' attitude that of acceptance and gratification?

E. Were psychosocial needs met?

F. Was the environment conducive to rest and relaxation?

G. Were physical changes managed properly?

H. Were levels of fatigue and exhaustion minimal?

 I. Was immediate, safe physical care of the newborn adequate?

 J. Were the delivery and immediate recovery accomplished with minimal trauma to the mother?

114

Vulval and Perineal Care

I. ASSESSMENT OF SITUATION

A. Definition

Cleansing the vulval and perineal area

B. Terminology

Smegma: thick, cheesy, ill-smelling secretion of the sebaceous glands of the perineal area

C. Rationale for Actions

1. To teach the patient to properly care for her own personal hygiene and that of her female children

2. To prevent or reduce infection

3. To provide a dry area for healing

4. To observe the perineum

II. NURSING PLAN

A. Objectives

1. To remove secretions and discharges
2. To examine the perineal area
3. To reduce irritation and odor
4. To prepare the area for local applications, such as a dressing, heat, and ice
5. To provide comfort
6. To teach self-care and genital hygiene
7. To complete a bed bath for a patient who is unable to bathe herself
8. To record the condition of the area and the type and amount of discharge

B. Patient Preparation

1. Explain to the patient the importance of vulval and perineal care.
2. Explain what the hospital routine will be and answer questions.

C. Equipment

1. Freshly cleaned washbasin
2. Clear warm water, soap, clean washcloths or cellulose squares
3. Container of medicated sponges, if prescribed
4. Receptacle or newspaper squares for soiled dressings and pads
5. Perineal pad
6. Tissue
7. Disposable gloves (may be used)

III. IMPLEMENTING NURSING INTERVENTION

A. Therapeutic Aspects

1. Pathogenic organisms may be transferred to susceptible surfaces by unclean or careless technique. Wash hands thoroughly before and after every procedure. Clean the washbasin with a cleanser, soap, and water, and rinse thoroughly. All equipment should be clean.
2. The female urethra is short, and vaginal discharge is a satisfactory medium for the growth of bacteria. If an indwelling (Foley) catheter is present, clean all exudate from it to prevent the exudate from traveling into the urethra and bladder and causing infection. Avoid tension on the catheter during cleaning to prevent pressure on the internal urethral meatus.
3. The urethral area is considered clean, and the anal area is considered contaminated. Each cleansing motion is made from the front to back of the perineum. With a washcloth and warm soapy water, make

three downward strokes, using different section of the cloth for each stroke. Avoid the rectal area. In a patient with an episiotomy, separate the labia and wash downward over the sutures (Fig. 114-1). Turn the soiled portion of cloth to the inside, and wash the right side of the vulva with a downward stroke. Again turn the soiled portion to the inside, and with a clean area, wash the left side of vulva. Discard the cloth, without returning it to the basin of water. Rinse the perineal area, using a clean, wet cloth, in the same manner.

4. Drying reduces irritation and promotes healing. Pat the area dry with tissues or a dry towel. Have the patient lie in lateral Sims's position, if possible. Wash and dry the anal area. Apply dressing, as indicated. If a perineal pad is needed, it must be applied from front to back to minimize contamination of sutures or perineal area.

5. Leave the patient in a comfortable position. Wrap the dressings or pads in paper and discard in a bathroom wastebasket, to minimize odor and unpleasantness in the patient's bedside environment. Clean the washbasin with cleanser, and return it to the holder.

6. As soon as the postpartum patient is ambulatory, she may do her own perineal care. She must have perineal care after each bowel movement and voiding. She should have an ample supply of washcloths in the bathroom and should be shown how to use the three backward strokes to cleanse herself. There should be a linen hamper for these cloths in the bathroom.

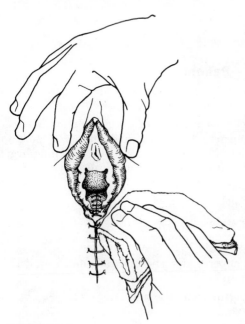

FIGURE 114.1

B. Communicative Aspects

1. *Observations*

    a. Postpartum lochia during the first 3 days is a discharge of red and white blood cells, cervical mucus, vaginal epithelial cells, and decidual tissue. Lochia does not clot. On days 1 through 3, the lochia is red pink and so charted. On days 3 through 6, the lochia is pink brown and charted as "serous." Later, puerperal lochia is pale and charted as "alba." The odor of lochia is fresh and fleshy. A foul odor indicates the presence of necrotic tissue or infection and should be reported immediately. Lochia is diminished in amount when the patient ambulates freely, has had a cesarean section, or is breast-feeding.

    b. The episiotomy should be noted for edema, inflammation, separation, or presence of hematoma

    c. When a catheter has been in place for 24 hrs, a transudate or exudate may cause local irritation. The condition of the urethra should be observed.

2. *Charting*

DATE	TREATMENT	TIME	OBSERVATIONS	SIGNATURE
5/15	Perineal care	0800	Lochia red brown. Approx. pad change q 2 hr. Episiotomy healing well.	F. White, R.N.

3. *Referrals*

    Not applicable

C. Teaching Aspects—Patient

1. Explain to the patient the principle and importance of front-to-back cleaning in giving self-care and female child care.

2. Discuss feminine hygiene in daily life, regarding the removal of odor-producing smegma by external washing, and the use of pure soap and clean water or wipes. Advise the patient that feminine hygiene sprays are not necessary at this time and may cause irritation.

3. On dismissal, ask the patient to report to the physician any bleeding, bright red spotting, or passage of clots.

IV. EVALUATION PROCESS

A. Were the nursing objectives met?

B. Was the patient's level of perception and understanding considered in teaching and communication?

C. Were charting and reporting complete and relevant?

115

Vulval-Perineal Preparation

I. ASSESSMENT OF SITUATION

A. Definition

The removal of hair from the skin around the delivery area in preparation for the birth of a baby

B. Terminology

1. *Episiotomy:* incision of the vulval-perineal area to facilitate delivery and prevent tearing
2. *Perineum:* muscle and fascia that lie across the pubic arch
3. *Vulva:* external female reproductive organs—the mons pubis, labia majora and minora, clitoris, the vestibule, urethral opening, and hymen

C. Rationale for Actions

1. To aid in the maintenance of a germ-free environment during delivery
2. To provide optimal visualization during the delivery process
3. To promote a cleaner environment for healing
4. To aid in healing of the episiotomy

II. NURSING PLAN

A. Objectives

1. To offer explanation and support to the patient as labor progresses
2. To remove all hair from the vulval and perineal area, to reduce the chance of infection
3. To protect the integument by taking care not to scratch, scrape, or cut the skin during shaving

B. Patient Preparation

1. Explain the need for the procedure to the patient.
2. Explain the procedure.
3. Explain the importance of relaxation.
4. Discuss the approximate period of time the pubic hair will grow back (6 wk).

C. Equipment

1. Preparation tray, including razor and blades, shaving cream or soap, and antiseptic solution
2. Preparation solution
3. 4 in X 4 in sponges
4. Disposable gloves
5. Warm wash cloths
6. Goose-neck lamp

III. IMPLEMENTING NURSING INTERVENTION

A. Therapeutic Aspects

1. Microorganisms are normally found on the skin and are harbored in the hair. Removal of the hair facilitates removal of germs.
2. The patient should be encouraged to relax during the procedure. A protective covering under the buttocks will protect the bed linen. The patient should be draped to avoid exposure and chilling (Figs. 115-1, 115-2).
3. Soap reduces surface tension. With the patient on her back and her knees flexed widely apart, the vulval area should be lathered, always working from front to back (Figs. 115-3, 115-4). The anal area is

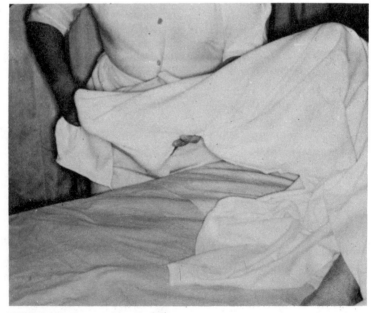

FIGURE 115.1

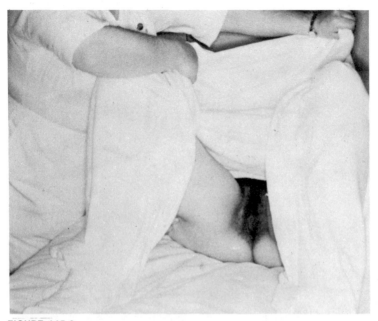

FIGURE 115.2

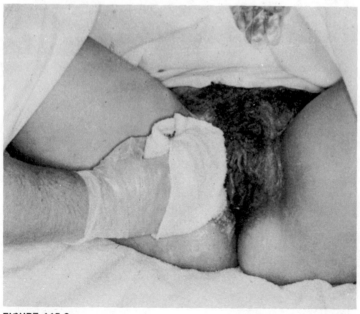

FIGURE 115.3

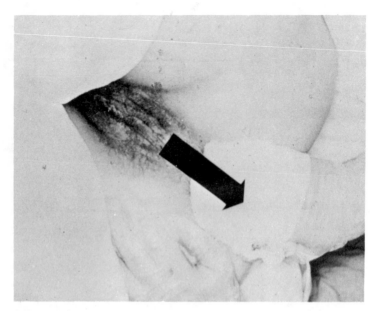

FIGURE 115.4

considered contaminated, so germs from that area should not be transferred to the vulval area.

4. Shaving the vulva should proceed with short downward strokes beginning at the top of the pubic area (Fig. 115-5). The area may be kept taut with the other hand. Care must be taken not to cut or nick the skin, especially around moles, warts, or old scars. Some physicians do not require the area over the mons pubis to be shaved because of its distance from the vagina and the discomfort caused when the hair grows back.

5. After shaving, the entire area should be rinsed with warm water and the preparation solution, using a new sponge for each front-to-back stroke, and dried in the same front-to-back manner.

6. With the patient on her side, the anal area is lathered and shaved with outward strokes. The upper buttocks may be held up and apart with a gauze sponge. Since the anal area is considered contaminated, care must be taken not to cut or nick the area, especially around hemorrhoids or folds of skin. The area is rinsed and dried as described above.

B. Communicative Aspects

1. *Observations*

   a. Observe carefully for any nicks or cuts in shaved area.

   b. Note any skin changes.

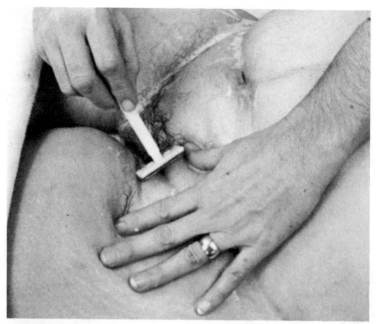

FIGURE 115.5

c. Observe the reaction of the patient.

2. *Charting*

DATE	TREATMENT	TIME	OBSERVATIONS	SIGNATURE
1/5	Vulval-perineal prep	1600	Entire vulval-perineal area shaved. No abnormalities noted.	G. Ivers, R.N.

3. *Referrals*

Not applicable

C. Teaching Aspects—Patient

1. Instruct the patient in the essentials of aseptic technique and cleanliness.

2. Explain the organs involved in delivery and the functional roles of each.

IV. EVALUATION PROCESS

A. Was all of the vulval-perineal hair successfully removed?

B. Was the patient protected from cuts and scraping during shaving?

C. Did the nurse offer emotional support?

D. Did the patient understand the need and procedure?

Suggested Readings

BOOKS

Armstrong M *et al:* McGraw-Hill Handbook of Clinical Nursing. New York, McGraw-Hill, 1979

Barrie J: Emergency Nursing. New York, McGraw-Hill, 1978

Beland I, Passos J: Clinical Nursing: Pathophysiological and Psychosocial Approaches, 4th ed. London, Macmillan, 1981

Bower F, Bevis EO: Fundamentals of Nursing Practice: Concepts, Roles and Functions. St Louis, CV Mosby, 1979

Brunner LS, Suddarth D: Textbook of Medical-Surgical Nursing, 4th ed. Philadelphia, JB Lippincott, 1980

Burrell Z, Burrell L: Critical Care, 4th ed. St Louis, CV Mosby, 1981

Conway BL: Neurological and Neurosurgical Nursing, 7th ed. St Louis, CV Mosby, 1978

Elhart D *et al:* Scientific Principles in Nursing, 8th ed. St Louis, CV Mosby, 1978

Eliopoulos C: Gerontological Nursing. New York, Harper & Row, 1979

Fielo SB, Edge S: Technical Nursing of the Adult: Medical, Surgical, and Psychiatric Approaches, 2nd ed. London, Macmillan, 1974

Given BA, Simmons S: Nursing Care of the Patient with Gastro-intestinal Disorders, 2nd ed. St Louis, CV Mosby, 1975

Hudak C, Lohr T, Gallo B: Critical Care Nursing, 2nd ed. Philadelphia, JB Lippincott, 1977

Jensen, M, Benson R, Bobak I: Maternity Care—The Nurse and the Family, 2nd ed. St Louis, CV Mosby, 1981

Jones D, Dunbar C, Jorovec MM: Medical-Surgical Nursing: A Conceptual Approach. New York, McGraw-Hill, 1978

Kintzel KC: Advanced Concepts in Clinical Nursing, 2nd ed. Philadelphia, JB Lippincott, 1977

Kernicki J, Bullock B, Mathews J: Cardiovascular Nursing. New York, GP Putnam, 1971

Larson CB, Gould M: Orthopedic Nursing, 9th ed. St Louis, CV Mosby, 1978

Leitch CJ, Tinker RV: Primary Care. Philadelphia, FA Davis, 1978

Lewis LW: Fundamental Skills in Patient Care, 2nd ed. Philadelphia, JB Lippincott, 1980

McInnes ME: The Vital Signs: A Programmed Presentation Including Material on the Apical Beat, 2nd ed. St Louis, CV Mosby, 1975

Meltzer L, Pinneo R, Kitchell J: Intensive Coronary Care, 3rd ed. Bowie, Maryland, Charles Press, 1977

Miller ME, Sachs ML: About Bedsores: What You Need to Know to Help Prevent and Treat Them. Philadelphia, JB Lippincott, 1974

Murray M: Fundamentals of Nursing. Englewood Cliffs, NJ, Prentice-Hall, 1976

Phipps WJ, Long BC, Woods NF: Medical-Surgical Nursing, Concepts and Clinical Practice. St Louis, CV Mosby, 1979

Reeder S et al: Maternity Nursing, 14th ed. Philadelphia, JB Lippincott, 1980

Sorenson K, Luckmann J: Basic Nursing—A Psychophysiologic Approach. Philadelphia, WB Saunders, 1979

Steinberg F: The Care of the Geriatric Patient, 5th ed. St Louis, CV Mosby, 1976

Taber WC: Taber's Cyclopedic Medical Dictionary, 14th ed. Philadelphia, FA Davis, 1981

Warner C: Emergency Care—Assessment and Intervention, 2nd ed. St Louis, CV Mosby, 1978

Wolff Weitzel MH, Fuerst EV: Fundamentals of Nursing, 6th ed. Philadelphia, JB Lippincott, 1979

Wood LA, Rambo BJ: Nursing Skills for Allied Health Services, 2nd ed. Philadelphia, WB Saunders, 1977

JOURNALS AND PAMPHLETS

Baya A, Hinshaw R: A Safe Way to Perform Intraclavicular Subclavian Vein Catheterization. Surg Gynecol Obstet 30: 1970 pp. 673-676

Dailey E, Andrews R, Vickers I: Silicone Gel Flotation Pads and Decubitus Ulcer Problems. The Nation's Hospitals and Nursing Homes 1: 1970

Foster Reversible Orthopedic Bed, Bulletin #F.B. 1253A. Oakland, CA Gilbert-Hyde, Chick Company

Isolation Techniques for Use in Hospitals, 2nd ed. 1975, US Department of Health, Education and Welfare. Atlanta, Georgia, Public Health Service, Center for Disease Control, 1975

Stryker Flotation Pads. Fort Worth, TX, Medical Rents, Inc

Index

Page numbers in *italics* indicate illustrations.